DAILY SOURDOUGH

healthy recipes
for every meal

LISA BASS

FROM FARMHOUSE ON BOONE

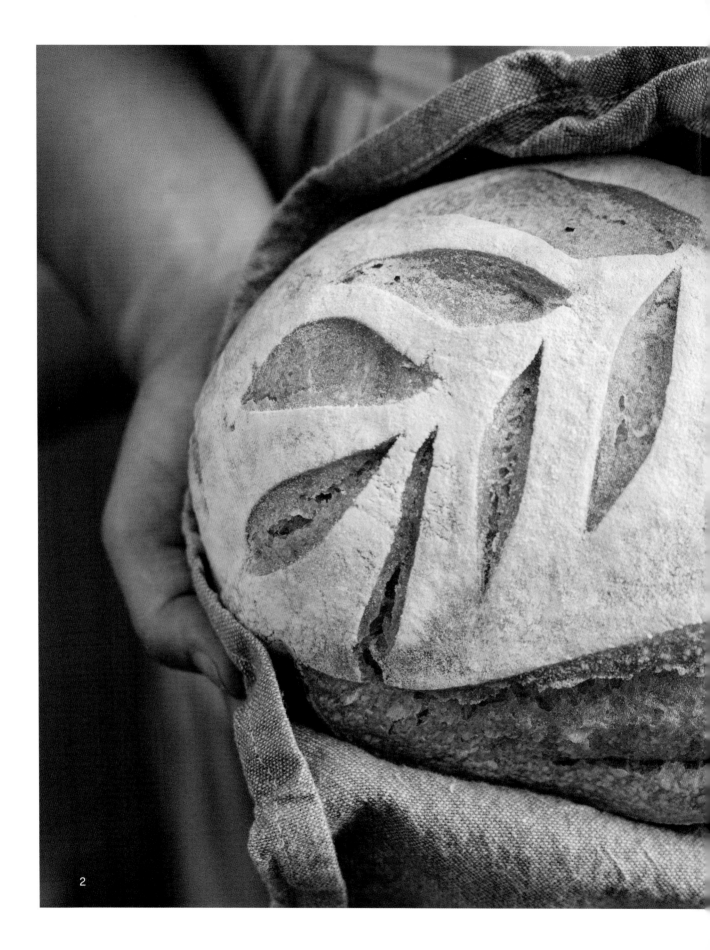

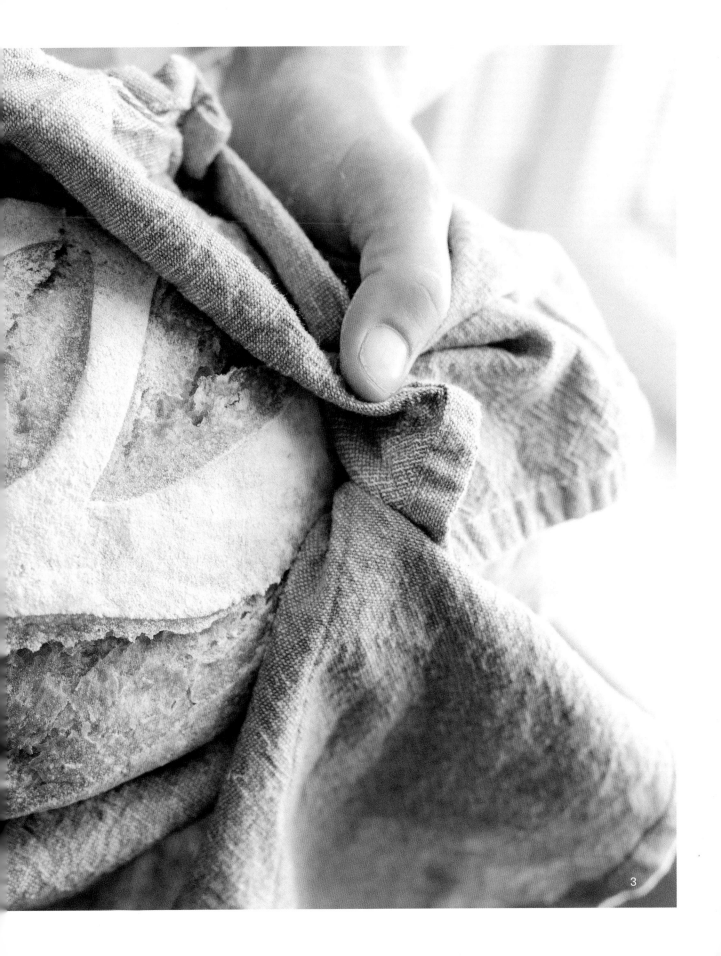

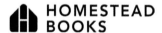

HOMESTEAD BOOKS

First publication in 2024 by Homestead Books, a subsidiary of Homestead Living, Inc.
Homestead Living, PO Box 2055, Stillwater, MN 55082

Cover design and layout by Allan Nygren of Mosaic Productions
Publishing Director: Jeremy Stevens
Writing and Development Coach: Jenny McGruther
Project management and proof review by Felicity Fields
Photography by Jessie Watts, Lisa Bass, Amy Knight, and Christy Faber
Photographic editing by Nathan O'Malley
Editing by Mikayla Butcher
Proofreading by Gleni Bartels
Indexing by Ken DellaPenta

For more information about our other products, please visit: www.homesteadbooks.com

ISBN: 978-1-963008-00-5

Dedication

To my husband, Luke: your unwavering support and partnership through all the years of learning and growing together made it possible for us to transition from our cozy town life to the fulfilling days on our small farm.

To my children: your laughter and love fill our home with joy. You are my inspiration and my motivation.

To my extended family: your encouragement and support have been a constant source of comfort and strength.

To the Homestead Living team: your expertise, dedication, and passion for this project have turned a dream into reality. Thank you.

To my writing and development coach and guide, Jenny McGruther: Your wisdom, guidance, and encouragement have been invaluable. You helped shape this book into something I am truly proud of.

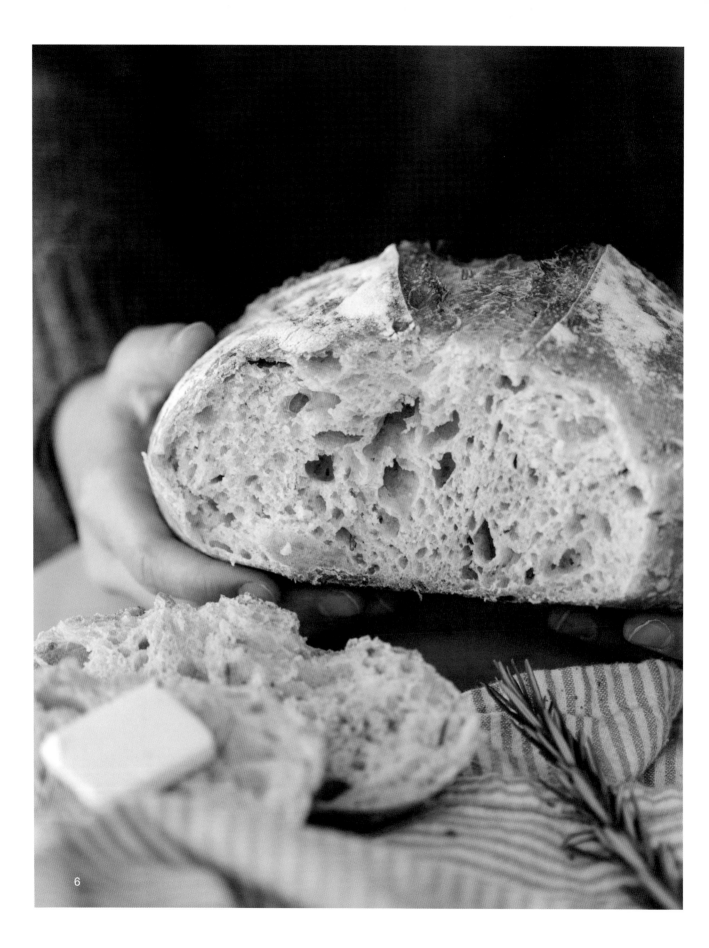

Contents

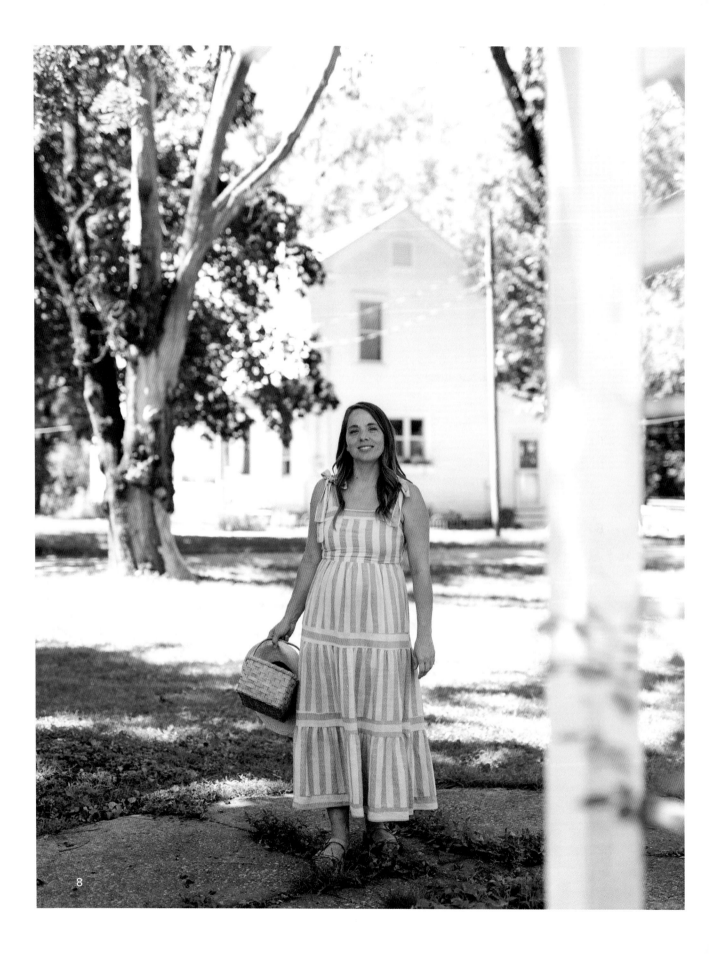

Introduction

I FELL IN LOVE with sourdough baking in 2008. Newlywed with a newborn baby girl, my husband and I moved into our first home—a 1920s bungalow. I didn't know much at twenty-three, but I did know that I wanted to craft a meaningful life. More than that, I wanted to build a family and give it the best start I could.

At that time, everything I knew about nutrition came from the USDA food pyramid and a handful of books leftover from the 1990s crash-diet culture. Fat was out. Butter was bad, and margarine reigned supreme. Whole grains were the foundation of a healthy diet. Meat posed a dire risk. Raw vegetables? Eat those in bulk, but only with fat-free bottled dressing (if you're feeling indulgent).

In essence, I had no clue. One thing I did know for certain was that I held a tiny 6-pound, 15-ounce baby girl in my arms, and her entire future depended on me. (No pressure.)

I came to my marriage without homemaking skills. I didn't know how to roast a chicken or even make meatloaf. So I pulled out the cookbooks I received at my wedding shower. I browsed their pages and figured out how to marinate chicken. Mixing a batch of no-frills chocolate chip cookies came next. The pages promised dutifully low-fat recipes that become dinnertime staples. If I came across easy meal ideas in a magazine, I'd clip them out and stuff them into a binder. Living on a bare-bones budget, my husband and I didn't have smartphones (or Wi-Fi), so my resources were limited. I learned what I could from old books and magazines or the occasional trip to the library. But they all said the same thing: Fat-free food was in, and the faster you got dinner on the table, the better. This approach lacked soul. There was no heritage to these recipes.

Sometime later, I came across *Nourishing Traditions* (2001, NewTrends Publishing). It opened my eyes. Maybe there was more to know than what mainstream nutritional advice offered. Perhaps traditional cultures could offer insight into thriving health and wellness. They might offer a path to health rooted in heritage and tradition. Generations of healthy families came before us. They didn't subsist on fat-free rice cakes or bland meals of boneless, skinless chicken breast and steamed broccoli. I started to question everything I knew about food, nutrition, and homemaking. What if our modern food culture had it wrong?

I learned that our society has a lot of fear surrounding food: fat, calories—you name it. Even more, we live in a hyper-sanitized society. Could all that emphasis actually be doing us harm? Why did we start pasteurizing milk? Why doesn't the average cook know that vegetables and salt become a probiotic superfood with enough time on the counter? I read enough to know that I had a lot to learn and a long journey ahead of me.

My little, blessed bungalow came with its own challenges. I learned to cook on a decades-old oven. I had zero pantry space for storing bulk goods. My tiny, antiquated fridge could hold only so much. But I committed. Learning these traditional skills was important to me. I wanted my children to grow up knowing what I had to work so hard to learn.

Our single income allowed for only a shoestring budget. There was no room for fancy equipment or pricey ingredients. In such circumstances, you learn to make do, and I did. I acquired the tools I needed one by one. With a growing family, certain purchases made sense. I saw them as investments in my family's health and our future. I bought a grain mill so I could make fresh flour, still rich and vibrant with its innate vitamins. Stainless steel bread pans meant I could bake sandwich loaves at home and stop buying them from the store. Big food-grade buckets stored grain, allowing me to save money by purchasing in bulk.

When I first learned the basics of bread baking, I used little packages of store-bought yeast. I made fresh bread with grains I ground at home. Then, shortly after I gave birth to my second baby, I tried making sourdough. I mixed a little water and flour together in a small jar. Within a few days, it started to bubble. Within a week, it was strong enough to make bread rise. It was my first (and only) sourdough starter, and it's been with me for well over a decade. I've nurtured it

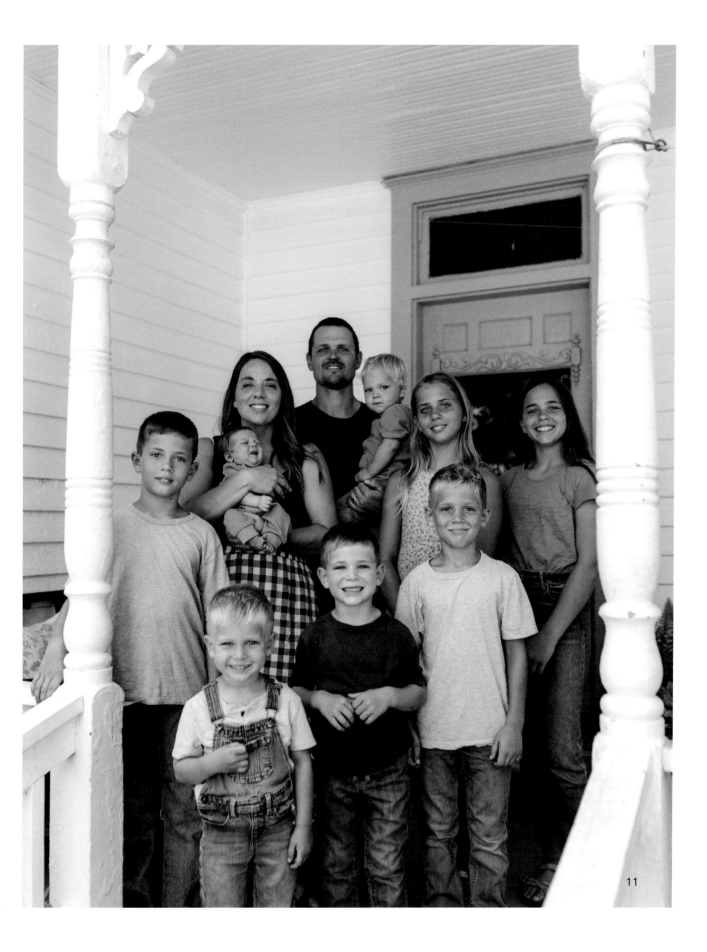

over the years. In that time, it has rewarded me with countless loaves of bread and plenty of pastries and treats, too. If you feed it regularly, your own starter can last a lifetime—even generations.

I started with a very basic loaf of whole-grain sourdough bread. I didn't trouble myself with complicated recipes or fussy equipment. My kitchen was too small for bannetons and scales and dough whisks. As for my time? My little children kept me busy. I didn't have time to worry about professional baking lingo like "hydration" or "autolyze." (And I still don't care much for them.) I also didn't have time to worry about perfecting complex techniques. I felt content just baking wholesome bread for my growing family.

That same sourdough starter has nourished our family for fifteen years. It has seen us through the births of six more babies and a move to a beautiful farm-house on our seven-acre homestead. It's part of our family now. At first, I made only the basics: sandwich loaves, pancakes, English muffins, and the like. Now? I love experimenting with new flavors and new styles of bread. To tell the truth, I work that trusty sourdough starter into just about any baked good I can—including cookies and cakes.

Sourdough allows for full creative expression. There's satisfaction in scoring a beautiful pattern onto a boule. There's pleasure in folding butter into layers of dough, knowing they'll turn into flaky croissants in the oven. I love the way a little rye flour changes the texture of an artisan loaf. I enjoy how buttermilk trans-forms sandwich bread and the yellow-gold color ancient grains lend to baked goods.

I encourage you to trust yourself and explore your own senses. Sourdough can be as simple or complicated as you want it to be. If all you want is a basic sand-wich loaf loaded with all the benefits of sourdough, I'm here for you. If you want to make great bread but don't want a degree in "baker's math," this book's for you. If you're an experienced home baker looking for a little inspiration, these recipes will get you to the next level.

Remember, sourdough should be simple. It has fed generations of families since the dawn of agriculture. I can promise you that these families kept it simple, too. Set your phone down, dive in, and celebrate the art of true from-scratch baking.

How to Use This Book

I wrote this book to provide the resource I never had as a new homemaker. My hope is to equip you with the knowledge and techniques you'll need to make great bread. When you're ready, I hope to help you expand to other baked goods, too. There's a whole world of sourdough beyond a loaf of bread.

For Sourdough Newcomers

If you're brand new to sourdough baking, start at the very beginning of this book. You'll need to know how to stock your pantry and which pieces of equipment are worth buying. Then, read through all you need to know about a sourdough starter and get the process going. Review that section as often as you need to as you get your sourdough starter ready. If you stumble upon a phrase or term you don't know, take a look at the glossary on page 17.

Once your starter is active and bubbly, it's time to make bread, so jump into the bread recipes first. Study the steps on baking bread on page XX. It will build your confidence, and you'll know exactly what you need to do to make great bread.

RECIPES FOR NEW BAKERS

SAME-DAY SOURDOUGH BREAD
   (PAGE 118)
BASIC SANDWICH BREAD (PAGE 144)
SOURDOUGH PANCAKES (PAGE 275)

Try a recipe and make it again and again until you've mastered it. You may struggle a bit at first. Remember that some techniques, such as shaping, take time to learn and perfect. Many of my first few loaves of sourdough seemed more like bricks than bread. Give yourself the space and time to learn.

Once you have a recipe down and see consistent results you love, try expanding your reach. If you're satisfied with your bread, try a few pastries next. Take it slow and enjoy every step. If you run into trouble, check out the guide to troubleshooting (page 331).

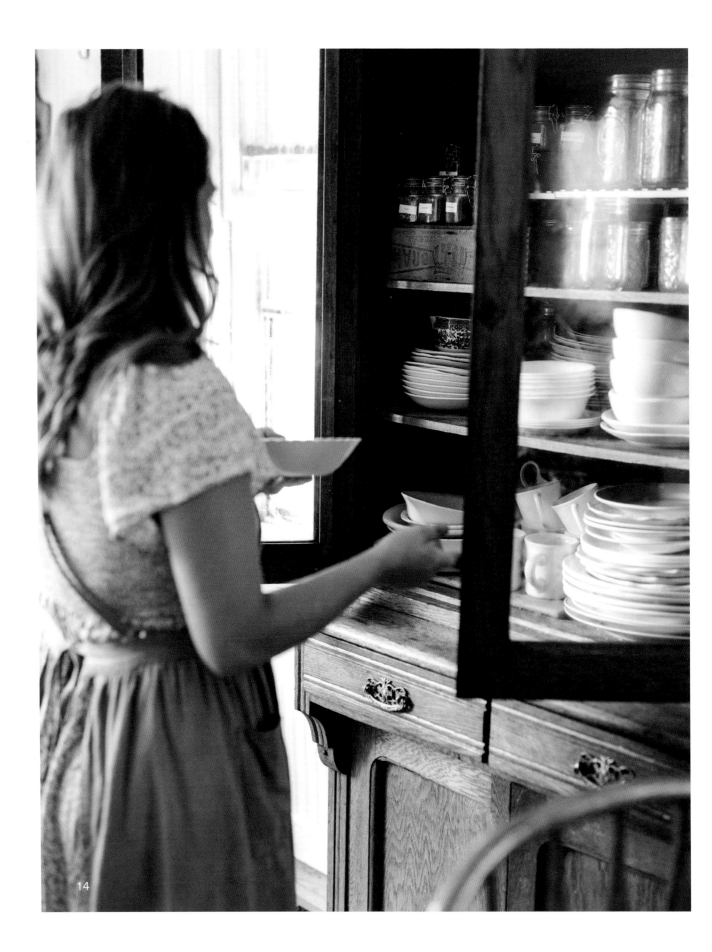

If You Already Have a Starter (But Are New to Baking)

Maybe you have a lively starter bubbling away in your kitchen already. Perhaps you have even made a few loaves, too. But if you've hit a stumbling block or want to perfect your technique, review the chapter on starting, maintaining, and proofing your starter (page 73) and review the guidelines for mixing, proofing, shaping, and baking bread (page 103). These two sections provide steady guidance that can help you nail down your technique. Additionally, review the recommended tools (page 38) to shore up any gaps in your kitchen. A stand mixer, Dutch oven, bread lame, and proofing baskets are my must-haves.

RECIPES FOR NEW-ISH BAKERS

JALAPEÑO-CHEDDAR BREAD (PAGE 137)

SOURDOUGH RYE BREAD (PAGE 132)

FUDGE WALNUT BROWNIES (PAGE 256)

Once you review those sections, try a few new techniques. Using alternative flours such as rye, spelt, or einkorn might be a nice way to level up your baking. Or, better yet, try adding inclusions to your bread. Dried fruit, toasted nuts, and chopped fresh herbs can transform a basic loaf into something special. Soon, you'll feel as if you have an artisan bakery at the heart of your kitchen.

For Experienced Bakers

If you're an experienced baker with a tried-and-true sourdough starter, dive right into the recipes. It's still a good idea to review the chapter on making a sourdough starter (page XX) and other basics. Once you're feeling confident, try some of the more technique-heavy recipes. Fortified doughs, those made with plenty of butter and eggs, are a good place to start. They're trickier to make and take a little longer to rise. Or challenge yourself by making flaky pastries. Sourdough gives them a delicious edge.

Whether you're a long-time baker with an heirloom starter handed down from your grandmother, or someone who has never touched an oven, slow down and enjoy the process. Revel in the pleasure of baking. Know that with every success and failure, generations of bakers are behind you. All you need to do is try.

RECIPES FOR EXPERIENCED BAKERS

SOURDOUGH BRIOCHE (PAGE 150)

CHOCOLATE CROISSANTS (PAGE 222)

RASPBERRY SWEET ROLLS (PAGE 213)

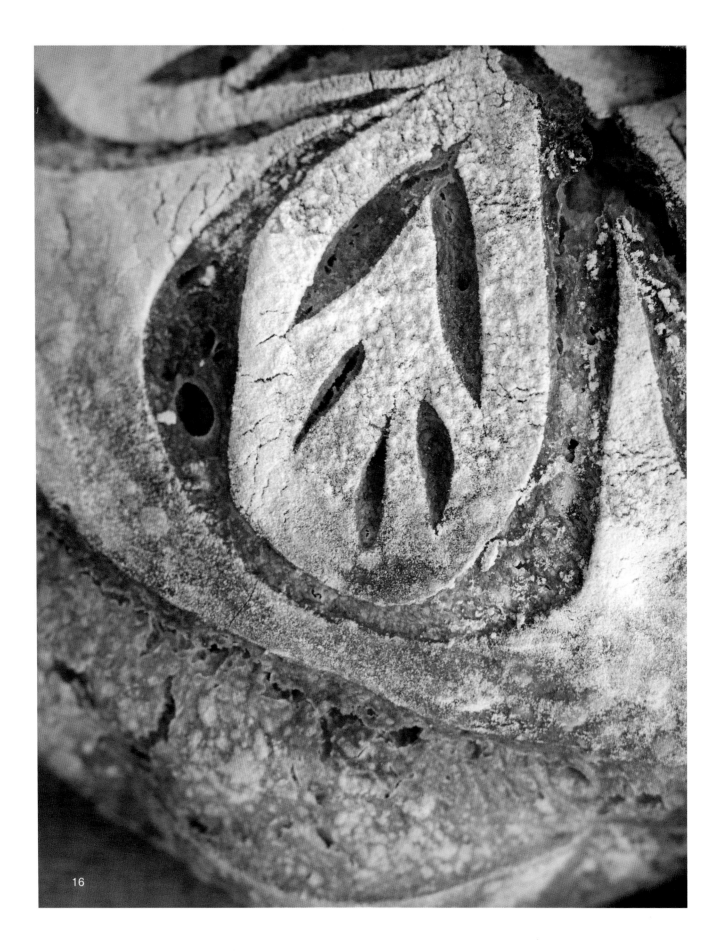

Glossary

Here are some key terms you will find useful throughout the book.

Autolyse
Autolyse is a technique that involves mixing only the flour and water together before letting it rest. This process enhances gluten development and improves bread texture and flavor.

Boule
From the French word for "ball," a boule is a crusty round loaf of artisan-style bread.

Bulk Fermentation (Bulk Rise)
Bulk fermentation refers to the first time bakers allow the bread to rise. The dough rises as a single large mass, and the process takes several hours. This step enhances flavor, texture, and gluten development.

Crumb
Crumb refers to the interior texture of a loaf of bread. The type of dough and the amount of carbon dioxide produced both influence the consistency of the crumb. Wetter doughs produce an airy crumb. Drier doughs and enriched doughs produce a tighter crumb.

Ears
The ear is the crusty flap that forms on artisan-style bread during baking. After you score your dough, it will expand in the oven and produce an ear.

Enriched Dough (Fortified Dough)
Enriched dough is bread dough made with added fat. Typically, this type of

dough includes eggs, butter, or milk. Enriched doughs are soft and tender. They also take longer to rise.

Feeding

Feeding is the process of removing a small bit of starter and then adding fresh water and flour. Feeding your sourdough encourages it to rise, making it ready for baking.

Float Test

This is a test to determine if your sourdough starter is active and ready for baking. To perform the test, take a small glass of room-temperature water. Add a quarter-sized dollop of active sourdough starter. If it floats, the dough is ready. If it doesn't float, it is not active and may need more time or another feeding.

Hooch

Hooch, a grayish liquid, occasionally appears on the surface of sourdough starter. The liquid is made of alcohol. It is a byproduct of fermentation. It is a sign that your starter is hungry, and you need to feed it. Pour off the hooch and feed your starter as you normally would.

Hydration

Hydration refers to the ratio of water or other liquid to flour in either bread dough or your starter. It can also describe the hydration of a starter. A starter with 100% hydration is one that is fed equal parts flour and water by weight.

Inclusions

Inclusions are additional ingredients you add to bread dough, such as cheese, herbs, fruit, and nuts. They add flavor, texture, and visual appeal to bread.

Kneading

Kneading is the process of working dough to develop gluten. Through repeated folding, pressing, and stretching, gluten strands form, creating an elastic dough. This step enhances texture and allows the dough to rise properly.

Laminated Dough

Laminated dough is a pastry dough created by repeatedly folding and rolling butter into a dough. This process produces a flaky, tender texture in baked goods like croissants and puff pastry. It creates distinct layers when baked.

Levain

Levain is a mixture of sourdough starter, water, and flour. It is allowed to ferment separately. Then, it's added to the remaining ingredients as a leavening agent.

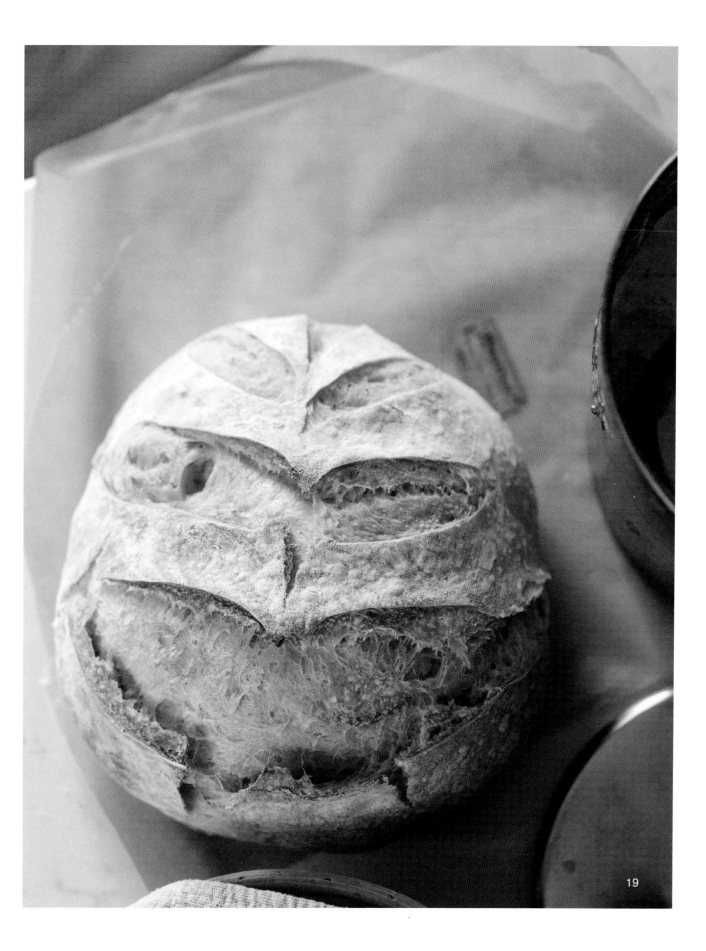

Naturally Leavened

Naturally leavened refers to bread or other baked goods that rise without using commercial yeast or chemical rising agents, such as baking soda or baking powder.

Oven Spring

Oven spring refers to the rapid expansion of a loaf of bread at the start of baking, usually within the first 10 minutes. The strength of the dough and the shaping process influence oven spring.

Proofing

Proofing can refer either to bread dough or to your starter. To proof a starter, you feed it with the intention of baking once it becomes active. For bread dough, proofing refers to the final rise before you transfer the dough to the oven.

Resting

Some recipes may call for a short period of rest before shaping your dough. Let your dough rest on the counter for the amount of time in the recipe. Resting allows the gluten to relax before final shaping. This technique minimizes the risk that your dough will tear when you shape it.

Retardation

To retard your dough is to intentionally slow down the fermentation process, usually by transferring it to the fridge. Cold temperatures slow the rate of growth for yeast and bacteria.

Shaping

Shaping is the process of manipulating your dough into the shape you want before baking.

Scoring

Scoring is the process of using a sharp tool (usually called a bread lame) to slice bread dough before baking. Scoring your bread helps encourage an even oven spring. It also prevents tearing while it bakes.

Expansion scores are deep cuts, about 1/2 inch deep. These cuts encourage the dough to expand when baking. Artistic scores are shallow cuts, about 1/4 inch deep. Artistic scores create attractive designs in a bread's crust as it bakes.

Sourdough Discard

Sourdough discard is the amount of sourdough starter you remove from the jar at a feeding. The yeast in sourdough discard is inactive, so it isn't appropriate for making bread rise.

Sourdough Starter

A sourdough starter is a mixture of flour and water that has been allowed to ferment. This mixture is acidic and contains wild yeast and bacteria. The bacteria give the bread flavor, while the yeast makes bread rise.

Stretching and Folding

Stretching and folding is an artisan bread-baking technique. It encourages the development of gluten. This strengthens dough and helps it hold its form. In bread baking, you grab and pull the dough up. Then, you fold it over itself. Bakers often use this technique instead of kneading.

Tension

Tension refers to the tightness of the surface of the dough. Your dough develops tension through proper shaping techniques. Tension supports the dough's structure during proofing and baking. This results in better oven spring and a desired loaf shape.

Windowpane Test

The windowpane test involves stretching a small piece of dough until it forms a thin, translucent membrane without tearing. This indicates sufficient gluten development.

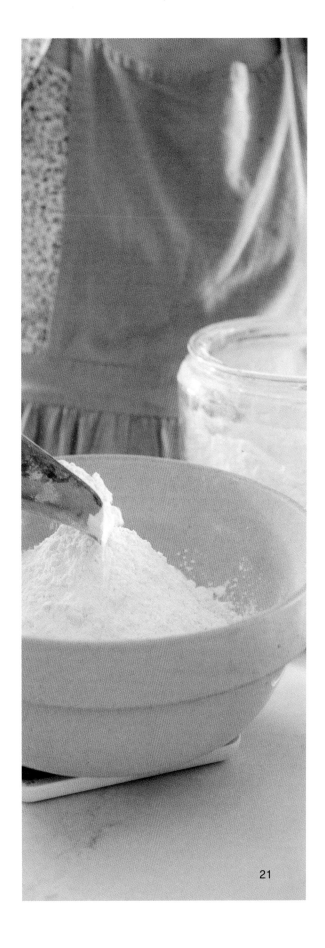

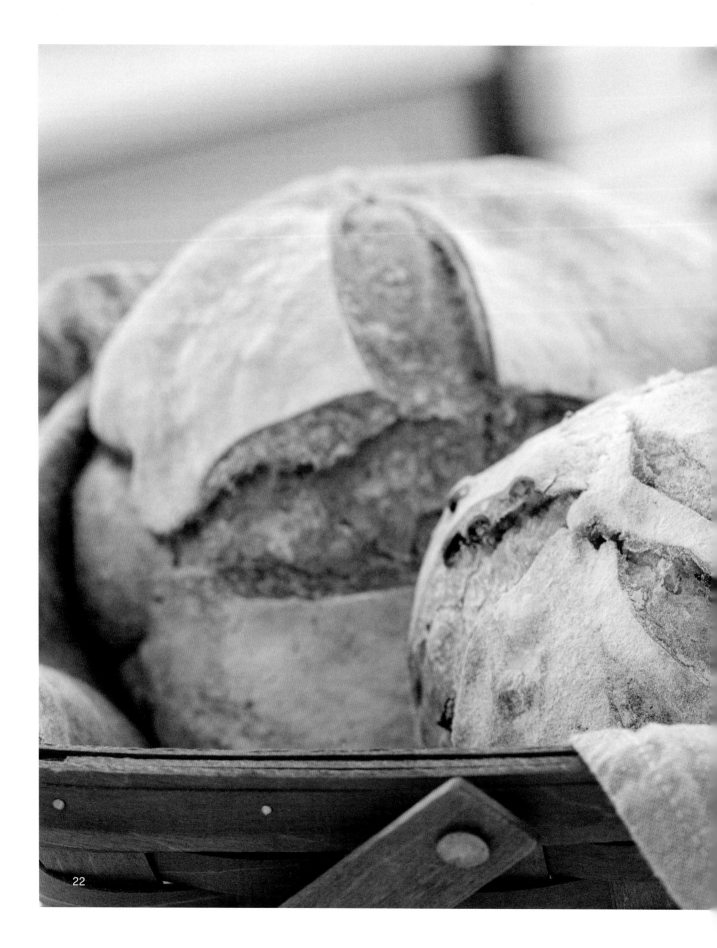

CHAPTER 1

Sourdough Basics

LONG BEFORE you could head to the local market and buy a packet of yeast, bread bakers relied on wild yeast. Wild yeast exist all around us: on our skin, in the environment, and on grain. When you grind grain into flour and mix it with water, it forms a nutrient-rich slurry that attracts yeast and beneficial bacteria. As the yeast gobble up the flour, they produce enough carbon dioxide to make bread rise.

It's an age-old method. Some of the earliest archaeological evidence of bread baking dates to the fertile crescent tens of thousands of years ago. Ancient Egyptians also mixed water and flour together until it bubbled with enough yeast to make bread rise. Medieval bakers used the same technique, and so did settlers in the American West. It worked because the process is easy, intuitive, and simple.

When baker's yeast arrived on the scene in the nineteenth century, it changed the way people baked. They no longer needed to tend and maintain careful pots of fresh yeast and sourdough starter. Louis Pasteur's discoveries in microbiology during the 1860s contributed to the understanding of yeast's role in fermentation, including its importance in bread making. This scientific breakthrough paved the way for the mass production and distribution of baker's yeast. Since then, baker's yeast has become a staple ingredient in bread making. It offers bakers convenience and consistency.

Quickly, that generations-old technique of sourdough baking lost its prominence. No longer did households keep little pots of starter on the countertop to make bread, not when baker's yeast seemed so convenient. In opting for the convenience of instant yeast, bakers lost the heritage of sourdough. It's a beautiful heritage, too—and worth reviving.

It takes effort to make a starter from scratch and plan to organize your baking. But it's worth every moment. Sourdough is a beautiful art form rooted in heritage and tradition that spans generations. Very little has changed since those first humans ground ancient grains into flour and mixed them with water to make bread. It's as simple a process now as it was then.

Why Sourdough?

Sourdough is an ancient baking

technique. It combines flour and water to leaven bread with the goal of capturing wild yeast and bacteria. These tiny, invisible microorganisms consume the starches in the flour. As they do so, the yeast produces carbon dioxide, which makes bread dough rise and, eventually, double. Just as the yeast make the bread rise, the beneficial bacteria in the starter release acid, which gives the bread flavor.

It is a slower process than baking with tidy packages of instant yeast. Wild yeast takes more time to develop and flourish. Sure, it takes a little more planning and a good dose of patience, but the end result is delicious. More than that, sourdough bread is more nutritious, too.

While I'll always love good bread, it wasn't the taste that drew me to sourdough. Rather, it was the nutritional benefits. Sourdough bread is more nutrient-dense and easier to digest than modern baked goods. I wanted to feed my family the most nutrient-dense foods I could, and sourdough hit the mark.

Minerals and Nutrition

Have you ever looked at the nutritional profile on the back of an expensive loaf of whole-grain bread at the health food store? Looks pretty impressive, right? Unfortunately, our bodies aren't actually able to absorb most of those minerals. Soaking, fermenting, and sprouting grains resolves that problem. So I take the time in my kitchen to find and prepare quality whole grains and organic flour. The hard work of baking seems wasted if you're not getting the most nutrition out of what you make. Sourdough allows you to make the most of your efforts.

Sourdough fermentation breaks down complex carbohydrates and proteins, making them easier to digest. It's loaded with B vitamins, especially folate. It also helps your body better absorb minerals, such as iron, zinc, phosphorus, and magnesium. That's because this technique deactivates certain compounds in grains that make minerals hard for your body to use.

Grains, beans, nuts, and seeds contain a high concentration of food phytates. Phytates are a plant's storage system for phosphorus. Phosphorus is an essential mineral required for germination, flowering, and root formation. Phytates provide a readily available source of phosphorus for their growth and development.

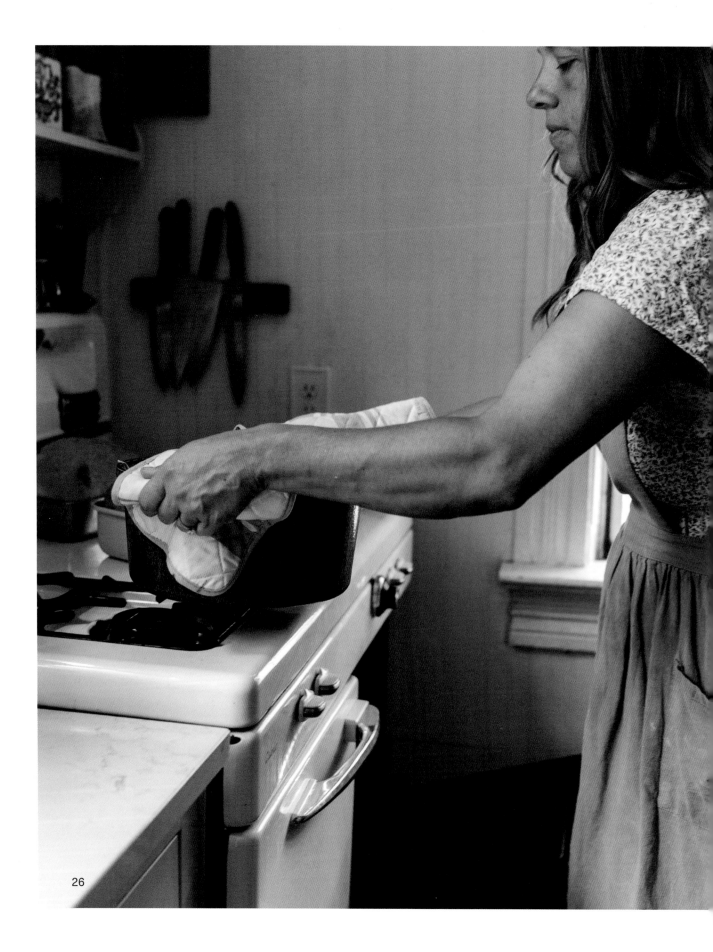

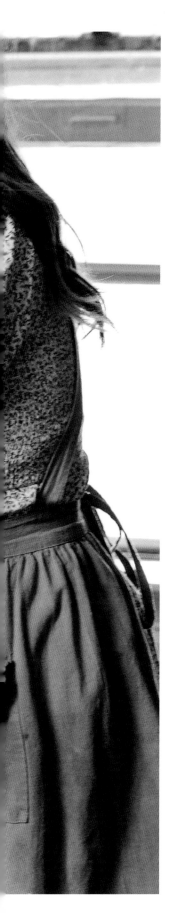

These "antinutrients" bind to minerals such as zinc, magnesium, and others. As a result, some of these nutrients are difficult to absorb. Sourdough fermentation helps break down phytates, releasing the trapped minerals so that you're better able to make use of all the minerals in whole grains.

The increased mineral value of sourdough extends only to whole grains. The grain's bran and germ contain most of its minerals. (The bran and germ are two of the parts that make up a grain.) When millers sift out the bran and germ to make white flour, they remove most of the grain's innate nutrition. So there's not much mineral value left in baked goods made with white flour. Sourdough is pretty amazing, but it won't increase minerals where they don't exist.

Metabolic Health

Better mineral absorption isn't the only benefit of sourdough. It also supports better blood sugar balance. Sourdough bread typically has a lower glycemic index (GI) than bread made with commercial yeast. During fermentation, beneficial bacteria break down the starches in flour. As they gobble up all that starch, they produce beneficial acids. That's why sourdough tastes sour. As a result, sourdough has a lighter impact on blood sugar balance. That's true of both sourdough made with white flour or whole-grain flour. But with whole-grain flour, your body will enjoy the added benefits of fiber and more minerals.

Digestion

The wild yeast and good bacteria in your sourdough starter break down complex starches. This process makes sourdough easier to digest than commercial bread. Sourdough fermentation also produces prebiotic compounds. These compounds serve as food for beneficial gut bacteria. As a result, many people find sourdough to be a great choice for gut health. The benefits are even more pronounced the longer you allow your dough to ferment.

Remember that fermentation doesn't remove the gluten. So if you adhere to a gluten-free diet for medical reasons, you'll need to do gluten-free sourdough recipes. The fermentation process can help break down gluten to some extent, and some people with mild sensitivities may find sourdough easier to digest. This is especially true when it is made with ancient grains or fermented overnight.

Longevity

All the acids that those beneficial microorganisms create do two things. First, they make sourdough bread taste delicious. Second, they make sourdough bread last longer. The acidic environment created during sourdough fermentation helps inhibit the growth of mold. It also inhibits the growth of some harmful bacteria. As a result, sourdough bread can have a longer shelf life. Best of all? It doesn't need preservatives or additives.

Flavor

Sourdough tastes amazing. It feels empowering to craft something so delicious completely from scratch. While sourdough's flavor isn't what drew me to baking, it fuels my passion. You might find it does the same for you, too. The slow fermentation process develops dimension and depth of flavor. It transforms ordinary grains into something with complexity.

Sourdough breads vary in flavor. That lack of uniformity is part of the appeal. The type of flour you use impacts flavor. It also depends on the strains of yeast and bacteria in your starter, how long you let your bread rise and so much more. Even the temperature of your home can impact the flavor of your bread. Sourdough bread can have a mildly sweet or nutty undertone or a robust and earthy flavor. Even home-baked bread made with commercial yeast can't replicate that kind of nuance or depth.

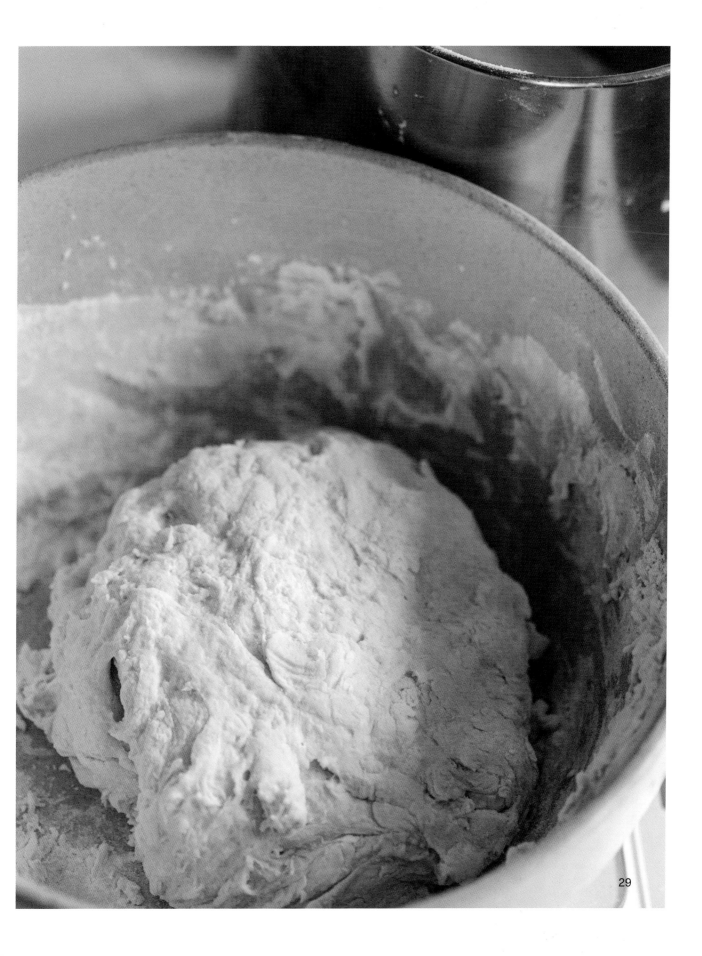

MY APPROACH TO SOURDOUGH

When I began baking with sourdough a decade ago, I had small children to raise, a garden to tend, and a home to keep. Time was a precious commodity, with little extra to spare. So I aimed for streamlined simplicity in my kitchen. Yes, I certainly wanted to feed my family nutrient-dense, traditional foods that could nourish them deeply. Still, all that needed to fit within the puzzle of hectic mornings and busy evenings.

My approach was practical: I needed to feed a growing family as best I could. That need led to a sort of homemaker's rhythm. I kept a big bubbly jar of sourdough starter in the fridge, fed on freshly milled grain before transitioning to all-purpose flour. Each morning, I'd pull out the jar. I'd spoon a little starter into a mixing bowl. Then, I'd whisk it together with a few extra ingredients from the pantry to make pancakes. It took less effort than making them from a mix, and they tasted better, too. Later, I'd add more flour to the jar of starter.

When the starter rose and bubbled, I'd make bread in the stand mixer. I didn't make fancy loaves, only simple, plain sandwich bread. It was the kind of bread that knew its job and did it well. On busy nights, I'd sauté some vegetables and brown a little meat in a hot cast-iron skillet to start dinner. While they sizzled away, I'd whisk herbs, melted butter, fresh eggs, and a few other staples into some extra starter. Pouring the sourdough batter into the skillet, I felt grateful: Dinner was done. That one-pan meal covered all the bases:

protein, vegetables, healthy fats, and fermented whole grains. I tucked the little ones into bed, their bellies full, and sighed with relief at the closing of the day.

The following morning, the cycle would start again. Sometimes, it proceeded with a few variations, waffles, perhaps, instead of pancakes. Or, occasionally, I might chop fresh herbs from the garden and knead them into the bread dough—if only to save them from waste. The practical need to feed my family led the charge and shaped those days. It was neither fancy nor beautiful, but it worked: simple sustenance prepared traditionally.

I also made do with what I had in my kitchen—a stand mixer, some good mixing bowls, wooden spoons, and a few loaf pans. At the time, I didn't own a banneton, a lame, a kitchen scale, a bench scraper, or even a cast-iron Dutch oven. I had never encountered the word "boule." The thought of calculating the hydration of a dough never occurred to me. With a decade of experience, I now use that same starter to make pastries and pizza. I also make airy artisan-style bread and even cakes. Still, the heart of my approach is simple and rooted in the practical desire to feed a family wholesome food.

So if you've stumbled upon sourdough but feel a little overwhelmed, know this: Simplicity is key. Start slow, begin with the basics, and expand your techniques a little at a time.

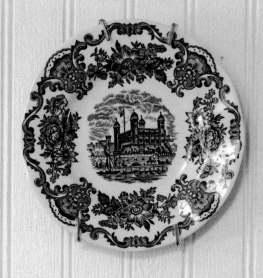

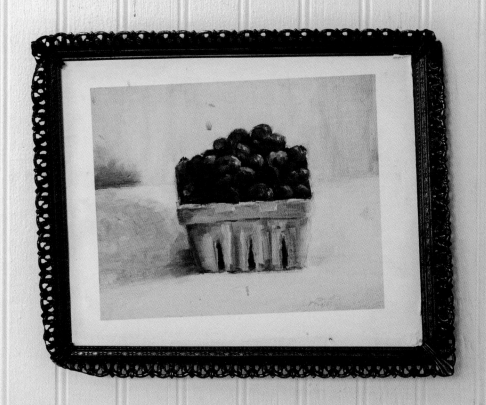

Keep It Simple

When it comes to sourdough, a simple approach works best. Remember, sourdough has nourished generations of families since the dawn of time. No one worried about digital scales and hydration percentages. Rather, baking was intuitive. The goal was simply to feed yourself and your family. I encourage you to take a simple approach, too. It's easy to overcomplicate things, making them feel harder and more complex than they really need to be. Sourdough is no exception.

Allow yourself plenty of time.

Creating a sourdough starter from scratch takes about a week. Sometimes, it takes a little longer. So mark out time in your calendar when your schedule is slow enough to allow you to spend 10 to 15 minutes of dedicated time in the kitchen every day. That's all it takes.

When it comes to baking your first loaf, remember to plan. Like many heritage cooking techniques, sourdough is a deliciously slow process. Sourdough starter takes longer to proof than packaged yeast. Dough takes longer to rise. Many sourdough recipes call for feeding the starter in advance and proofing the dough overnight. Good things are worth the wait, and sourdough baking is a constant reminder of that. Just take it slow and plan ahead.

Start with something familiar.

If you've ever baked before, start with something you know. Maybe it's a loaf of sandwich bread (page 144), a quick bread, such as Blackberry Muffins (page 193), or something as simple as brownies (page 256). Your prior baking knowledge will guide your hands. You'll feel at ease using sourdough techniques. If you still feel uncertain, baking a No-Knead Sourdough Bread (page 120) is always a good place to start.

Precision is helpful (but not essential).

When I first started baking, I relied on measuring cups and my own eyes. I didn't even own a kitchen scale and still baked beautiful breads. You can, too. Over time, I learned that measuring in grams is convenient in many cases. Grams are extremely precise, so they lead to consistent results. You also dirty only a single bowl rather than a slew of measuring cups and spoons. I'm a fan of anything that cuts down on dishes. Despite the advantages of a scale, I still rely on my trusty measuring cups for most baked goods.

If you favor a more rigorous approach, start by measuring in grams with a digital scale. If you don't have a scale yet, using cups and measuring spoons is fine. Both methods yield beautiful, crusty loaves of bread and gorgeous pastries. They also make delicious treats your family will love. Do what works best for you.

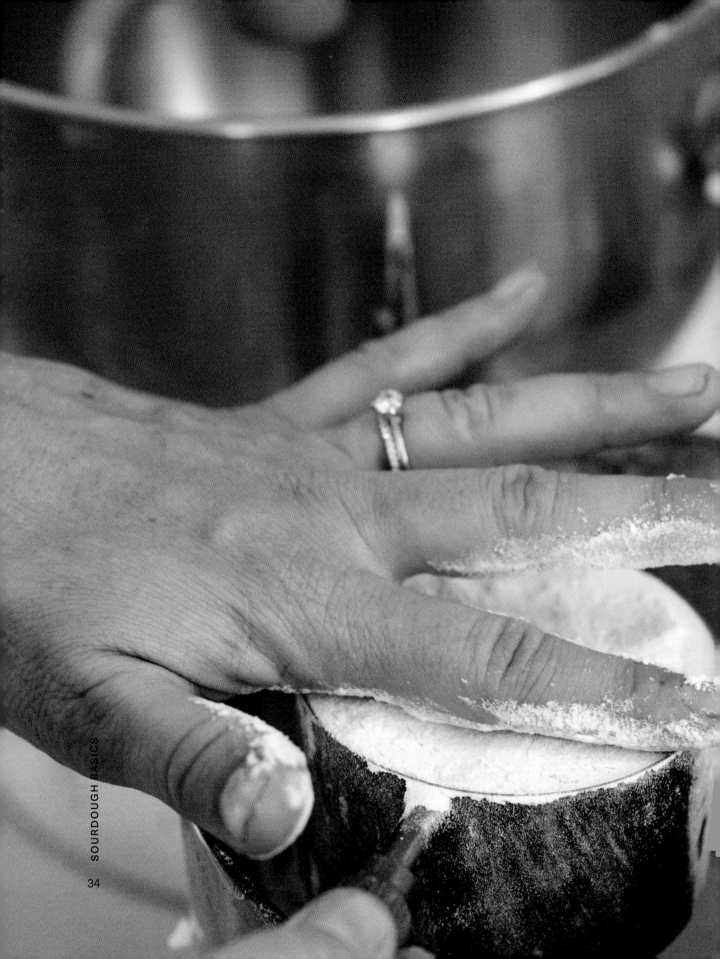

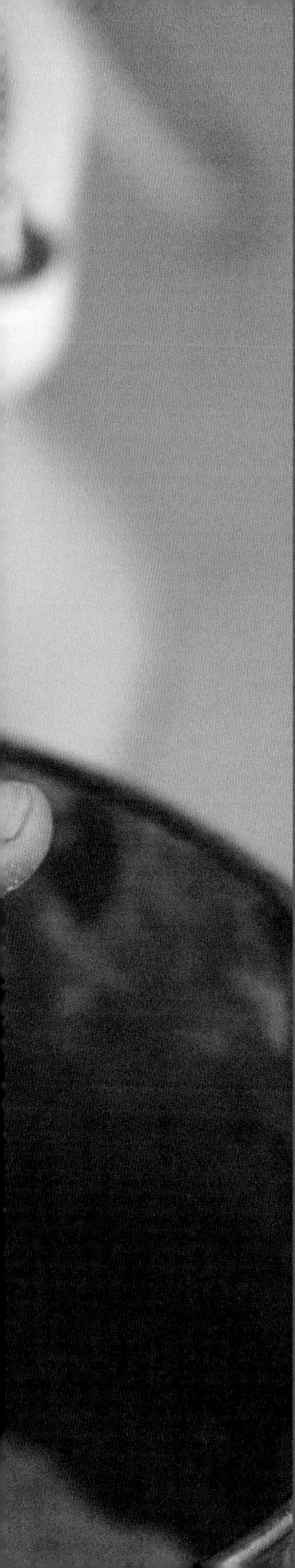

HOW TO MEASURE FLOUR

From a technical perspective, you should measure flour by first sifting it to fluff it up. Then, spoon it carefully into a measuring cup and level it off with a kitchen knife.

But I am not a technical baker. I care more about the practicalities of feeding my family wholesome foods than I do about ultra-precise measurements. I'm no fan of painstakingly measuring ingredients spoonful by spoonful. It's just too much fuss for me. Instead, I dunk my measuring cup into a jar of flour before shaking it off (sometimes I use my finger) until it's level. It's efficient and practical.

Using my method, you'll find that the flour is slightly more compacted and dense. Each cup weighs somewhat more than if you had sifted and spooned it into your measuring cup. The chart below gives you a good idea of how much ingredients weigh using my method.

TYPE OF FLOUR	WEIGHT OF 1 CUP (IN GRAMS)
ALL-PURPOSE	140
BREAD	140
WHOLE-WHEAT	140
WHITE WHOLE-WHEAT	140
ALL-PURPOSE EINKORN	130
WHOLE-GRAIN EINKORN	140
OAT	110
RYE	140
WHITE SPELT	140
WHOLE-GRAIN SPELT	140
KHORASAN WHEAT	140
SOURDOUGH DISCARD	250
ACTIVE SOURDOUGH STARTER	200

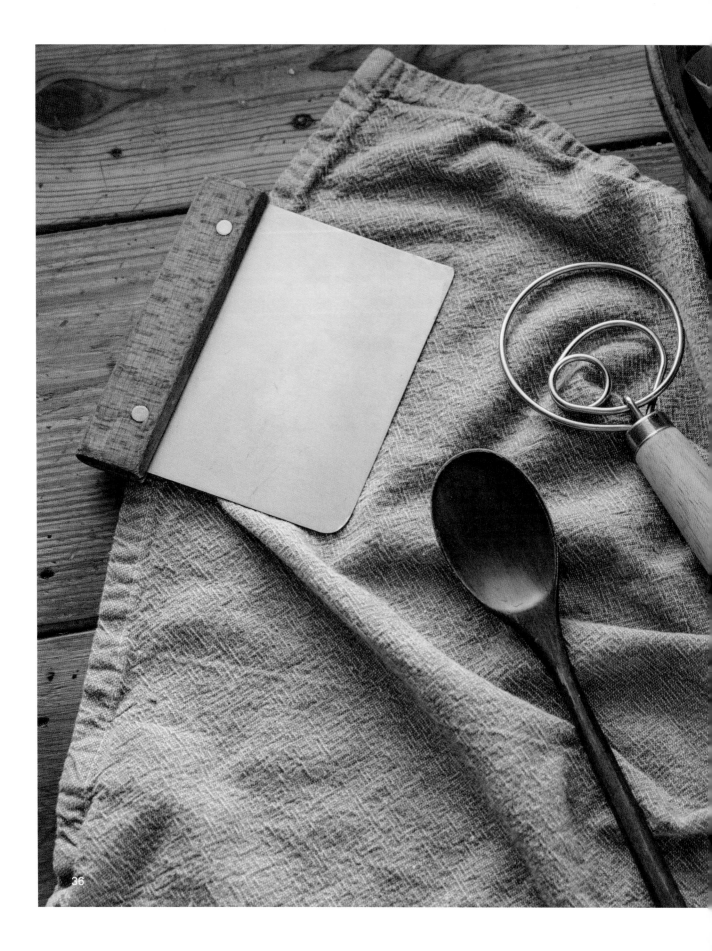

CHAPTER 2

Notes From a Farmhouse Kitchen

WHEN I FIRST STARTED BAKING, I had nothing. Well, almost nothing. The tiny kitchen in my little Midwestern bungalow was just large enough for a stand mixer and a few extra tools. My pantry could hardly hold a week's worth of groceries, let alone countless jars of specialty flours. Later, when we expanded to the farmstead, I had a little more room. As my love of baking grew, so did my tools and pantry.

If you're new to baking, invest in a few essentials: good mixing bowls, quality flour, and a Dutch oven. As your skills and interest grow, you can invest in your tool set and add new ingredients to your pantry. Simple is good.

Helpful Tools

You don't need much to bake great bread. Generations of bakers have successfully made gorgeous loaves of bread and beautiful pastries without fancy equipment. They used little more than good ingredients and a few tools. I had no banneton baskets, food scales, Dutch oven, or scoring tools when I started. Instead, I relied on a sturdy stand mixer, a few loaf pans, and my own two hands. While you don't need much to get started, there are a few tools I find particularly helpful. If you already bake, you may already have a few essentials tucked away in a cupboard in your kitchen. If not, consider picking up a piece or two from a local kitchen shop or online.

Digital Kitchen Scale

Good baking benefits from precision. Precision leads to consistent results from loaf to loaf. The best way to guarantee precise measurements is to weigh your ingredients. If you plan to bake frequently, invest in a digital scale.

Choose a scale that measures in both ounces and grams. It should also be easy to tare the scale, which means to set it to zero. You'll use this feature when you need to set a mixing bowl on top of the scale, into which you measure your ingredients. Ideally, choose a scale with a surface that's easy to wipe clean, as you will inevitably spill flour and other ingredients on it during baking. Remember that even the best kitchen scales have trouble accurately weighing small increments. They especially struggle with amounts under 5 grams, so you'll still need a set of measuring spoons.

Measuring Cups and Spoons

Using volume measures may be less precise than using a scale, but this method worked for me for years and works for many other home bakers, too. Measuring cups and spoons are helpful for scooping ingredients and are necessary for smaller quantities that scales can't accurately measure.

Mixing Bowls

I use mixing bowls with nearly every bake. They're helpful for combining and storing ingredients. If you can find mixing bowls with lids, that's even better. Many sourdough recipes call for letting the dough rest overnight on the countertop or in the fridge. Lidded bowls help prevent your batters and doughs from drying out. Choose glass or stainless steel nesting bowls for easy storage. Look for a set with sizes ranging from 1 to 5 quarts.

Stand Mixer

While you can mix your doughs and batters in a big mixing bowl with a wooden spoon, a stand mixer speeds up the process. In a busy kitchen, it's nice to let the mixer do the heavy lifting while you finish a meal or work on other tasks.

Stand mixers come with dough hooks, whisks, and paddle attachments. These tools expand how you can use the mixer. A dough hook mixes and kneads bread more efficiently and quickly than most of us can manage by hand. Whisks are good for beating air into batters, egg whites, and cream. The paddle attachment is a middle ground between the two. Use it when making batters or cakes or when creaming butter and sugar together.

> **THE ESSENTIALS**
>
> IF YOU CAN ONLY AFFORD A FEW ITEMS, INVEST IN THESE ESSENTIALS:
> - MIXING BOWLS AND SPOONS
> - MEASURING CUPS AND SPOONS
> - A BREAD LAME
> - A DUTCH OVEN

When I do not have a stand mixer and am kneading by hand, I use stretching and folding until the dough reaches the correct consistency. Throughout this book, you'll see instructions for using a stand mixer. However, know that you can use the stretch-and-fold technique instead.

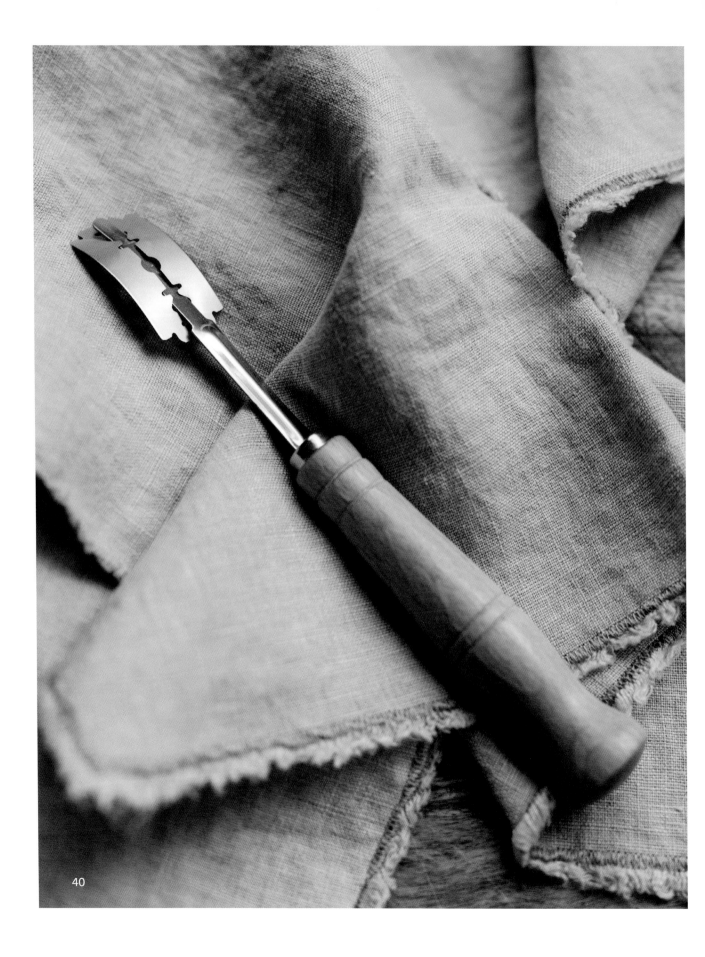

Lame

Right before you place your bread in the oven, you need to slash or score the dough to help control the expansion of the bread during baking. This technique allows the bread to rise properly and creates an attractive pattern on the crust. A bread lame (pronounced "lahm")—a long, often wooden, stick with a metal razor blade attached to it—is one of my favorite ways to do this. Its sharp blade produces deep, clean cuts that are hard to replicate with a knife, and it's easy to replace when it grows dull with use.

In the absence of a lame, you can use a small sharp knife to score your bread with simple slashes. Knives are duller and less delicate than a lame, so achieving intricate scoring patterns is more challenging.

Bannetons and Proofing Baskets

Bannetons and proofing baskets hold the shape of your loaf during its final rise before you transfer it to the oven to bake. Because wetter doughs have a higher water-to-flour ratio, they tend to lose their form without a container. Similarly, bread made from heritage grains, such as einkorn or spelt, have a weaker gluten structure, making it difficult for them to hold their form after shaping.

Proofing baskets are perfect for the task. They come in various shapes, though round ones are the most popular. Rattan bannetons tend to be the best quality and the longest lasting, but you can also find them in wicker or even plastic. Many come with linen or cotton liners. Dusting the liners with flour before each use helps the dough release from the basket when you turn it out to bake. If you opt not to use liners, you'll need to season your banneton (see sidebar). A medium round basket or a kitchen bowl lined with a floured tea towel makes an acceptable substitute.

> **HOW TO SEASON A BANNETON**
>
> Bannetons benefit from seasoning to create a nonstick surface, just like a cast-iron skillet. To season your banneton, spray it with water and dust it generously with flour. Dump out the excess flour, and then let it dry completely. Repeat the process once or twice before you use it for the first time. Spray it again and dust it with flour once more before each bake.

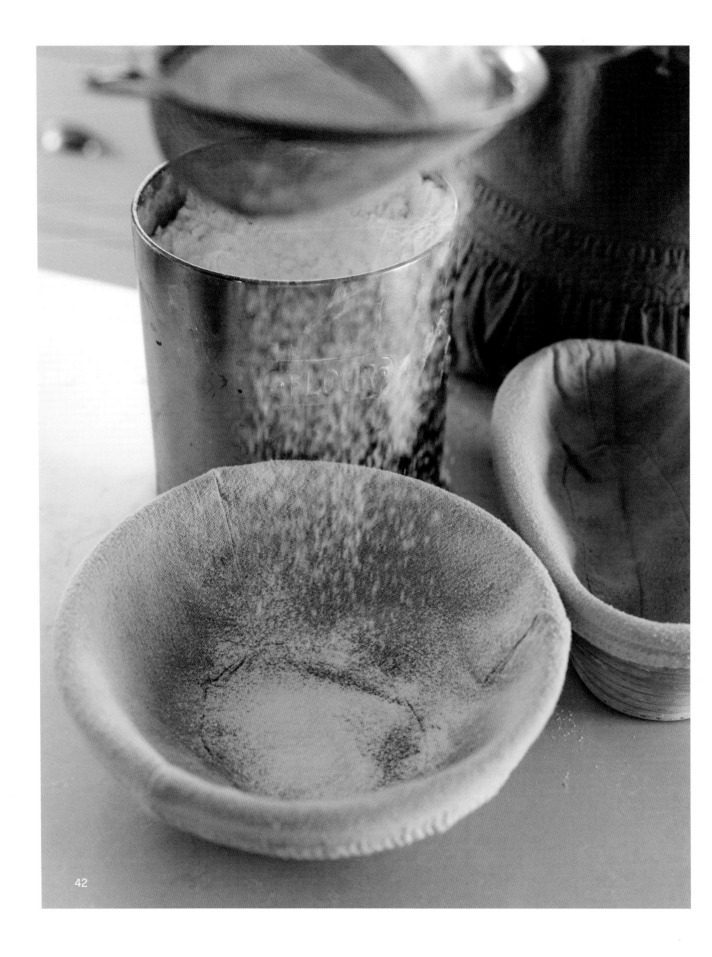

Tea Towels and Proofing Linens

I always keep a trusty tea towel, which is a versatile baking tool, at the ready. Drape one over a mixing bowl of dough to keep it moist and pliable as it rises. Line your proofing basket with a floured towel to help the dough release when you turn it out, and gently cover the dough with another towel to protect it from dust and debris.

Cotton or linen towels work the best. Choose thin, smoothly woven cotton towels, such as flour sack towels. Avoid towels made of nubby cotton terry cloth. They'll catch your dough in every nook and cranny, and tear it when you turn it out of the proofing basket. While more expensive than cotton, linen lasts longer and is less likely to stick. You can order both linen and cotton tea towels from any kitchen or baking supply store. If you have a mind to make your own, pick up a few yards of cotton or linen at your local fabric store.

Cast-Iron Skillet and Dutch Oven

Castiron can last for generations. If you care for them well, they will never wear out and you can pass them on as heirlooms to your children.

A well-seasoned cast-iron skillet transfers easily from the range to the oven and is perfect for a wide variety of uses. Use it to sauté vegetables for sourdough skillets (page 279), make pancakes (page 275) or crêpes (page 270) if you don't have a crêpe pan, or bake treats, such as double chocolate sweet rolls (page 220).

For baking boules, nothing beats a Dutch oven. When you preheat a Dutch oven, it becomes scorching hot and maintains that heat well. This ability to retain and distribute consistent heat helps high-hydration loaves keep their form and cook evenly, which translates to deliciously crusty loaves.

Keeping the lid on the Dutch oven during the first 20 minutes of baking captures the steam the bread releases as it bakes. This humidity slows down the formation of the crust, allowing the bread to rise more fully. As a result, you can produce airy loaves with a soft crumb and crisp, crackly crust.

Cast-iron skillets and Dutch ovens are affordable, given their longevity and versatility. Enameled cast iron is pricier but doesn't require seasoning or special maintenance. It makes a good choice for your Dutch oven. Plain, uncoated cast iron works best for your skillet.

But you can still make great bread without a Dutch oven. Bake your boules on a baking sheet lined with parchment paper or a pizza stone. You can also make delicious bread in a loaf pan, especially for sandwiches.

To emulate the humidity of a Dutch oven if you're using a pizza stone or a baking sheet, try this hack: Fill a cast-iron skillet with a cup or two of water and set it on the bottom rack of your oven. Then place your bread on a baking sheet or pizza stone set on the middle rack. As the bread bakes, the heat will cause the water in the skillet to steam. It may not spring up quite as high as one baked in a Dutch oven, but it'll still develop a delicious crackly crust.

Baking Pans and Bakeware

When it comes to baking pans, buy only what you need and only what you plan to use frequently. A muffin tin helps muffins hold their shape while they bake, and you can make popovers in it, too. Rimmed baking sheets are perfect for biscuits and cookies. Pie plates are essential for making pies and just as good for cobblers. Cake tins and brownie pans are necessary if you plan to make either. Loaf pans are suitable for both quick breads and sandwich loaves.

I love glass bakeware as well as stoneware and stainless steel. Glass cleans up well and distributes heat evenly, whereas stoneware is great for retaining heat so food stays warm even out of the oven. Stainless steel loaf pans are always a favorite, too. These are all made with nontoxic materials, so you don't have to worry about the potential health hazards that come with certain nonstick pans.

Pizza Stone

A pizza stone is a flat piece of stoneware that fits on your oven rack. Like cast iron, it retains heat well, which translates to even cooking. It also absorbs excess moisture, giving bread and pizzas a crisp crust.

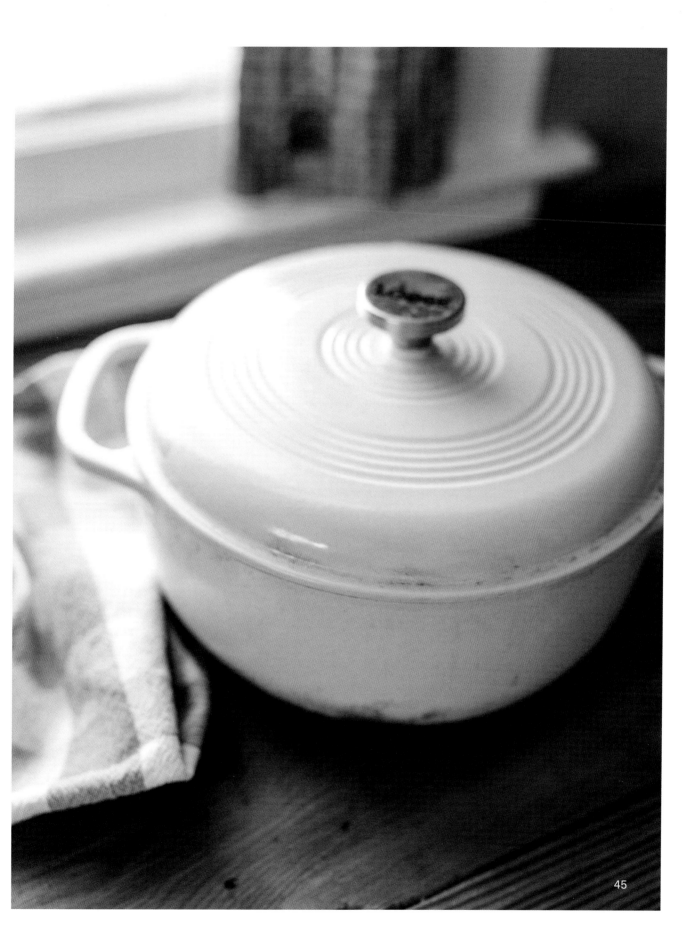

Look for a flat, rectangular pizza stone, which is more versatile than round stones. If you cannot find a pizza stone, a baking sheet lined with parchment paper will do for most applications. You may find that your crusts aren't quite as crisp, but they will still taste delicious.

Grain Mill

Baked goods made from freshly ground grains have a rich, distinct flavor that's hard to get from pre-ground flour. Commercially processed flour often loses micronutrients due to the heat and oxidation from milling, transportation, and prolonged storage. By contrast, freshly milled flour generally contains more micronutrients than store-bought whole-grain flour. As a result, baked goods made with freshly milled flour are more flavorful and nutritious.

Still, a grain mill can be costly. For most people, using pre-ground store-bought flour works fine. Grain mills designed for home usage produce only whole-grain flour. It might not be worth the investment if you prefer to bake with all-purpose or bread flour. If you love whole grains and are committed to making the most nutritious bread, consider picking one up.

Cooling Racks

When making bread and other baked goods, you want to promote both even cooking and even cooling. These small, elevated metal racks allow air to circulate on all sides of your bread and cookies as they cool. In contrast, if you let your baked goods cool directly on a plate or countertop, they will cool unevenly, making the bottom crust moist and sometimes even mushy or tough.

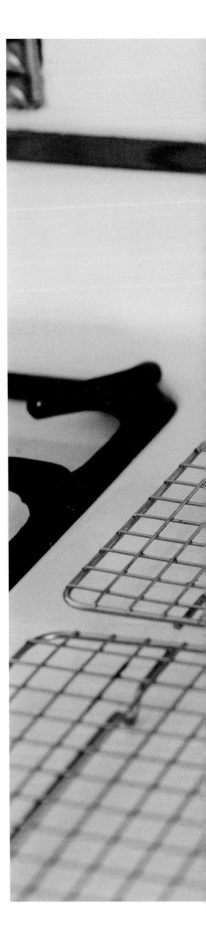

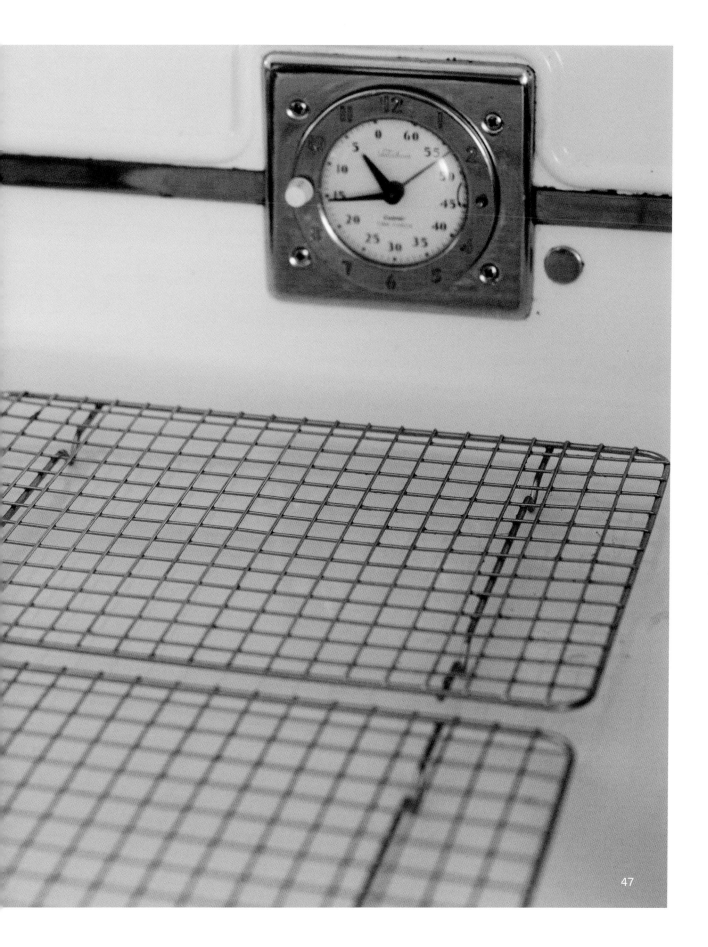

Bench Scraper

Bench scrapers (sometimes called bench knives) help you manipulate dough on your working surface. They are ideal for separating dough into smaller pieces for shaping. You can also use them to lift pieces of dough off your countertop.

Many bench scrapers have a rectangular stainless steel blade and a wooden or plastic handle that makes them easy to grip. Stainless steel scrapers are best for separating and cutting dough. You can also find flexible scrapers made from plastic or silicone. Many flexible scrapers have both a straight and a curved edge. Use the curved edge to scrape every last bit of batter out of a mixing bowl. Then, cut the dough into smaller pieces and lift them off your countertop with its straight edge.

Rolling Pin

Rolling pins help press your dough into an even thickness. The technique is especially important for pie crusts, sweet buns, and rolls. There are three primary varieties of rolling pins.

- Traditional pins are typically made from wood. They are a straight cylinder with an even width from end to end. Their straight design makes them a good, versatile option for various purposes. Traditional pins with handles are popular. However, those without handles allow better control over the dough's thickness for more uniform results.

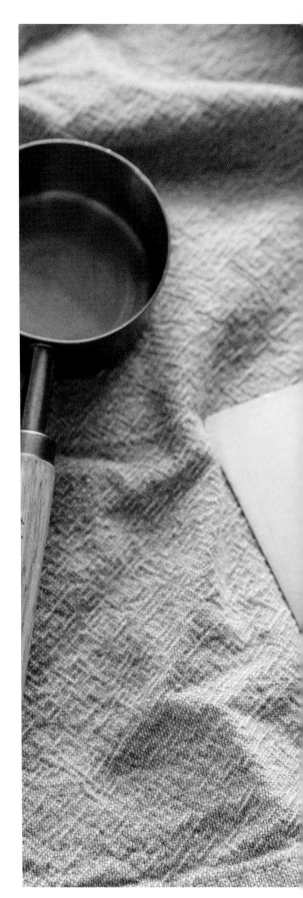

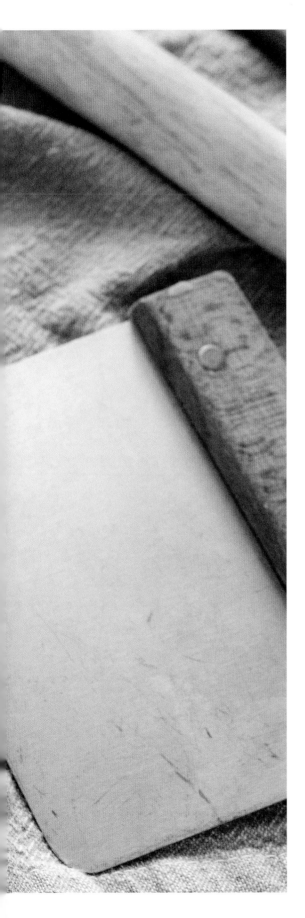

- French rolling pins look like traditional pins but are tapered on either end, with a thicker center. This shape makes it easier to control the thickness of the dough in various areas. These versatile pins are good for shaping round dough, such as pie crust.

- Marble rolling pins are shaped like traditional pins, but dough tends to stick less to the smooth surface than it does to wooden pins. Unlike wood, marble also stays cool when handled, which keeps your dough from getting too warm.

Pasta Maker

If you plan to make sourdough noodles (page 284), a pasta maker produces finer, thinner noodles than if you were to cut them by hand. Pasta makers are also excellent for rolling out paper-thin sheets of dough that make lovely crackers when you bake them.

Stainless steel hand-crank models are popular. You clamp the device on to the table and then you slowly work the dough through rollers, gradually narrowing the space between them until the dough is so thin you can see light through it. Some stand mixers, such as KitchenAid, also sell good pasta-making attachments.

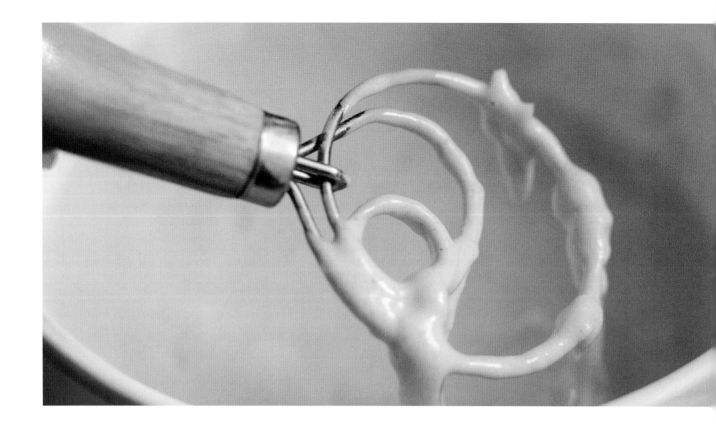

If you rarely make pasta and don't want to invest in a pasta maker, you can simply roll out your dough thinly and cut it by hand for charming, rustic noodles.

Danish Dough Whisk

A Danish dough whisk is a wooden-handled tool equipped with a metal curlicue on one end. Use it for mixing dough, especially wet, shaggy bread dough. If you're making pastries, a dough whisk is helpful for working cold butter into flour. Due to its design, it gently incorporates the ingredients together. There's little risk of overworking the dough, which can happen with electric mixers. They're designed to mix dough efficiently, are easy to clean, and minimize the mess that sometimes accompanies hand mixing. A sturdy wooden spoon is a good (though less efficient) stand-in for a Danish dough whisk.

Hand Tools

Having a few other versatile tools is helpful when baking.

- Ice cream scoop—good for dishing out muffin and cookie dough into even scoops.

- Pastry blender—work cold butter into flour for utterly flaky biscuits and pie crusts.

- Pizza cutter—slice pizza or even strips of dough for sweet rolls and sticky buns.

- Long-handled spider strainer or slotted spoon—lift pretzels or bagels from their baking soda bath.

- Pastry brush—coat your pastries and bread with egg wash to make them shiny and brown like professional baked goods.

- Biscuit cutter—use the sharp edge to cut out biscuits cleanly, encouraging them to rise tall. If you don't have one, you can use an inverted mason jar, though its dull edge may mean less loft in your biscuits.

Heat-Resistant Gloves

Things get mighty hot when you're baking bread—especially if you bake your loaves in a cast-iron Dutch oven like I do. Keeping a pair of heat-resistant gloves in your kitchen keeps things safer. It's easier to lift the scorching lid of a Dutch oven with properly protected hands. Even if you're taking extra care as you plop proofed dough into a preheated Dutch oven, you can still burn yourself. So hand protection is smart.

Plastic Wrap, Plastic Bags, and Waxed Cloth

While your dough rises, especially during bulk fermentation, you need a way to keep it moist. If your mixing bowl doesn't have a tight-fitting lid, cover it with a square of plastic wrap to prevent the dough from drying out and crusting over. Similarly, plastic bags laid gently over rising loaves of bread help keep the moisture in. If you avoid single-use disposable plastic, buy a few pieces of waxed cloth, such as beeswax wrap, and mold them over your mixing bowls for a tight-fitting seal. The best part? They're reusable.

Parchment Paper

I often use parchment paper when baking everything from bread to cookies. Parchment paper acts a barrier between your baked goods and the pan, redistributing heat, minimizing hot spots, and promoting even baking.

When baking bread, place the dough on parchment paper after its final rise. Transfer the dough to the oven by gently lifting the parchment and drop it into the preheated Dutch oven. (The parchment helps keep the loaf from sticking to the bottom of the Dutch oven.) When baking cookies and other treats, line the baking sheet with a slip of parchment paper for easy cleanup.

Farmhouse Pantry

To make great-tasting sourdough, you need to start with great-tasting ingredients. Remember that expensive ingredients are not always synonymous with *quality* ingredients. Simple, wholesome ingredients such as whole grains and minimally processed flour add a delicious depth of flavor to your baked goods. Additions like punchy extra-virgin olive oil and creamy yellow grass-fed butter lend a richness to breads and pastries. Emphasize fresh vegetables, fruits, and herbs at the peak of their season, which are not only plentiful and affordable but also boost the nutritional value and taste of your bakes. The quality of your bread can only be as good as the ingredients you put into it.

When baking sourdough, there are a few staples that I could never do without. They take your baking to a new level, infusing it with rich and unforgettable flavor. You might find they're essentials in your kitchen, too. When it comes to wholesome foods, invest in the best quality that fits your budget.

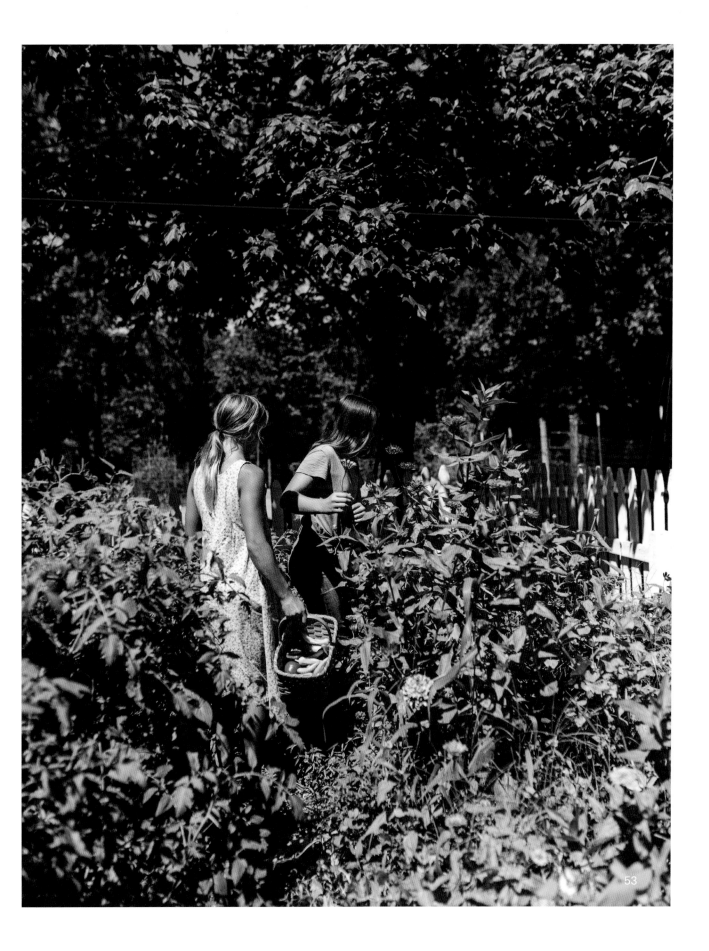

Grains and Flour

Flour is the foundation of good bread. To bake excellent sourdough, you must have a firm understanding of flours and grains. Though all grains provide starch, fiber, and small amounts of vitamins and minerals, each variety offers unique flavors and baking properties. For instance, the quality of wheat varies from season to season, rye introduces a rustic edge, and ancient grains add more nutrition.

Similarly, flour varies depending on the grain from which it is milled. It took me time to determine which grains I preferred and how these differences manifest in baking. So take your time, too. Explore various grains and flours and soon you will feel familiar with their qualities.

Whole Grains

Whole grains taste delicious, with their subtle sweetness and light nutty undertones. They can add texture and depth of flavor to baked goods. I keep a bag of cereal mix in the cupboard. It contains a variety of grains such as wheat berries, oats, barley, and rye. I use it to make multigrain bread. Additionally, I buy bags of whole grains in bulk and mill them myself in my grain mill. Wheat and einkorn are among my favorites.

Bread Flour

Bread flour is a type of white flour, as it does not contain the grain's bran or germ. Bread flour, usually made from hard red wheat, has more protein than all-purpose flour. This makes it the top choice for baking most types of bread, especially artisan styles. Its high protein content is the bedrock for gluten development, which is crucial for the bread's structure and texture. A robust gluten network allows the dough to trap the gasses produced by yeast during fermentation. This results in light and airy bread with a deliciously chewy crumb.

Unbleached bread flour with a high protein content (typically 12 to 14%) is my first choice for many breads. The high amount of protein lends to better gluten development. High-hydration loaves, which are looser because of their higher water-to-flour ratio, benefit the most from the structure that bread flour provides.

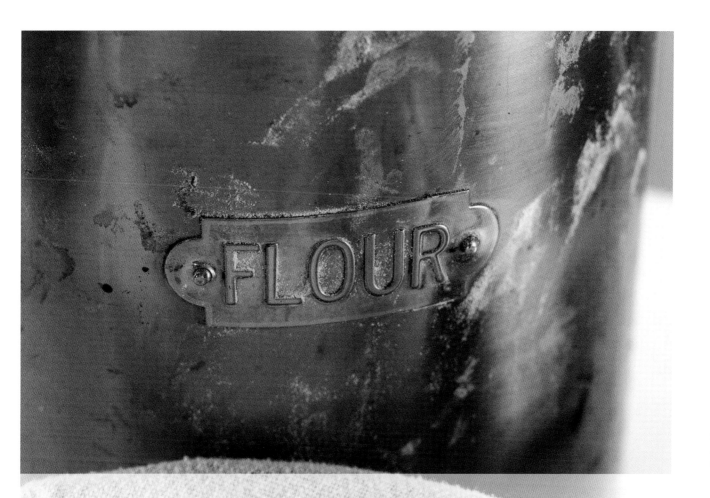

BLEACHED OR UNBLEACHED?

For generations dating back to ancient Rome, the color of your bread marked your social class. At the time, white flour required more labor to produce, which made the softer, whiter loaves affordable only to the wealthy. Plain brown bread was for the poor classes. Whiter bread meant better bread, regardless of nutrition, and this trend continued into the early twentieth century.

Ingenious millers wanted to give people exactly what they preferred. So they whitened their naturally creamy-colored flour by bleaching it stark white. In the early days, this process involved highly reactive chemicals, such as nitrogen oxide and chlorine gas. Now, benzoyl peroxide is more common.

Even though unbleached flour requires less processing, it, oddly, costs a little more than bleached flour. I find it well worth the price.

All-Purpose Flour

Besides bread flour, I keep a big glass jar of all-purpose flour in my pantry. You can use it for everything from bread to pastries and even pasta. It is softer than bread flour, with a lower protein content that hovers between 8 and 11%. That's enough protein to give a little to bread, but not so much that it runs the risk of making your pastries tough. This balance makes all-purpose flour exceptionally versatile. If you have room for only one kind of flour in your kitchen, it's the one to buy.

Whole-Wheat Flour

Millers produce whole-wheat flour by grinding the entire wheat kernel— including the bran, germ, and endosperm (see page 58). It retains essential nutrients like fiber, protein, vitamins, and minerals that are otherwise lost in the refining process of white flour. Whole-wheat flour is usually made from hard red wheat, the same variety used in making bread flour. Its coarse texture and rich flavor make it a great addition to bread, lending it a rustic quality and brown appearance.

You can find whole-wheat flour at almost every supermarket as well as online. Some millers combine whole-wheat flour with white flour. Carefully inspect the label to make sure it contains 100% whole wheat. If you have your own grain mill, you can grind hard red wheat berries at home to make your own. Wheat berries are available at natural markets, specialty stores, and online.

White Whole-Wheat Flour

A variation of whole-wheat flour, white whole-wheat flour (sometimes called white wheat flour or whole-wheat pastry flour) shouldn't be confused with white flour. Like whole-wheat flour, millers grind the entire grain, but they use white wheat, which has a lighter color and milder flavor than red wheat. It's a good choice for bakers who want to emulate the mild taste and paler color of white flour while retaining the nutrition and flavor of whole grains. Despite its light color, it contains plenty of fiber, various B vitamins, and many minerals.

White whole-wheat flour behaves similarly to regular whole-wheat flour, but it may produce slightly lighter and more tender results. This is because of its finer texture and milder flavor. Use it in breads, cookies, biscuits, pancakes, and anything that calls for white flour.

If you wish to grind your flour from scratch, buy soft white wheat berries for pastries and hard white wheat berries for bread. If you don't have a grain mill, you can buy it online at most natural foods markets. Look for labels that describe the flour as "100% whole grain."

Einkorn Flour

Einkorn is an ancient variety of wheat with a rich nutritional profile and, when baked, a creamy golden color. It has a higher protein and fat content than modern wheat but a soft texture, making it particularly good for pastries and quick breads. The gluten content of einkorn differs from that of bread flour, so einkorn breads don't have the lofty structure you find in other loaves Still, it tastes wonderfully delicious with a delicate sweetness and rich, nutty profile.

As with wheat flour, you can buy whole-grain einkorn and all-purpose einkorn flour. If you have a grain mill, you can buy einkorn berries and grind them fresh to make whole-grain flour. Good quality all-purpose einkorn flour has a soft texture and a pale, creamy color. Whole-grain einkorn flour is flecked with bits of amber brown, thanks to the inclusion of both the bran and germ.

Spelt Flour

Like einkorn, spelt is an ancient grain related to wheat. Its rich, complex flavor lends a delicate, nutty note to baked goods. Spelt flour contains slightly more protein than wheat, but its gluten structure is weaker. This makes it less likely to produce a light, airy loaf, but its soft texture is excellent for cookies and pastries. If you want to bake bread, consider combining it with stronger flour, such as bread flour, for better structure.

Most natural foods markets and many grocery stores sell spelt berries and flour. You can also buy them online if you can't find them locally. Whole-grain spelt flour has a creamy color flecked with gray. White spelt flour is also widely available.

ANATOMY OF A GRAIN

A staple for thousands of years, grains hold all the power of life within their tiny kernels. Grains are seeds. They stay dormant until the right circumstances allow them to sprout and grow into plants. Each kernel holds all the nutrition those very young plants need—primarily starch. Fortunately, they also provide plenty of nourishment for us, too.

Whole grains, such as wheat or rye berries, comprise three distinct parts. These are the bran, the germ, and the endosperm. Whole-grain flour contains all three components. White flour contains only the endosperm. Millers sift out the bran and germ to make it.

The bran is the husk, the brown outer layer of a grain. It acts as a shell, protecting the more fragile components within the kernel. The bran is exceptionally nutritious. It contains fiber, various B vitamins, and minerals. It also contains phytic acid, which can bind minerals and prevent their absorption. Sourdough fermentation helps break apart phytic acid. This process makes those minerals easier to absorb.

The germ stores the bulk of the grain's micronutrients. It contains a small amount of fat, fiber, various B vitamins, and vitamin E. It also has many minerals and antioxidants. When the grain sprouts, the germ grows to form a seedling and, eventually, a plant.

The endosperm acts as the food storehouse for the grain. It contains protein and carbohydrates, which provide nourishment for the sprouting plant. When we bake the grain into bread, these nutrients not only fuel us but also provide elasticity to the dough and bulk to the baked loaf.

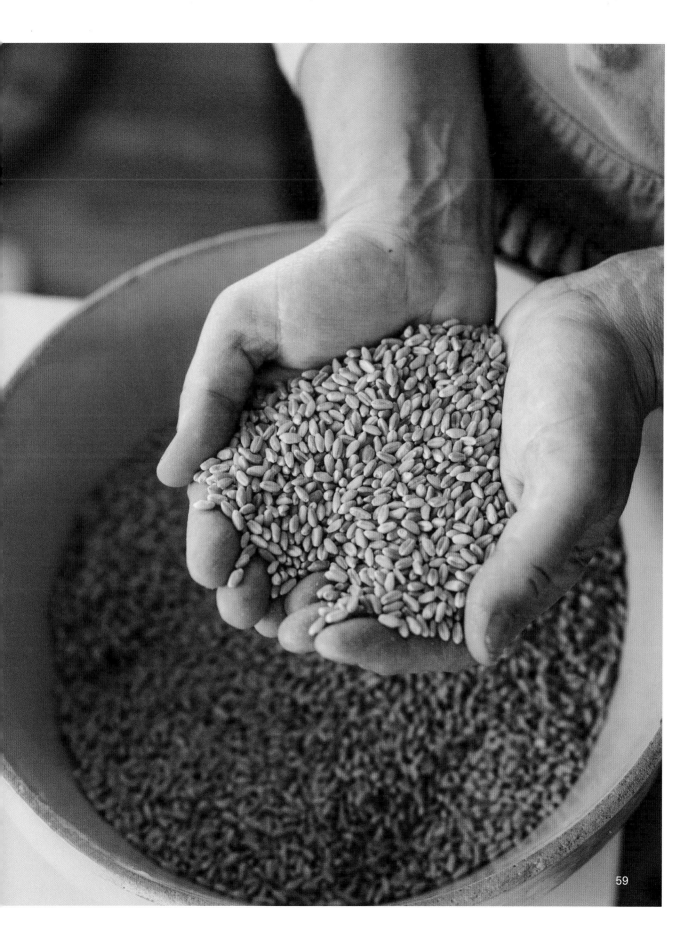

Rye Flour

Rye is a dusty gray grain with a malty, earthy flavor, making it the perfect choice for rustic loaves. Because it contains much less gluten than wheat flour, rye flour produces denser loaves with fewer air bubbles. It's also a more nutrient-dense option than wheat, since it is rich in fiber and minerals like manganese, magnesium, and phosphorus. Rye's lower glycemic index means it supports better blood sugar balance than wheat as well.

Many health food stores stock rye berries and rye flour. Rye flour contains all parts of the grain, including the fiber-rich bran and nutrient-dense germ. Light rye flour is similar to white flour, with a milder flavor and softer texture.

Oats Flour

Oats are a gluten-free grain. As such, they lack the sticky protein structure that gives bread its ability to rise high and develop an open, airy crumb. For this reason, oats don't make a good foundation for bread. Rather, use them as an accent grain. Chewy rolled oats lend a toothsome texture and sweet, earthy notes to wheat-based doughs.

I like to use old-fashioned thick-cut rolled oats in baking. They tend to be a little thicker than the quick-cooking kind, which can fall apart when exposed to too much liquid. Thick-cut rolled oats, by contrast, keep their chewy texture. I like to work them into bread doughs and batters, but you can also scatter them on top of a loaf of bread just before it heads into the oven. The oats lend a pretty, rustic appearance to homemade bread.

Khorasan Wheat Flour

Khorasan wheat, often marketed as Kamut (which is simply a specific brand), originated in the Fertile Crescent thousands of years ago and has gained popularity thanks to a rising interest in ancient grains. Distantly related to durum wheat, Khorasan wheat is a large, plump grain with a rich nutritional profile that appeals to health-minded consumers. Like many ancient grains, Khorasan wheat is higher in protein than modern wheat. It also contains more vitamins, antioxidants, and minerals—especially zinc and selenium. Like einkorn,

Khorasan wheat is a good source of beta-carotene, which gives the grain a beautiful amber-gold hue.

Its deliciously nutty flavor translates well to gorgeous, rich-tasting pizza crusts and focaccia. Shop for Khorasan wheat flour in health food stores, natural markets, and online.

Brown Rice Flour
Brown rice flour is coarse, and it's perfect for dusting bannetons and tea towels. Its rough texture and lack of gluten make it an excellent barrier between your rising dough and the banneton. As a result, your dough is less likely to stick.

Fats and Oils
Fats and oils infuse your baked goods with flavor and support their structure. They also lend tenderness and moisture. They make biscuits light, cookies tender, and pie crust flaky. At the farmhouse, we skip the margarine and vegetable oil. Instead, we stick to traditional cooking fats, such as butter, olive oil, and lard. They have nourished healthy people for generations. That's good enough for my family, too.

Butter
Butter is a perennial favorite of bakers. It adds richness to everything from cookies to pastries, making them more enjoyable and satisfying. Butter also plays a crucial role in creating tender and moist baked goods. It coats flour particles and inhibits gluten formation. This results in a softer texture and improved moisture retention. It ensures that cakes, cookies, and other treats remain moist and delicious.

Butter's properties vary depending on its temperature. Cold butter is excellent for making flaky pastries and pie crusts. Soft, room-temperature butter is ideal for cookies and cakes. It holds on to air bubbles when whipped, turning baked goods fluffy and tender. Melted butter is excellent for brushing over pastries and bread. It coats their crusts and encourages browning.

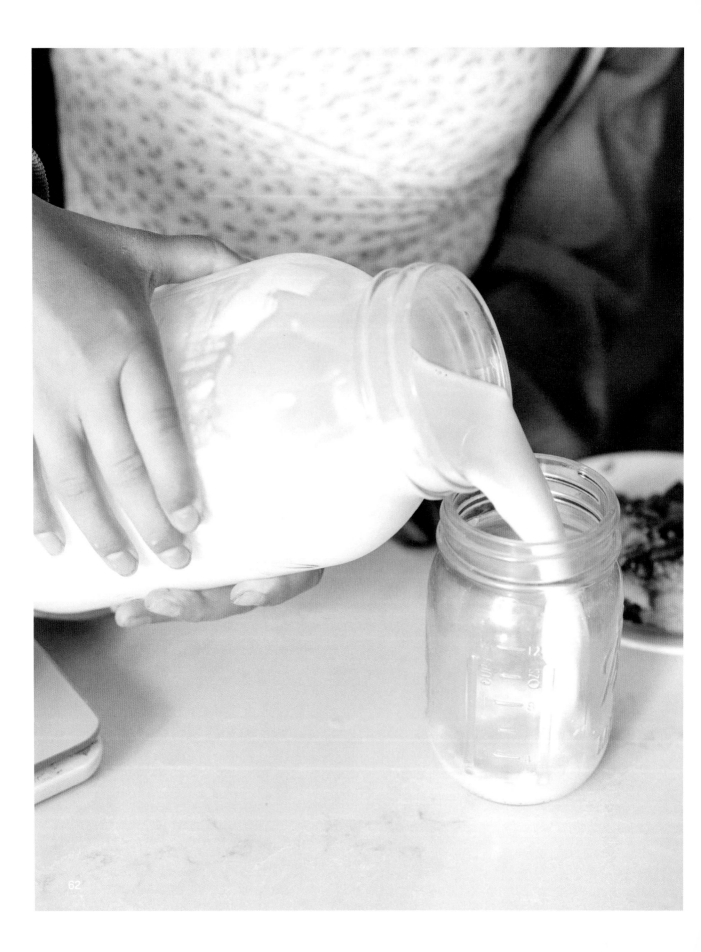

I use unsalted butter in baking, because it allows me to control the salt content of my baked goods more effectively. Additionally, cultured butter is always a good choice. Cultured butter is made from fermented cream. It has a richer and more complex flavor than butter made with sweet cream. Baked goods made with cultured butter taste divine.

Look for butter made from the cream of grass-fed cows. It has a richer nutritional profile and more flavor than conventional butter. Grass-fed butter typically contains higher levels of healthy fats, fat-soluble vitamins, and antioxidants. This is because the cows' natural diet is rich in these nutrients. It is widely available in grocery stores.

Extra-Virgin Olive Oil

Like butter, extra-virgin olive oil adds flavor and tenderness to baked goods. I often swirl a little olive oil into mixing bowls to prevent dough from sticking as it rises. It also contributes flavor to ciabatta (page 140) and other breads. Look for extra-virgin olive oil with a flavor that you enjoy. They all taste a little different depending on the region where the olives were grown. The olives also taste different depending on when the growers harvest and press them. Extra-virgin olive oil is the most flavorful and contains the most antioxidants.

Coconut Oil

Coconut oil is a favorite in my kitchen. It's versatile and easy to use. It makes a great alternative to butter if you're cooking for someone with a dairy sensitivity. Coconut oil mainly contains saturated fats, which make it last longer in the cupboard. Its high smoke point also makes it a good choice for high-heat applications such as frying.

Most coconut oil tastes and smells like coconut, but you won't notice it much in your baked goods. Some companies bleach and deodorize their coconut oil. Look for minimally processed options. Cold-pressed, extra-virgin, and virgin coconut oil are good choices.

Lard

Lard is rendered pork fat, and it has a vaguely bacon-like flavor. Its high smoke point makes it excellent for frying foods such as donuts. It also makes lovely pastries since it is hard when cold and soft at room temperature.

Most lard sold in the grocery store is hydrogenated so it stays hard at room temperature and lasts longer. Makers must disclose this on the label. You only want non-hydrogenated lard. If you find a jar of lard that doesn't mention hydrogenation, you should be fine.

Dairy and Eggs

At the farmhouse, we like to keep our food as close to home as we can. We keep chickens for eggs and opt for fresh, raw milk and cream from healthy grass-fed cows. They just taste better. The eggs from hens raised with plenty of room to roam and forage taste delicious with their rich golden-orange yolks. Farm-fresh milk has a beautiful sweetness and an incomparable creaminess. These foods are also more nutrient-dense than those from animals held in close quarters as is done in conventional farming. That flavor (and all those nutrients) will translate to your baking. As a result, your breads and treats will be more nutrient-dense and taste better, too.

Sweeteners

Sugar, maple syrup, honey, and other sweeteners make your food taste delicious. They also help your baked goods retain moisture and stay tender. A little bit can add depth to bread and encourage it to brown. In larger amounts, they sweeten treats like cookies and cakes. They also add volume and structure to these baked goods. It's a good idea to keep a few different sweeteners in your kitchen.

Sugar

Sugar does more than sweeten baked goods. It also provides moisture, promotes tenderness, and supports their structure. Granulated sugar is the most popular choice, as it's affordable and has a neutral flavor. I also often bake with brown sugar. It adds moisture to baked goods, and its rich, caramel-like flavor is hard to beat in cinnamon rolls and other sweets. Powdered sugar

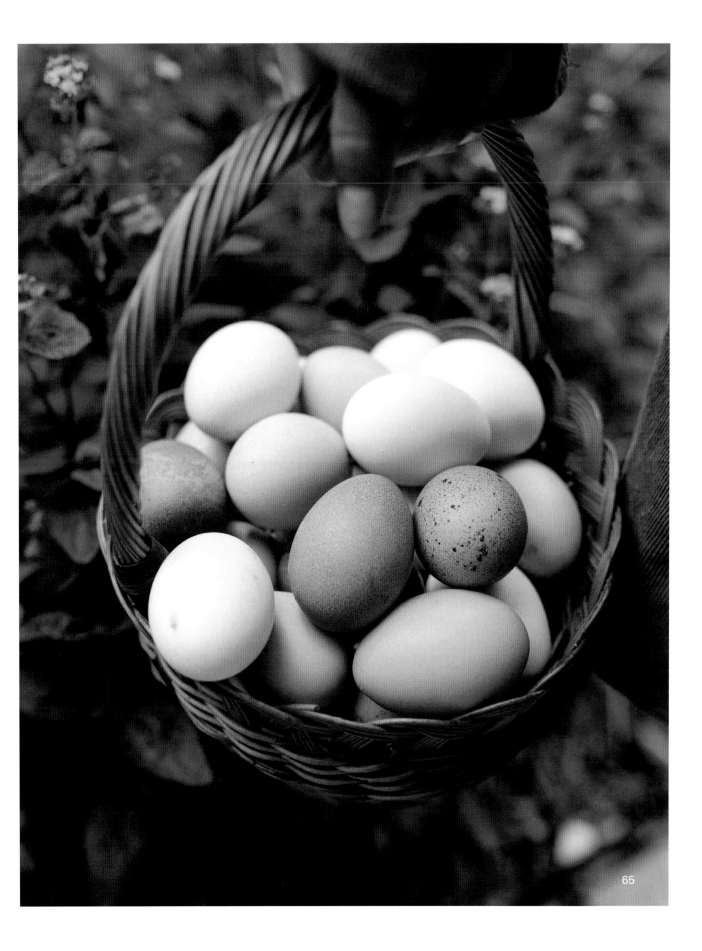

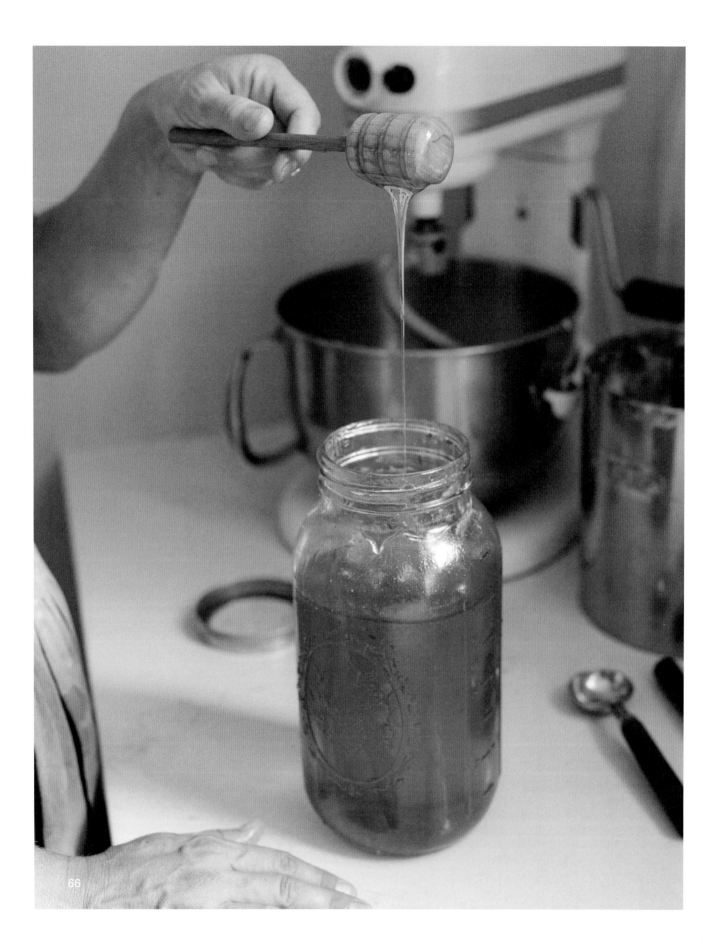

is perfect for frostings and glazes. I keep a jar in the cupboard for special occasions.

I also like to use minimally processed sweeteners, too. Rapadura sugar is a favorite. It's like granulated sugar in texture but has the rich, molasses-like flavor of brown sugar. Coconut sugar, made from the sap of the coconut palm, is a great substitute for cane sugar. These minimally processed options retain more of their mineral content than granulated sugar, which, in part, accounts for their deeper flavor.

Maple Syrup

Maple syrup's rich, woodsy notes and toffee-like sweetness make it a natural match for warm winter spices like cinnamon and cloves. As a liquid sweetener, it adds moisture to baked goods without making them too dense. It is also easy to whip into soft cream cheese or butter for frostings and glazes.

Pay attention to labels when purchasing maple syrup. "Grade A" indicates that it's pure maple syrup without any additives. You might also notice other indicators on the label, too. Golden maple syrup is the lightest, with a lovely, delicate, tawny straw color. It has a sweet flavor with delicate notes of vanilla. Amber maple syrup tastes of caramel with light woodsy notes. Dark maple syrup has a robust flavor with a toffee-like intensity. The darker the maple syrup is, the richer and more intense its flavor.

Honey

Honey's flavor varies widely from light and floral to rich and chocolate-like. It depends on the flowers that the bees feed on. Wildflower honey tastes like flowers. Orange blossom honey reminds me of fresh citrus fruit. Buckwheat honey has a rich, nutty flavor that's hard to resist. My favorite is local honey. It tastes sweet and delicate, with notes of wildflowers and orchard blossoms.

Just a little honey adds depth to bread, especially in combination with whole-grain flour. Sometimes, I'll swirl a little into whipped cream and serve it with berries. I'll also fold it into the batter for French Toast (page 232).

Salt

Sure, salt enhances the flavor of your foods, but it does a lot more than that. Notably, salt strengthens bread dough by tightening the gluten framework. The tighter gluten structure traps carbon dioxide produced by the wild yeast in your starter. This allows the dough to expand and rise properly. Salt also helps control yeast fermentation. It regulates the rate at which these microorganisms eat the sugar in the flour and produce carbon dioxide. This controlled fermentation process ensures that the dough rises evenly and at a consistent rate. As a result, bread baked with salt tends to have better volume, an even texture, and a well-developed crumb structure.

You can find plenty of different types of salt at the market. Iodized salt is budget-friendly and widely available. However, it can give baked goods a subtle but unpleasant metallic flavor. I prefer to use minimally processed salt that retains its natural array of minerals. You can find salt that has been mined from ancient sea beds and sea salt that is harvested from briny ocean water. Both work fine. Finely ground salt is the right choice for most recipes, as it dissolves easily. By contrast, coarse salt can give many baked goods a beautiful finishing touch. For example, pretzels benefit from this salty crunch.

Other Pantry Favorites

I keep the farmhouse pantry stocked with jars of dried fruit, nuts, and chocolate. The kitchen is brimming with spices and herbs. Some are fresh from the garden, and others are dried. Fruit, nuts, chocolate, herbs, and other add-ins bring dimension to your baking. These inclusions transform even the simplest bread into a treat. The best part is that once you get the hang of sourdough basics, you can start making unique types of bread and baked goods. Sometimes, all it takes is some toasted almonds, dried apricots, or chopped fresh basil straight from your garden to transform a plain loaf into a memorable one.

Chocolate

I love working chocolate into my baked goods. I use it in cookies, muffins, and croissants. I prefer semi-sweet chocolate for baking. It's only lightly sweet and has a deep, robust flavor. Chocolate chips are a great option to stock in your kitchen, but I find chocolate chunks to be indulgent and far superior for baking. I usually make my own by coarsely chopping a bar of dark chocolate and mixing it into cookie batters.

The best chocolate has a rich flavor and glossy finish. Look for chocolate with a high cocoa content, preferably above 60%. High cocoa content indicates a richer taste and smoother texture. Pay attention to the ingredients list, too. Avoid chocolates with additives or artificial flavors. Opt for brands with simple, natural ingredients that you recognize easily.

Dried Fruit and Nuts

Dried fruit is perfect for baking because it doesn't add moisture. Raisins, dried figs, and dried apricots are delicious with their concentrated, complex sweetness. They're easy to incorporate into batters and doughs. Similarly, nuts are also an excellent addition to baked goods because they don't add a lot of moisture. You can incorporate them into batters and dough without making any adjustments to your liquid ratio. Toasting nuts helps them bloom, bringing out complex notes of caramel. It's a simple step that ensures spectacular bread, cookies, and other treats.

You can find dried fruit and nuts in most grocery stores. If you're buying from the bulk bins, double-check for freshness. It's perfectly acceptable to ask the store's staff the last time they restocked the bin. If you have allergies, take extra care with bulk bins, as they're prone to cross-contamination.

Some manufacturers add sulfur dioxide to dried fruit to preserve its color and increase its shelf life. Unfortunately, some people have negative reactions to this additive. When buying dried fruit, look for "unsulphured" varieties. I find it works better in baking, giving baked goods a better flavor profile.

Fresh Fruits and Vegetables

Summertime bursts with abundant produce. We pick berries and fruit from the orchard near our house, and my garden brims with zucchini, tomatoes, and so many other vegetables. Naturally, I work to include them in almost everything I make. After all, I don't want them to go to waste.

Fresh fruits and vegetables add moisture and bulk to baked goods. Recipes made with them tend to use less liquid. It's essential to use the best-quality fruits that you can. It's tempting to use aging produce in baked goods, where their texture is less critical. Remember that your baked goods will only taste as good as the ingredients that go into them. Quality, freshness, and flavor matter. Together, they can make the biggest impact on your cooking.

Herbs and Spices

Herbs and spices add flavor and depth to breads and baked goods. Garlic's sweet, pungent flavor perfectly matches sourdough's acidity. Cinnamon brings a comforting warmth to morning pastries. Rosemary can enliven a loaf of bread.

You can buy individual spices or mixes. I often find that spice mixes are helpful to have on hand. This way, you don't have too many tiny bottles cluttering up your cupboards. Keeping a single bottle of pumpkin pie spice mix takes up less space than individual bottles of cinnamon, allspice, nutmeg, and cloves. It's more affordable, too.

Look for spices that are vibrant in color and aromatic. This indicates freshness and potency. Avoid spices that appear dull or have a lackluster aroma, as they may have lost their flavor over time. Consider purchasing them from reputable sources that specialize in spices and herbs, which are more likely to offer high-quality and fresh products than what you might find in the grocery store. Choose spices stored in airtight containers or bags that protect them from light, heat, and moisture. Finally, consider buying spices in smaller quantities. This is especially important for spices you rarely use. You don't want them to linger in your cupboard and go stale.

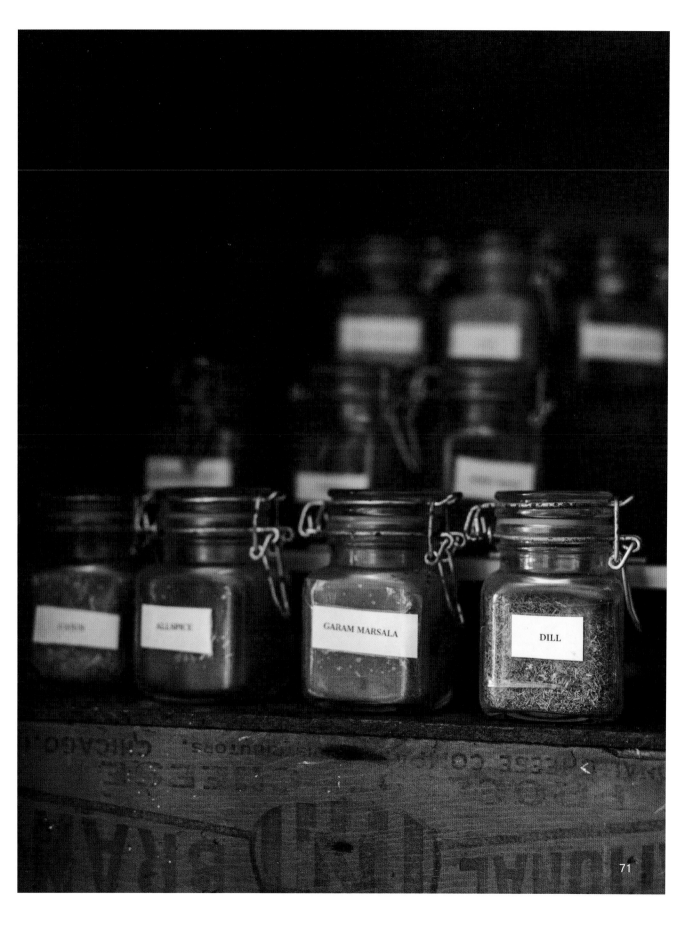

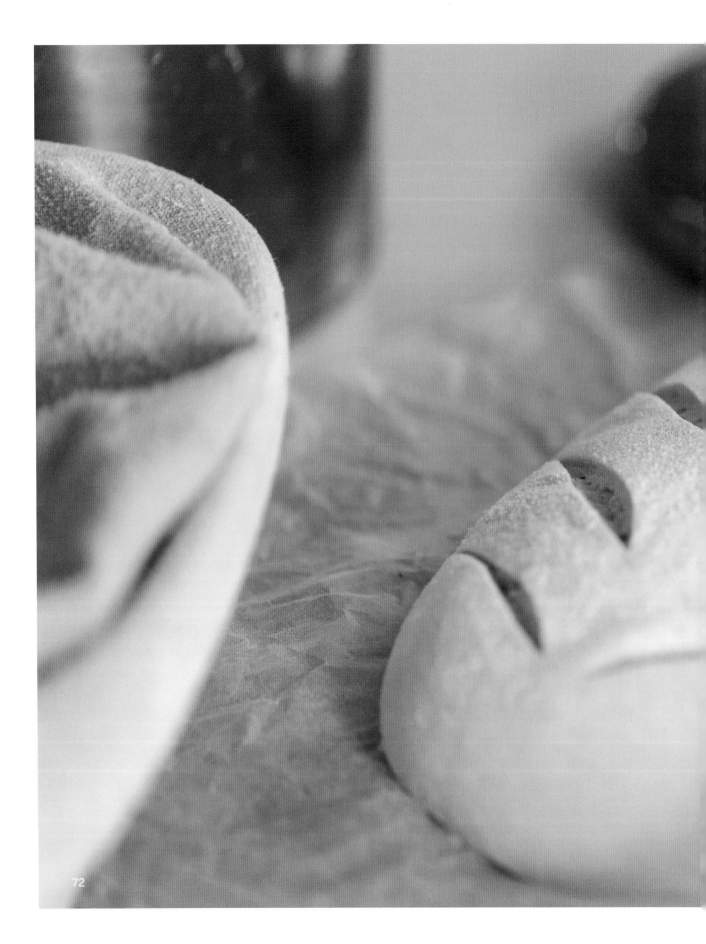

CHAPTER 3

Getting Started

TO GET STARTED, all you need is flour, water, and a jar to mix it in. Sourdough is simple, I promise. Nomadic people roamed the desert of the Fertile Crescent ten thousand years ago and still made bread. So can you. After all, you even have a kitchen with an oven at your disposal. Here's a secret worth sharing: Bread baking is essentially the same now as it was then.

All bread making relies on fermentation. You can use packets of yeast or your own homegrown sourdough starter. The process works the same way. Yeast gobble up the sugars in the grain, and as they do so, they release carbon dioxide. Kneading and handling the dough helps gluten develop. This traps the air bubbles and makes your bread rise.

Wild yeast and beneficial bacteria are naturally present in our environment. They surround us. They're on our hands and countertops, on grains and flour, and just about everywhere. Engaging in this generations-old baking technique, you can capture and cultivate your own little colony of yeast. It's a simple process that has provided staple nourishment for generations.

What Is a Sourdough Starter?

At its simplest, a sourdough starter is a slurry of flour and water that's been allowed to ferment. It's teeming with beneficial bacteria and wild yeast. They work in symbiosis to colonize the flour-and-water mixture, growing in numbers. A typical sourdough starter contains about fifty strains of lactic-acid bacteria. It also contains about twenty species of yeast. Some research suggests that sourdough starters may host an even more microbially diverse array of bacteria—up to three hundred strains.

These microorganisms are imperceptible to the naked eye. You can't see them, but you can see what they do. They complete their entire life cycle within the matrix of flour and water. They grow, reproduce, and eventually die. As they do so, they use the carbohydrates in the flour as fuel. This process releases beneficial acids and carbon dioxide. The bacteria creates acid that gives sourdough its characteristic sour flavor. The yeast emits carbon dioxide to leaven the bread.

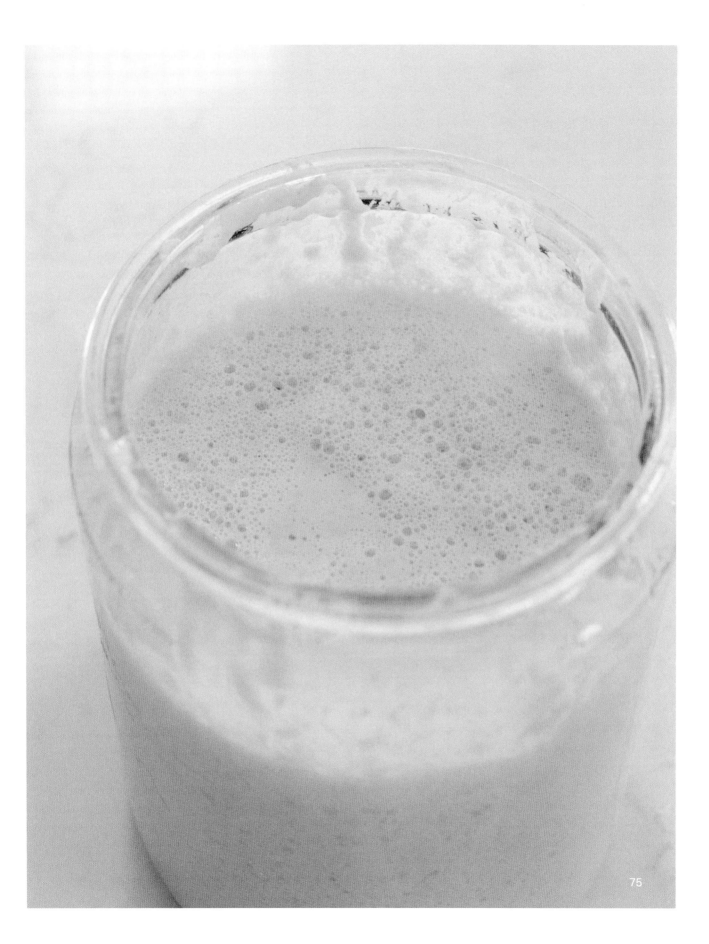

What's in It?

With just two simple ingredients and enough tender care and attention, you can make countless loaves of bread. When you're tired of bread, you can make pancakes and pastries, buns, and pie crusts, too. It's so versatile that you can make just about any baked good with sourdough starter.

Grains are rich in carbohydrates. As a dry good, the nutrients in flours and whole grains are held in a kind of stasis. When the conditions are right, they wake up. A little water does just that. Combining the two creates the perfect environment for wild bacteria and yeast. Growing a culture of bacteria and yeast may seem better suited to a lab than a kitchen. Many of us grew up in a climate of fear about bacteria. It was definitely the enemy—especially in the kitchen. While that's true for some bacteria, sourdough starter is different. It's brimming with healthy bacteria. These bacteria and yeast serve a purpose. They're good. Still, for many of us, it can be uncomfortable to leave food sitting out to grow bacteria on purpose, but trust the process. It's a generations-old tradition that's easy to embrace once you get the hang of it.

Like any new hobby or project, getting started takes effort and consistent attention to detail. The whole process takes about a week. Some bakers find it takes two or three weeks—especially those that keep a cold kitchen or start the process in winter. Every day, you'll carefully mix flour and water in a jar, discarding a bit from the previous day, hoping it comes together. It always does, and with time, the process becomes intuitive. That fussy week or two you spent nurturing your first starter fades to a simple, easy rhythm.

The Flour

You can feed your starter with any flour you happen to like. Wheat, spelt, einkorn, and Khorasan wheat make great choices. Some grains work better than others. All grains are rich in carbohydrates that provide important fuel for the microflora that will eventually take root in your starter and flourish. The rhythm of mixing flour and water works the same way regardless of which type of flour you choose. I reach for unbleached all-purpose flour more often than not. The same goes for discarding and feeding your starter. The yeast just needs a constant source of food, and this can come in many forms.

White Flour Starters

White flour is the perfect choice for beginning bakers. You can find it at every grocery store. You probably have a jar tucked away in your cupboard right now. Starters made from white flour, such as all-purpose or bread flour, tend to be less fussy and more reliable. Once established, they rise consistently and predictably. That's a win for beginning and expert bakers alike. The flavor is slightly sour like yogurt or buttermilk but mild compared to whole-grain starters, which appeals to a lot of people.

Whole-Grain Starters

Starters made with whole-grain flours develop deep, malty flavors. Whole-wheat starters often taste like beer, with a pleasant yeasty flavor. Starters made with rye develop a robust acidity. These subtle, nuanced flavors influence how your bread will taste. Whole-grain starters lend a greater complexity to baked goods.

Whole-grain flour contains more vitamins and minerals than white flour. It also contains a higher level of food enzymes. Both the enzymes and micronutrients in whole-grain flours speed up the fermentation process. This results in faster rising times that can be a bit unpredictable. Whole-grain flour is a great choice for experienced sourdough bakers.

Ancient Grain Starters

All grains are a food source for wild microbes that turn flour and water into sourdough starters. Einkorn, rye, spelt, and Khorasan wheat work just as well as wheat. The gluten structure and baking qualities of ancient grains can differ from modern wheat. Keep those properties in mind when creating a starter from them. When made with whole-grain flour, their flavors are deeper and more sour. Those made from refined flour tend to be sweeter.

The Water

Water brings sourdough starter to life. Once you stir water into flour, you create the perfect environment for yeast and beneficial bacteria to grow. These microorganisms need food, warmth, and water.

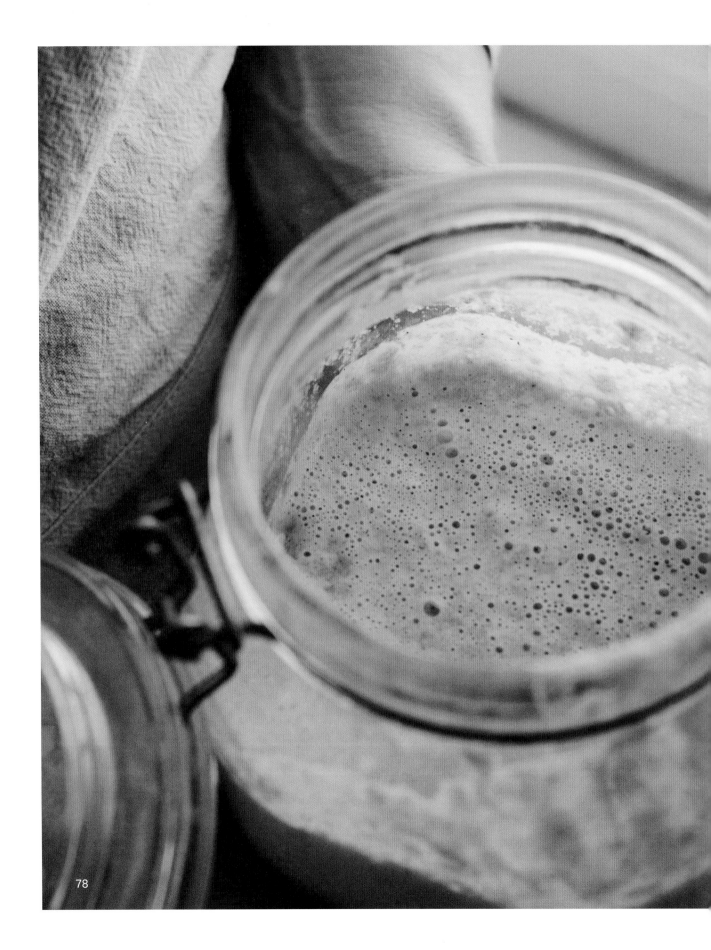

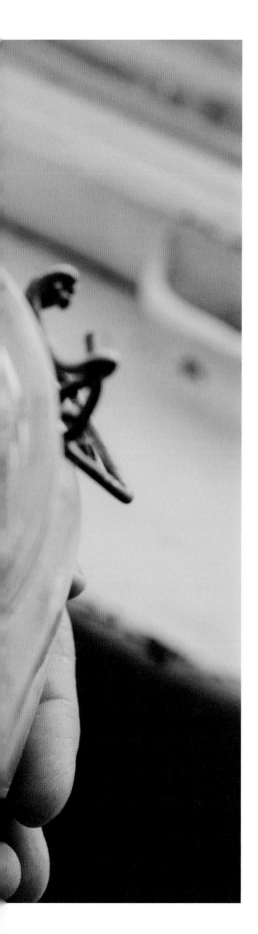

Filtered water works best. If you have a well or spring, that works, too. The real trick is to avoid treated tap water. Tap water often contains disinfectants such as chlorine and chloramine. These additives ensure that municipal drinking supplies are both clean and safe. Unfortunately, they can also hinder the growth of good bacteria and yeast in your starter. While many people have success using chemically treated tap water, if your starter isn't taking off, this could be why.

Water temperature is important, too. If it's too hot, you risk killing the fragile bacteria and yeast in your starter. If it is too cold, you might find that your starter responds more slowly and is less active. Room-temperature to lukewarm water works best. Fortunately, that's a wide range from 70 to 105°F.

An Heirloom Starter

One of the best ways to ensure success in any endeavor is to build upon what is already successful. Using an established starter to kick-start the process is a smart choice. If you're lucky enough to have a friend who bakes sourdough bread, you might ask for a few tablespoons of starter. If not, you can buy freeze-dried sourdough starter in packets online and at many natural foods markets. Even a little bit of an established starter can speed up the process of creating your own. But it's not necessary, and you can create a very successful starter without the added boost. When I began baking, I made my own from scratch, and it's served me well for over a decade.

How to Make
a Basic Sourdough Starter

Making your own sourdough starter is an exercise in patience. You can't rush it. The whole process takes about a week, possibly two, of diligence and dedication. Pick a time in advance when you know you'll be close to home. Make sure your schedule allows enough time to dedicate to a new hobby.

Then, pick a spot in your kitchen that's neither hot nor cold. Instead, it should keep a rather even temperature throughout the day. Temperature matters just as much as flour and water. If your home is on the cooler side, it is going to take longer for your starter to grow. Setting it on a window-sill or in a warmer place may help the process, but keep it away from cool breezes and drafts. On the other hand, if it is fairly warm in your home, your starter may grow faster and may need more frequent feedings.

Once you have your time and place sorted, select a vessel to store your starter. It should be large enough to allow the starter to double (or triple!) in volume, so err on the side of bigger rather than smaller. I'm fond of a half-gallon glass jar with a loose-fitting glass lid. You can also use a mixing bowl covered with a tea towel or even a mason jar with a loose lid. You just want to allow any gasses that build up during fermentation to escape.

INGREDIENTS

Flour, such as all-purpose, bread, or
   whole-grain

Water

Heirloom starter, optional

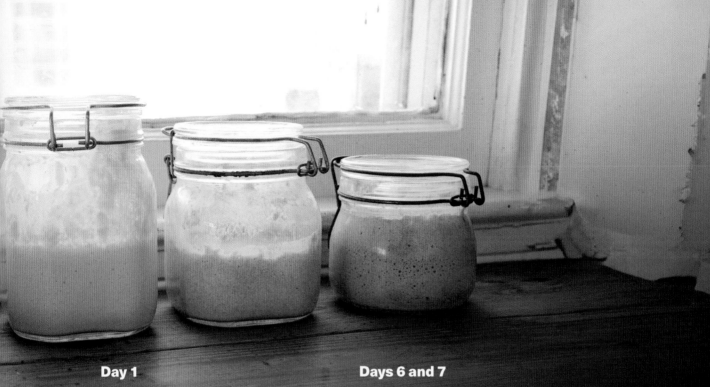

Day 1

Mix 1 cup (140 grams) flour with 1 cup (236 grams) water. If you are using an established starter, mix it in when you add the water to the flour. Stir vigorously, making sure to scrape down the sides of the jar and incorporate everything. Set it aside in a warm spot in your kitchen, away from drafts. Let it sit undisturbed for 24 hours.

Day 2

Discard half of the flour-and-water mixture. Then, add 1 cup (140 grams) flour and 1 cup (236 grams) water, stir vigorously, and cover once more.

Days 3 through 5

You may see bubbles appear or other signs of activity by day three. You should certainly see these signs of life by day five. Continue discarding half of the sourdough in the jar. Then, vigorously stir in 1 cup (140 grams) flour and 1 cup (236 grams) water.

Days 6 and 7

By now, your starter should be plenty lively with loads of bubbles at each feed. It might even rise a bit. You should also see signs that it is rising predictably each time you feed it. On these days, you'll need to increase the frequency of feedings.

Discard half of the starter as you normally would, and then stir in 1 cup (140 grams) flour and 1 cup (236 grams) water into the jar. Then, 12 hours later, repeat the process.

By the end of day seven, your starter should be active enough to bake bread. Sometimes the process takes a bit longer. If your starter is not doubling within a few hours of each feed, continue feeding it every 12 hours until it does.

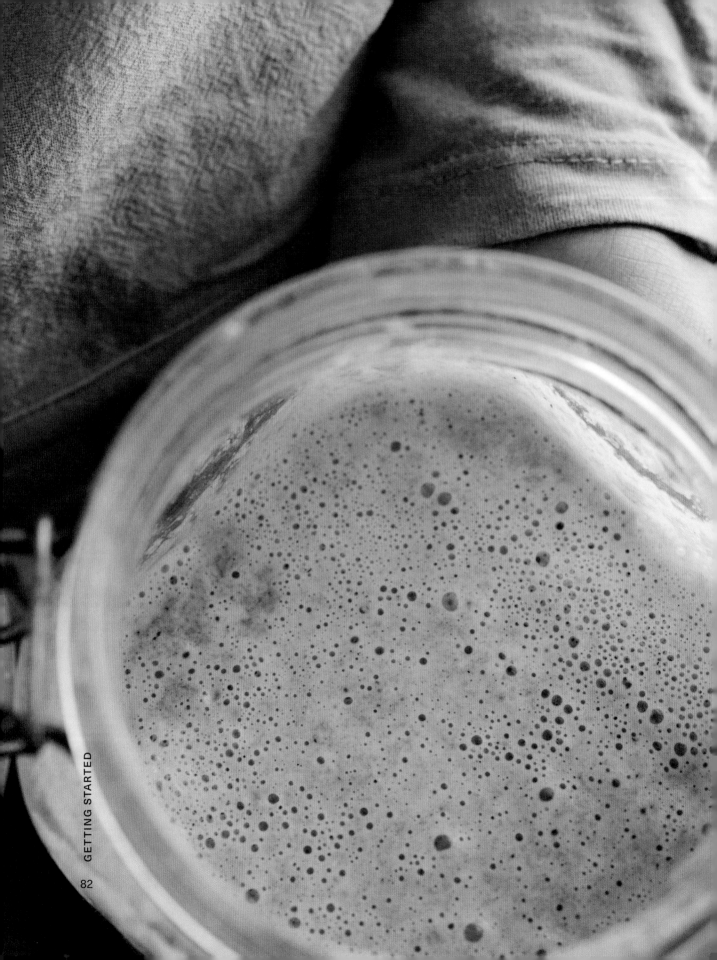

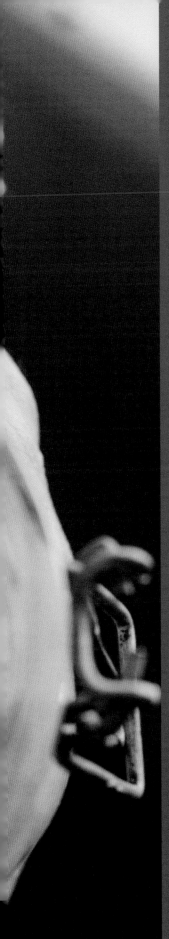

WHY DO I NEED TO DISCARD MY SOURDOUGH?

It feels wasteful to mix flour and water each day and discard half of what's already in the jar. But it's an important step. When you add flour and water, you discard half in order to create a healthy, mature starter. Without discarding a little each day, your sourdough starter would grow exponentially. Within a few days, it would spill out of the jar.

Additionally, in order for your starter to thrive, you must always feed it an amount equal to its volume. If you add too little, the culture will starve. Then you won't have the lively, bubbly yeast activity that makes truly great bread. Discard half of your starter before you feed it. This ensures that you're adding the perfect amount of flour and water to sustain it. Without discarding a portion at each feed, you would end up with a lot of extra starter by the end of the process. None of it would be mature.

Even when your starter matures and you move on to regular feedings, you will still need to discard some. Discarding keeps your starter both lively and manageable.

You do not have to discard every time you feed your starter, as long as you are feeding it in proportion to its volume. If you keep feeding without making anything or discarding, you are going to end up with a lot of starter. It will get out of control.

If you find that you have more than you can manage, you can always give some away. Or use the sourdough discard to make pancakes (page 275) or snickerdoodles (page 250). One of our family's favorite weeknight meals is a farmers' market sourdough skillet (page 279) made with sourdough discard. I keep a lot of extra starter on hand for all those recipes. These quick-cooking recipes are staples in our home.

Is Your Starter Ready for Baking?

A healthy starter should visibly rise and double in volume within 4 to 12 hours each time you feed it. Many starters will triple in volume. When you feed it, wrap the jar with a rubber band or stick a bit of tape to the outside at the level of the starter. This little trick makes it easier to see if your sourdough starter is rising and by how much.

A healthy starter will also have many bubbles and a somewhat elastic structure. When you stir it, you may see strands of starter form a sort of glutinous web to accommodate all those bubbles and air pockets. These air pockets make a well-fed starter less dense. There is such a striking difference in density that an active sourdough starter will float in water, while an unfed starter will sink.

Lucky for you, you can use this difference to your advantage. It's called the "float test." This test is a nifty trick that helps you determine when your starter is strong enough to make bread rise. Get a small glass of room-temperature water. Add a quarter-sized dollop of active sourdough starter. If it floats, it is ready. If it sinks, give it more time or feed it if you haven't already done so.

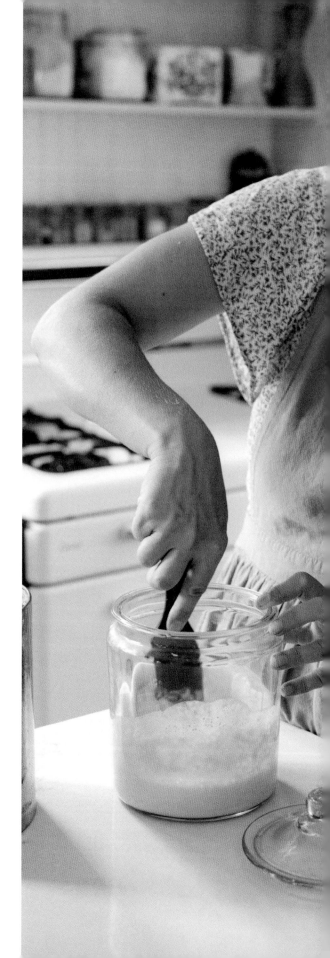

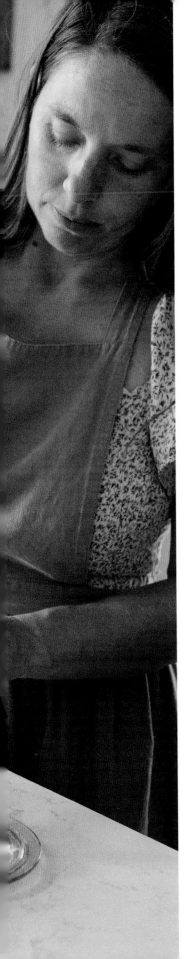

How to Feed Your Starter

Once your starter doubles reliably with each feeding, you can start baking. However, you can't just let your starter sit on the countertop and forget about it. Like any living thing, it needs attention, care, and plenty of food and water, so you must feed it regularly to keep it happy, brimming with life, and ready to make bread.

Just as you created your starter from little more than flour, water, and plenty of patience, that's all you need to feed it. There are no extra ingredients or any fancy techniques. It's a simple process. I don't worry about precise measurements here. Rather, it's all about developing good intuition. If you have too much, make some pancakes or pizza crust before feeding it. If you keep an eye on your ratios, your starter will be happy.

INGREDIENTS

Flour

Water

◆ Estimate the amount of starter in your jar. Then, mix equal parts flour and water together so that the slurry of water and flour is approximately the same as the leftover starter in your jar. Stir it into your jar with the remaining sourdough starter.

◆ For example, if you have 2 cups (454 grams) of starter in your jar, remove 1 cup (227 grams) and use it to make one of the sourdough discard recipes in chapter 8. Then, mix 1/2 cup (70 grams) flour and 1/2 cup (118 grams) water together. Stir the flour-and-water mixture vigorously into the jar's remaining starter.

◆ If you're planning to bake, let your starter sit out at room temperature until doubled—between 4 and 12 hours. If you have no plans to bake, transfer the fed starter immediately to the fridge. It will keep for 1 week before you need to feed it again.

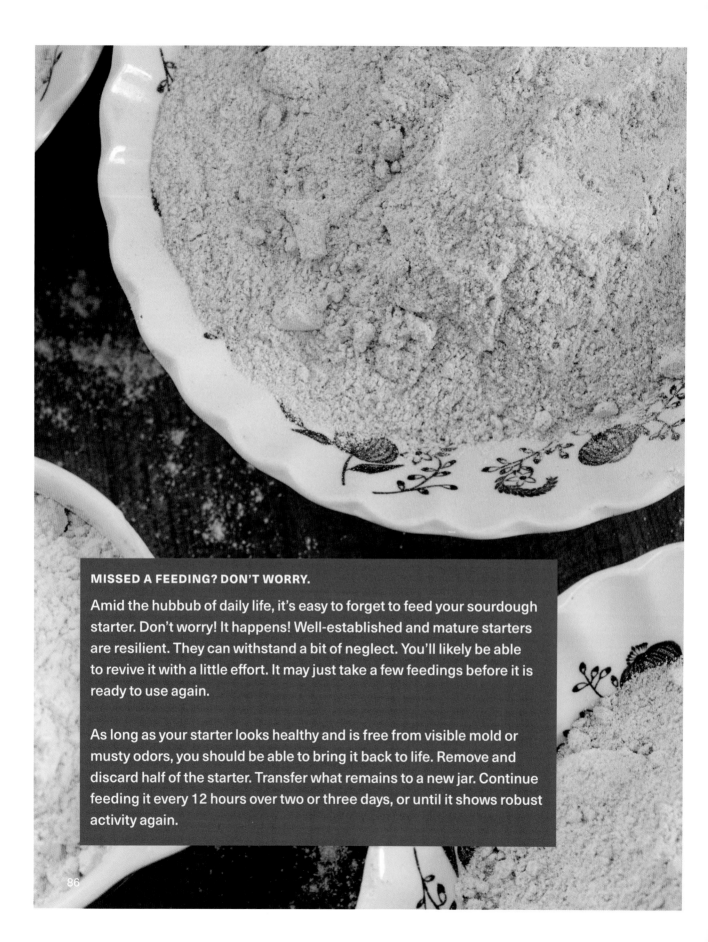

MISSED A FEEDING? DON'T WORRY.

Amid the hubbub of daily life, it's easy to forget to feed your sourdough starter. Don't worry! It happens! Well-established and mature starters are resilient. They can withstand a bit of neglect. You'll likely be able to revive it with a little effort. It may just take a few feedings before it is ready to use again.

As long as your starter looks healthy and is free from visible mold or musty odors, you should be able to bring it back to life. Remove and discard half of the starter. Transfer what remains to a new jar. Continue feeding it every 12 hours over two or three days, or until it shows robust activity again.

How to Proof Your Starter For Baking

Before you bake bread, you must proof your starter. That is, you need to ensure it's bubbly and lively. It should have enough yeast activity to make your bread rise. A dormant sourdough starter, or one that shows little activity, won't have enough active yeast to make your bread dough rise. If you recently fed your starter within the last 12 hours, you may not have to proof it. Just use the bubbly, fed starter when it's at its peak.

Proofing your starter takes about five minutes of active time in the kitchen and about four hours total. So plan ahead and account for this time when scheduling your bakes. Some starters will need more time, and others less. Mature starters need less time than young starters. Starters made with white flour typically need a little more time than those made with whole-grain flour. Lastly, starters kept in cold kitchens will need more time than those kept in warm ones.

Proofing your starter follows the same method as feeding it. Eyeball how much is in your jar, and then feed your starter an equal amount of flour and water.

INGREDIENTS

Flour

Water

◆ Estimate the amount of starter in your jar. Then, mix equal parts flour and water together so that the slurry of water and flour is approximately the same as the leftover starter in your jar. Stir the fresh flour-and-water mixture into the remaining starter in your jar. You should always feed your starter a mixture of flour and water that is equal to its volume. For example, if you have 1 cup (227 grams) of starter remaining in your jar. Then mix in 1/2 cup (70 grams) flour and 1/2 cup (118 grams) water.

◆ Cover your starter and let it sit on the countertop until doubled. Then, take out the amount you need for the recipe and spoon it into a bowl. Now, mix equal parts flour and water together so that it's equivalent to what you removed. Stir the fresh water and flour mixture into your jar, and transfer it to the fridge.

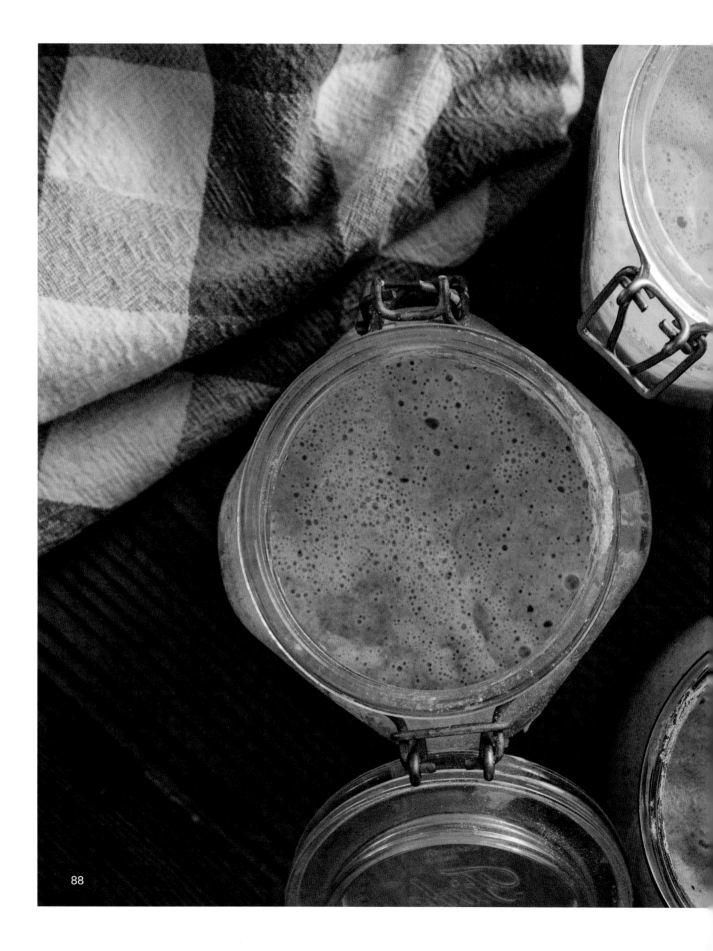

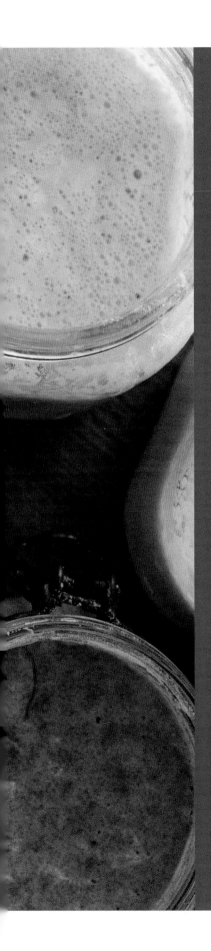

KEEPING IT SIMPLE

Now, some people prefer precision. They measure their sourdough discard on the scale and replace it with an exact measure of flour and water. I've never been one for complicated rigidity. To me, sourdough is one of the most flexible things I have in my kitchen. The trick is to not overcomplicate the process. You have to find what works for you when it comes to maintaining your sourdough starter. It mostly comes down to how often you plan to use it.

Your starter will work fine even without taking exact measurements. Some bakers may find this technique unreliable. But I have eyeballed the amount of flour and water I feed my sourdough starter for over a decade. If you'd rather be exact and use a kitchen scale or measuring cups, you can. Between a bustling kitchen and a busy home life, I find that exacting precision should take a back seat to what is practical and functional.

If you don't feed your starter enough, it may not become bubbly and active, in which case, simply add more flour and water. You can't really feed it too much, though. If I am running low on starter, I will add more to build it up again. A mature starter is not a fussy thing; rather, it handles these variations with ease. Often, it thrives. In fact, I find it comes back more active than ever after I've reduced it down to almost nothing and fed it large amounts of flour and water.

How to Store Your Starter

Sourdough starters are much like houseplants. In addition to regular care, they also need to live in a dedicated spot in your kitchen. Flexible things that they are, you can keep yours on your countertop, in your fridge, or even in your freezer. It all depends on how often you bake and how much space you have.

Storing at Room Temperature

Before refrigeration, bakers kept their starters in big crocks at room temperature. This method still works now, just as it did for generations. It won't take up valuable space in your fridge. If you bake frequently and have time to feed it every day, then this method is a good choice for you. During weeks of heavy baking, I often find that keeping my starter on the counter works best.

Remember that temperature affects how fast all the microbes in your starter grow. If you keep your starter on the counter at room temperature, feed it at least once a day. You might need to feed it more often if your kitchen is particularly warm. Otherwise, you may find that it becomes super acidic, and its yeast activity starts to lag.

Storing in the Fridge

For most people, the best place to keep your starter is in your fridge. Cold temperatures slow down the fermentation process. The fridge acts like a pause button, halting the activity of all those microbes. It's my favorite way to store my sourdough because it requires less maintenance. Unlike keeping your starter at room temperature, which requires daily feedings, you need to feed a refrigerated starter only once a week or on days you plan to bake.

Once your starter is mature, you might even be able to neglect it a bit. A well-established starter is resilient. It can withstand a month or two in the fridge without feeding, however, it may take some dedicated maintenance to bring it back to an optimal condition for baking.

CAN I USE MY STARTER DIRECTLY FROM THE FRIDGE?

It depends on what you are making! If your recipe calls only for sourdough discard, then you can pull that jar straight out of the fridge and dive in. If you need an active sourdough starter, you'll want to pull it out of the fridge, feed it, and wait until it has doubled. Most starters should double within about four hours, although some take longer.

I have gotten away with making bread, bagels, cinnamon rolls, and so many other things with my starter straight out of the fridge. I'm sure the results were slightly less than perfect, but we couldn't tell the difference. They just take a little longer to rise since the yeasts need to wake from their dormant state. The reason I can do this is partly because my starter is very mature and resilient. With time, yours will be, too.

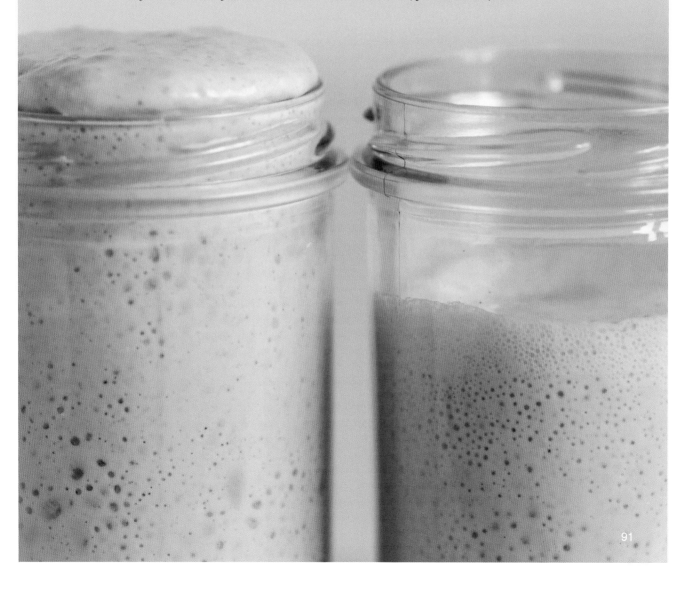

Storing in the Freezer

Sometimes, you need to store your starter for a longer period of time. Perhaps you're going on a vacation or visiting family. Or maybe you're overwhelmed with work, and tending to a starter is just one too many tasks to manage. That's okay. You can freeze it.

Freezing can damage some fragile microorganisms in your starter, but most will survive just fine. All they need is a little attention before the starter thrives once more. Make sure your starter is fully mature before you toss it in the freezer. It should double with each feeding and be robust enough to successfully leaven a loaf of bread.

To freeze your starter, feed it as you normally would. Allow it to proof, and when it doubles in size, spoon about 1/4 cup (57 grams) into a small container. Silicone muffin tins and ice cube trays work especially well for this job. Transfer it to the freezer and allow it to stay there until completely frozen for at least 6 and up to 24 hours. Carefully remove the frozen starter from the mold. Then, transfer it to a freezer-safe, ziplock bag. Label the bag and freeze it for up to six months.

When you're ready to begin baking again, allow the frozen starter to thaw in the fridge overnight. Then transfer it to a jar and feed it. Frozen starters typically need a little extra attention before they revive fully. Keep it on the counter and feed it every 24 hours or until it doubles again within a few hours of each feed.

Even if you don't plan to go on vacation or leave your starter for an extended period, freezing a little still makes sense. It's a fail-safe. Things go wrong. A family member might knock the jar off the counter, where it shatters to bits and splatters gooey starter everywhere. A busybody houseguest might clean your kitchen, discarding all the murky things in jars as a "favor." Either way, you're left to salvage what you can. Keeping a little starter in the freezer provides a foolproof backup plan in case of emergencies. You won't have to restart the process completely. If you're lucky and your starter chugs along with no emergencies, you can always give that frozen starter to friends along with some care instructions. They'll treasure it.

Dehydrating Your Starter

Drying your starter is also an effective strategy for storing it long-term. Drying an active sourdough starter puts the natural yeasts and bacteria into a dormant state. It's a nifty way of preserving it. When you are ready to use it, you can reactivate it to start baking.

As with freezing a starter, the trick is to use a mature, well-fed starter. First, feed the starter. Then, take about 1/2 cup (113 grams) of proofed starter from the jar. Spread it into a paper-thin layer on a square of parchment paper. If you have a food dehydrator, you can slip the starter onto a tray and let it dry at a low temperature. If not, place the parchment paper in a warm, dry spot in your kitchen with good airflow. Ideally, you can also choose a place where it's unlikely to be disturbed, such as on top of the cupboards or on a shelf in the pantry covered with a light tea towel. Let it stay there until it dries completely and flakes easily. This takes about 24 hours in a dehydrator and 48 hours on the countertop. Break it apart by hand and transfer it to a jar with a tight-fitting seal. Tuck it into the cupboard, where it will keep for about a year.

Reviving a dehydrated starter is a little trickier than reviving a frozen one. First, grind it into a powder. Follow the method for making a starter from scratch on page 80. Add a tablespoon or two of the powdered starter to the flour-and- water mixture on day one. Within about five days, your starter should be active and bubbly once more and ready for several baking projects.

Lean into Your Senses

Amid measurements, feedings every 12 to 24 hours, and watching for signs of life, it's easy to feel overwhelmed. You might even feel tempted to toss your starter in the compost bin and head to the store for a packet of yeast. Stay the course, because it's worthwhile. Soon, you will find yourself settled into a rhythm that feels good and works for you.

Many factors can influence your sourdough starter. They include the flour you use and the temperature of your water. This is especially true in its infancy. The process takes time and calls on both patience and intuition.

Think of it like growing a garden. At first, it is hard to know if you are watering enough or too much. Is the plant getting enough sun or not enough? Is the soil healthy, or is it missing key nutrients? As with any living thing, it is going to take time to learn how to care for it.

Remember that all-purpose flour is often easiest for beginners. Room-temperature, filtered water seems to work best for most people. Cold slows down fermentation, while warmth speeds it up. As you continue to nurture and feed your starter, lean into your senses, and you'll soon develop a baker's intuition. Above all, be patient.

Appearance

A healthy sourdough starter made with white flour, such as all-purpose or bread flour, will have a creamy color. Starters made with whole-grain flour vary in color. Rye flour produces a grayish starter, while whole wheat produces a tawny brown.

When the starter is at its peak, it will double or triple in the jar. You'll see bubbles all along the walls and surface. When you stir it, you'll see a web of glutinous strands develop as the air pockets in the starter collapse. A starter that needs feeding and is at the low point of its activity will sink toward the bottom of the jar. Its texture will be thick and creamy, like pancake batter.

If you notice a pink tinge or little dots of fuzzy mold on your starter, start over in a clean jar with fresh flour and water.

If you see a dingy liquid that resembles dishwater at the surface of your starter, don't feel alarmed. Sourdough bakers call this liquid "hooch," and it's a sure sign that your starter needs feeding. Simply pour it off, discard half the starter, and feed as you normally would. You'll find it revives quickly with this treatment.

Aroma

Naturally, sourdough starter should smell sour, but a delicious kind of sour. Think of the beautiful tangy aroma you find in buttermilk or yogurt—sour but sweet, too, and vaguely milky. The activity of lactic-acid bacteria gives sourdough this aroma as well as its distinct flavor. Your starter should also smell of yeast and grain. You might notice a delicate aroma of malt, especially if you use whole-grain flour to feed your starter. It may also border on beer-like, and these are all good signs that the wild yeast in your starter are active and happy.

Occasionally, starters may smell boozy and reminiscent of old moonshine. If alcohol is the first aroma you smell, your starter is hungry. The yeast are telling you it's time for a feed. Similarly, your starter may occasionally smell of acetone or nail polish. This aroma often arrives with the appearance of hooch at the starter's surface. Again, your starter is simply telling you that it needs a good feeding, so pour off any liquid, and then discard half of the starter before refreshing it with fresh water and new flour.

Very rarely, some bakers find that their sourdough has spoiled. Instead of smelling pleasantly sour and yeasty, it might smell putrid or like rotten food. If you recoil when you open the jar, it's a good sign that you should discard what you have and start over. This typically happens only when you neglect a starter for a very long time. If your starter smells musty or moldy, start over with a clean jar and fresh water and flour.

Activity

A healthy starter bubbles up and rises consistently within 4 to 12 hours of each feed. A mature starter typically takes less time to rise than a young one. Starters will also rise faster in a warm kitchen than in a cold one. A healthy and robust starter will rise and double on a consistent schedule. Those are good signs it will make excellent, lofty bread.

Starters that show activity and rise without doubling need a little more time to mature. You may need to move it to a warmer spot in your kitchen. Or try feeding your starter more often—at least once a day but no more than every 12 hours until it doubles.

Sometimes, a starter will experience a frenzy of activity within the first day or two of its life. You'll see plenty of tiny bubbles all throughout the starter. All that activity leaves inexperienced bakers feeling a flurry of excitement. Then, suddenly, all the activity stops, and the starter goes dormant. These false starts, while rare, can leave you feeling as deflated as your starter. They indicate a microbial imbalance in your starter. Some bakers find that if they continue feeding it on schedule, it will eventually revive itself. You can also start over with an heirloom starter because it already contains a good balance of healthy bacteria and yeast. As a result, it can help establish the right balance of yeast and bacteria in your starter, too.

Your starter communicates with you through these wordless signs. Trust your intuition and your senses. When you pay attention to appearance, aroma, and activity, your starter will respond. Your baking will soon improve. Sourdough baking is scientific, involving weights, measures, and microbial analysis. It's also a timeless art that relies on insights gained from practice, experience, and trust.

How to Use Your Starter in Just about Any Recipe

Once your starter is bubbling, and you've baked a few beautiful loaves of bread, you'll want to try adding a little sourdough starter to your favorite recipes to see what happens. It gives a greater depth of flavor to just about any baked good. Bread tastes more robust. Pizza tastes more complex. Even cakes and sweets taste somehow richer and brighter.

Before I began baking with sourdough, I baked with the little packets of yeast you find at the grocery store. I made plenty of bread and a few other treats, so we certainly had our favorites, and I wasn't about to give them up. So I did my best to adjust my favorite yeast-bread recipe to make it work with my new sourdough starter. After plenty of trial and error, I had a recipe that worked just as well as the original. Once you know the tricks to converting your yeast and non-yeast recipes, you can start making anything and everything into a sourdough version.

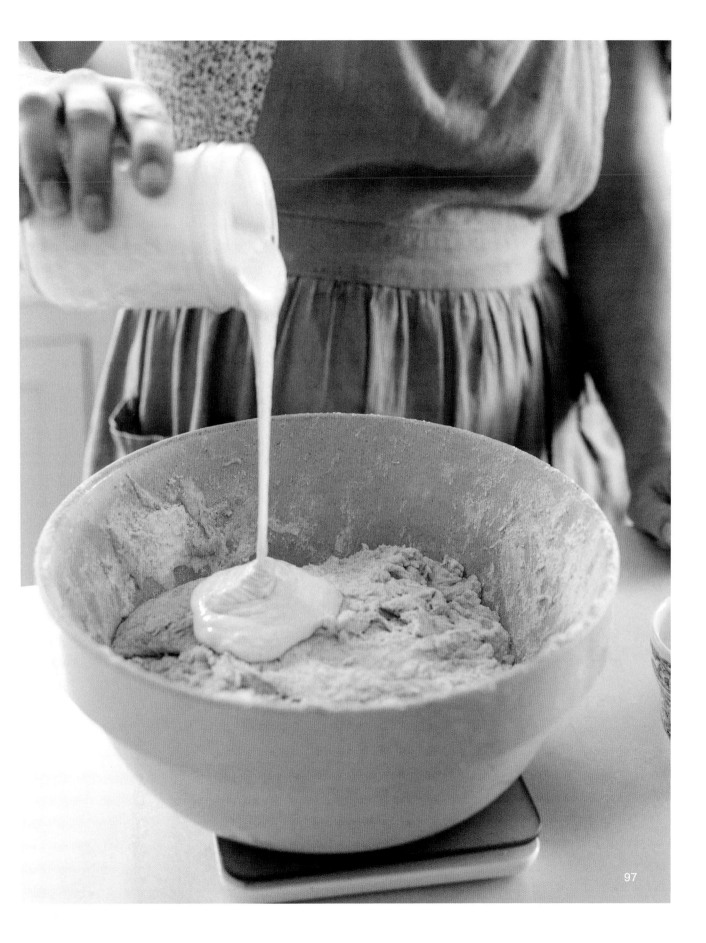

Yeast Breads

Sandwich breads and crusty baguettes rely on yeast to rise. The yeast can come from a packet or from your very own starter. Converting a recipe for yeast bread to sourdough isn't quite as easy as skipping the packet of yeast and adding starter instead. You must consider how active your starter is and how much liquid and flour the recipe needs. You also need to make additional accommodations for rise times.

Packaged yeast will come to life the instant you add water and a little sugar. It will fizz and foam within minutes, so you need to use an active, bubbly starter when the wild yeast are at their peak. One package (7 grams) of active dry yeast is equivalent to 1/2 cup (113 grams) of active sourdough starter. You also need to accommodate for the difference in timing. Whereas packaged yeast takes only a few minutes to proof, sourdough starter needs several hours.

Pay careful attention to hydration—the ratio of water to flour in your bread recipe. Since sourdough starter already contains a little flour and water, you will need to use less of both in your recipe, so make sure you calculate how much less your bread recipe needs. If you're adding 1/2 cup (100 grams) of active sourdough starter to a recipe, you'll also be adding the equivalent of about 47 grams of flour and 79 grams of water. Deduct these amounts from the amounts flour and water you add to the recipe.

YEAST BREAD CONVERSION CHEAT SHEET

1. Always use an active, proofed sourdough starter when replacing packaged yeast.

2. One packet of yeast is equal to 1/2 cup (100 grams) active sourdough starter.

3. A half cup (100 grams) active sourdough starter contains about 1/3 cup (47 grams) flour and 1/3 cup (79 grams) water.

4. Reduce the flour in the recipe according to the volume of starter you're using.

5. Omit the yeast from the recipe. Then, add the sourdough starter.

6. Proceed with the instructions as you normally would.

7. Allow more time for your dough to rise (usually twice the amount).

Last, make sure to allow plenty of time. The yeast in sourdough starter works more slowly than active dry yeast. You'll need to allow more time for your starter to proof, your dough to rise, and for the final proof before it goes into the oven. Estimate that the time the recipe requires will double.

For Quick Breads

You can use sourdough discard in most baked goods, including quick breads such as muffins and banana bread. These baked goods rise not because of yeast, but because of a chemical reaction between baking soda and acidic ingredients, such as lemon juice, buttermilk, or even sourdough starter. Think of the way baking soda (alkaline) bubbles when mixed with vinegar (acid). The air bubbles created in that chemical reaction are what leavens quick breads. Baking powder is a combination of acid and alkaline ingredients, and it reacts when you add liquid.

Quick breads are a great use for sourdough discard. When converting quick bread recipes to sourdough, you can skip the acidic ingredients unless you wish to include them for flavor. Sourdough discard is acidic enough on its own to create the reaction you want.

Limit the amount of sourdough starter you use. Too much can make your muffins and quick breads taste too acidic and make your baked good tough. Use up to 1/2 cup (125 grams) of sourdough discard. This seems to be the magic measurement, providing just enough to give baked goods great flavor and a good rise.

As with converting yeast bread recipes, you will also need to reduce the amount of flour and liquid in your recipe. A half cup (125 grams) of sourdough discard contains about 1/3 cup (47 grams) flour and 1/3 cup (79 grams) water. So you'll need to reduce the amount of flour in your recipe by 1/3 cup (47 grams) and the liquid in your recipe by 1/3 cup (79 grams).

QUICK BREAD CONVERSION CHEAT SHEET

1. Sourdough discard works best.

2. Measure the sourdough discard, adding no more than 1/2 cup (125 grams).

3. Reduce the amount of liquid and flour in the recipe in proportion to the amount of starter you use.

4. Add the sourdough discard to the wet ingredients, and then add the wet ingredients into the dry ingredients to mix your batter.

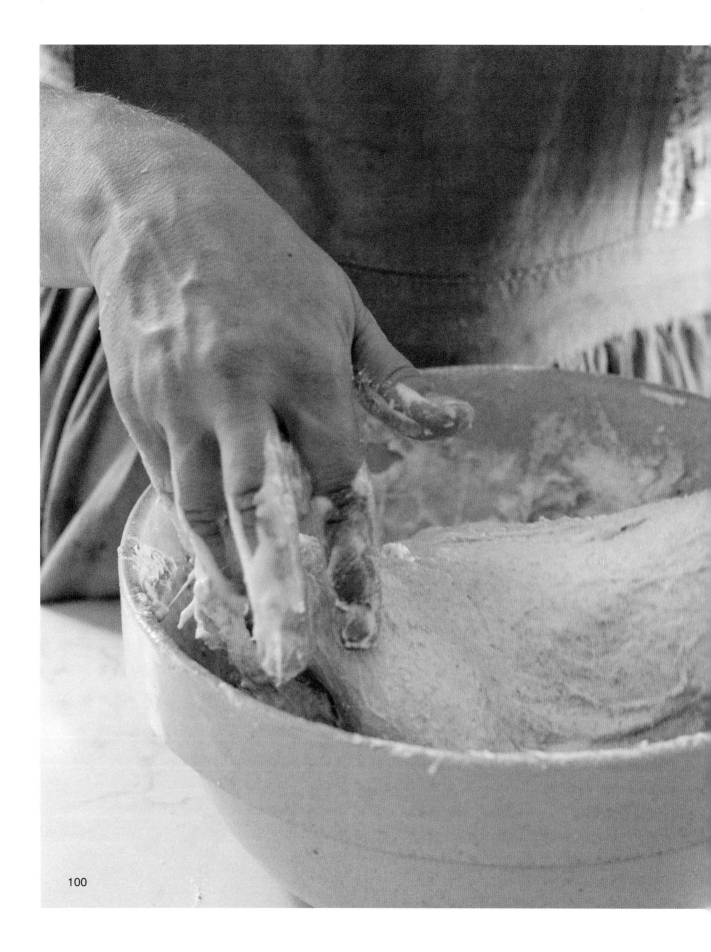

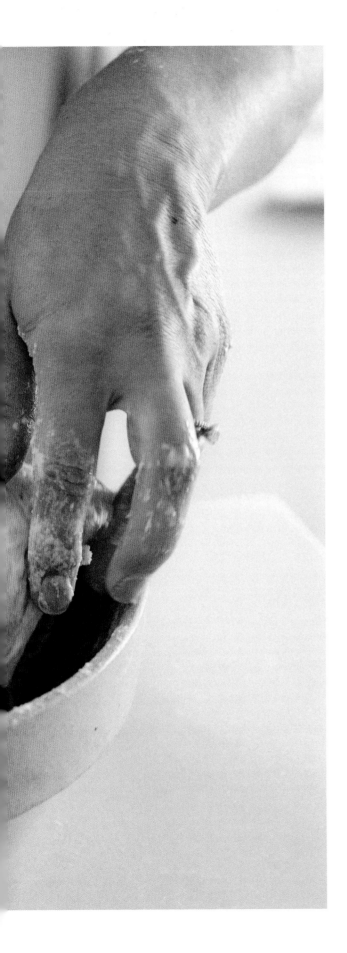

The order you mix your ingredients matters, too. In general, add sourdough discard to your wet ingredients, such as eggs, milk, water, butter, and oil. Then, when it's fully incorporated into the wet ingredients, work in the dry ingredients, such as flour, baking soda, salt, and spices. This approach gives you the best texture, and optimizes the chemical reaction between baking soda and your starter.

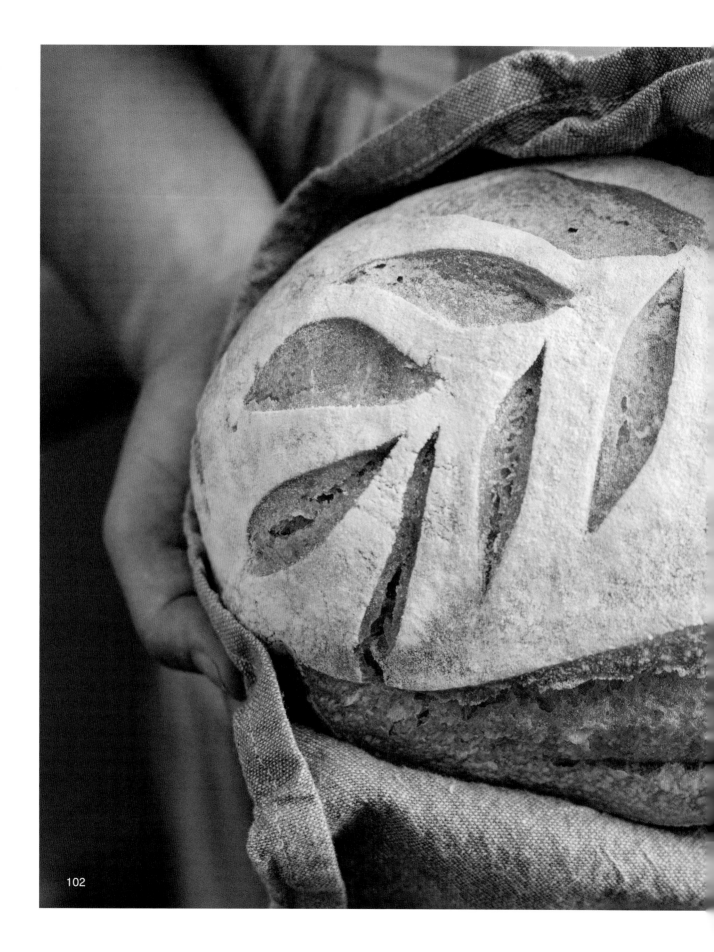

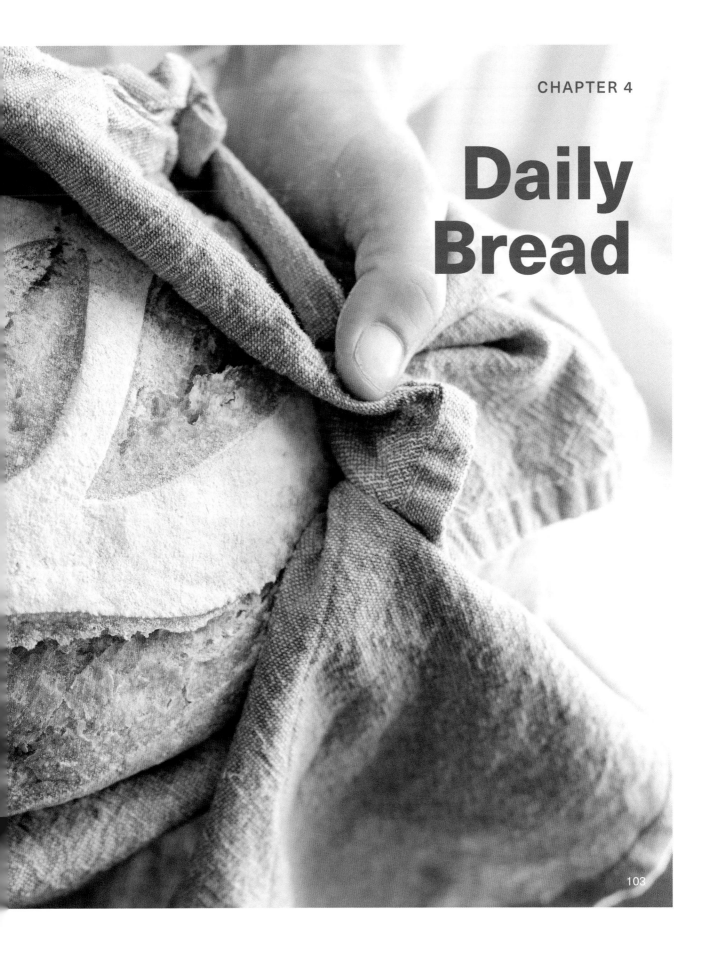

Daily Bread

MOST DAYS, THE AROMA of freshly baked bread perfumes my kitchen. It's ever present, a reminder of patience, diligence, and care. The starter needs feeding, and the dough needs shaping. Hungry children are ever ready to grab a hunk of bread and fresh raw-milk cheese. I like the meditative rhythm of it. Baking bread grounds me. In a fast-paced world, it's comforting to know that you can return to a practice that has nourished families and warmed kitchens for millennia.

Sourdough baking is just that. While the world moves on, sourdough remains much the same now as it did for generations: bubbly sourdough starter alive with wild yeast, flour, water, and salt. All the rest is time and technique. If you're a new baker, give yourself plenty of grace. Your first loaf (and possibly second and third) might not be perfect. Remember, sourdough baking is both an art and a science, with plenty of room for both error and growth. As you practice your technique, the first few loaves may be knobby or lopsided. Remember, they're still delicious. You can transform them into croutons, bread puddings, or even bread crumbs, if they're not suitable for slicing. It's all good food.

Simple Steps for Making Good Bread

Feed Your Starter

All good bread starts with a well-fed starter. Before you bake, proof your starter. Now, the conventional wisdom about feeding and proofing your starter is to remove, or discard, half of your starter every time before you feed it. I have found that it is not necessary to remove half of the starter or discard every time before feeding it. You can keep as much or as little starter as you'd like.

The only goal for a healthy starter is to feed it flour and water in an amount equal to its bulk. For example, if you have a 4 cups of starter, you would want to feed it equal portions of flour and water that add up to 4 cups. If you don't want to feed it 4 cups of flour and water and end up with 8 cups of fed starter, you'll want to reduce your starter down before you feed it.

Sometimes I keep large amounts of starter so I have enough to use the discard to make pizza crusts and pancakes, and sometimes I keep a tiny amount.

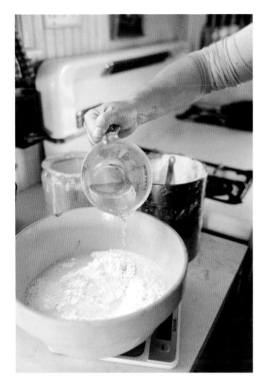

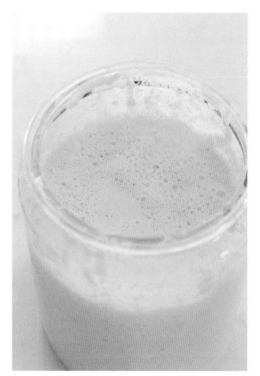

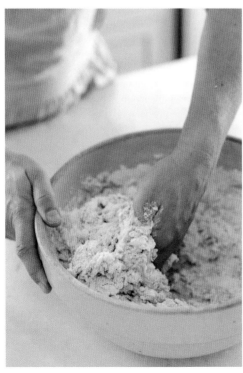

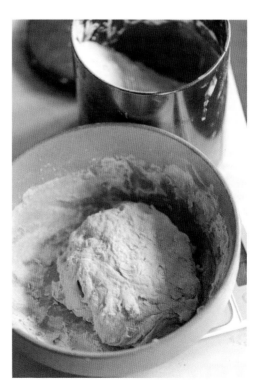

However much starter you have, it will need to be fed and active before you can bake bread with it. After you've added the same amount of flour and water that's currently in your starter, you'll wait for it to proof or activate.

When the starter has doubled in size and is bubbly, it's ready for baking. This process takes anywhere from 4 to 12 hours. Young starters will take more time to proof than well-established starters. Similarly, your starter needs more time in a colder kitchen than a warm one.

Mix the Dough

Mix the dough by combining the ingredients, either all at once or sequentially. The method depends on the recipe. Incorporate bulky ingredients, like nuts and dried fruit, into the dough after it initially comes together. You can add herbs at any time.

You can mix dough by hand in a large bowl with a wooden spoon or a specialized kneading tool, such as a Danish dough whisk. Most of the time, I prefer working with a stand mixer. It makes mixing and kneading easier, usually with superior results.

Note that just as bread and baked goods have different textures, your doughs will have different textures as well. In this book, I'll describe how the dough should feel in the recipe. However, there are two types of dough that will be useful to remember: Rough doughs are doughs that have just started to come together. They are rough and uneven. Shaggy doughs are wet and fully mixed so that you don't see any signs of flour inside your dough.

Knead

Kneading helps your dough build structure by developing the gluten framework. As you work the dough, the gluten strands become stronger. This gives the bread structure and elasticity. It's why flour, starter, and water transform from a gloopy mess into a smooth, pliable dough.

You can knead bread by hand, but I recommend using a stand mixer equipped with a dough hook. This hands-off approach takes less time and produces consistent, beautiful results.

INCLUSIONS: HOW TO MAKE YOUR BREAD YOUR OWN

Once you have baked a few successful loves, it's fun to experiment with new flavors. The easiest way to transform a loaf of bread into something new is to add inclusions. The term "inclusions" is simply the technical way bakers describe extra ingredients you add to the dough. Think of shredded cheeses, minced fresh herbs, dried fruit, or toasted nuts.

A basic loaf of whole-wheat sourdough transforms into a cozy, wintry delight with the inclusion of cinnamon, toasted walnuts, and golden raisins. Lemon zest and rosemary can give a basic white bread a beautiful, vibrant flavor. Some of my favorite combinations include jalapeños and cheddar cheese, parmesan and herbs, as well as dried fruit and toasted nuts.

Technique makes a difference, too. You can add herbs, and lighter add-ins, with the flour, starter and water. Add heavier, bulkier inclusions, such as nuts, dried fruit, vegetables, and cheese, when you stretch and fold the dough. Just sprinkle them over the dough, and then complete the stretches and folds as you normally would.

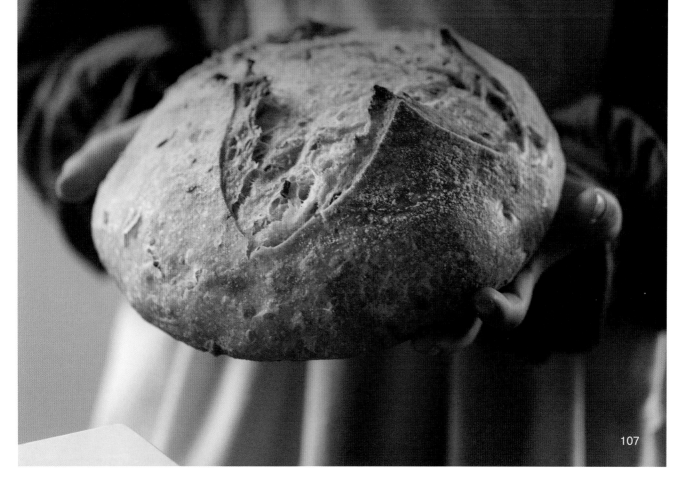

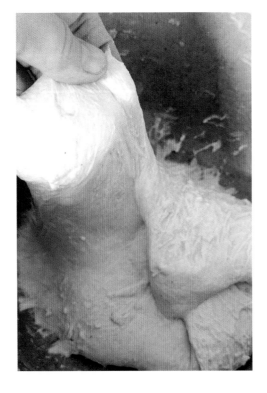

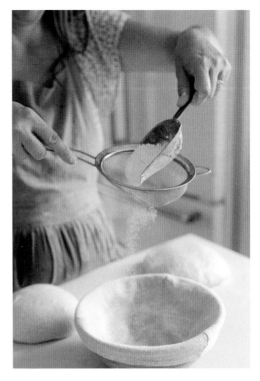

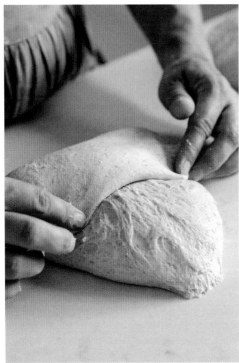

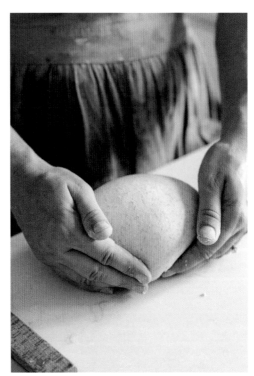

Window Pane Test

When your dough is smooth and pliable, pinch off a little portion about the size of a golf ball. Hold it with both hands. Use gentle pressure to stretch it slowly between both your hands, taking care not to tear it. As you stretch the dough, check for translucency. If the gluten is well-developed, the stretched dough should become thin enough so that light shines through. This makes it look like a window pane.

Bulk Fermentation

Sometimes called the bulk rise, bulk fermentation is a crucial step for bread makers. It allows the wild yeast and bacteria in your starter to do their work. During this step, all those microorganisms will eat the carbohydrates in the bread. The beneficial bacteria in your starter will produce various acids that give your bread flavor. The yeast will produce carbon dioxide, helping your bread rise and become tender and fluffy. Additionally, bulk fermentation allows the gluten to develop. It improves the texture of the dough and makes it easier to handle when shaping.

In general, let your dough rise until doubled in bulk. The time it takes dough to double varies and can take anywhere from 8 to 24 hours. Doughs made with young starters often needs more time than those made with well-established starters. Cold kitchens can lengthen the bulk rise, while warm kitchens may speed it up. Above all, sourdough is flexible and personal. As you get to know your starter, bulk fermentation will become more predictable.

It's crucial to keep the dough tightly covered during bulk fermentation. Otherwise, it will dry out and form a crust. This hinders gluten development and can easily ruin your loaf. Many mixing bowls come with tight-fitting lids that are perfect for bulk fermentation. You can also wrap the bowl tightly with plastic wrap. An eco-friendly alternative to plastic wrap is beeswax wrap, which is made with waxed cotton.

Stretch and Fold

During the bulk fermentation, many recipes for artisan-style bread call for stretching the dough and folding it onto itself. This technique replaces kneading and helps develop the gluten network and improves the dough's structure. It also helps aerate the dough. This allows for the open crumb structure and airy texture so desired in artisan bread.

Grab the edge of the dough in the bowl and pull it gently upward. Wiggle the dough a bit as you stretch it. Then, fold the dough back into the center. Turn the bowl a quarter turn, stretch, and fold the dough again. Then, repeat the process until you've gone around the bowl. This is one round of stretches and folds. Most recipes that incorporate this technique call for a series of stretches and folds, each separated by 15 to 30 minutes. I find it helpful to keep a bowl of warm water on the counter while I stretch and fold the dough. I dip my fingers in the water before grabbing hold of the dough to prevent it from sticking.

Rest

Some recipes may require a short rest before shaping your dough. You simply let your dough rest on the counter for the time the recipe requires. Resting the dough allows the gluten network to relax. This makes the dough more manageable and less likely to tear during shaping.

Shape

When you shape the bread, you help develop its structure and mold it into its final form. This could be a round boule, a pretty little sandwich loaf, or a long baguette. Properly shaped breads look more appealing and professional.

Shaping does more than make your bread look nice. Shaping develops tension, especially along the outer portion of the dough. This tension becomes the bread's crust. That surface tension holds the shape of the bread and allows for a smooth, controlled final rise.

To shape a boule, start by gently flattening the dough into a rough circle on a lightly floured surface. Then, fold the top edge of the dough down toward the center, pressing lightly to seal. Repeat this folding process with the bottom edge, slightly overlapping the top fold. Next, take one side of the dough and fold it toward the center. Then, repeat with the opposite side to create a round shape.

With the seam-side down, cup your hands around the dough. Rotate it on the countertop, applying gentle pressure to shape it into a tight ball. Finally, transfer the shaped boule to a floured proofing basket (seam-side up) or parchment-lined baking sheet (seam-side down). Allow it to rise before baking. This will achieve a beautifully rounded loaf with a crisp crust and soft interior.

Final Proof

The final proof is the last time your dough is allowed to rise before you bake it into bread. After shaping the dough, you'll transfer it to a banneton or proofing basket. For free-form loaves, set it on a square of parchment paper. Allow the dough to rise one more time. During the final proof, all the bacteria and yeast in your starter continue to eat up the flour's carbohydrates. This process contributes more flavor and creates air bubbles. Additionally, the dough has a chance to relax after shaping. This promotes oven spring, helping it rise and expand in the oven.

You can tell your bread is ready to bake and is finished proofing by gently pressing a fingertip on the dough. If it bounces back immediately, the dough needs more time. If a slight indentation remains, then it's time to bake.

Score

As bread bakes, the pressure created during the oven spring can cause the crust to tear. This happens when the dough expands rapidly, as it always will once it hits a nice hot oven. Tears are not only unsightly, they can also result in erratic expansion, poor crust formation, and uneven crumb. To prevent tearing, bakers score their loaves by slicing into them with a sharp tool, such as a lame, a razor, or even a serrated bread knife. They do this immediately before transferring the dough to the oven. These cuts are both beautiful and functional.

A properly scored loaf will expand evenly instead of tearing randomly as the bread puffs up in the oven. Scoring controls that expansion and can often look quite beautiful. Expansion scores are singular cuts 1/2 to 3/4 inch, into the dough. These pragmatic cuts help the bread expand in a controlled fashion without tearing. By contrast, artistic scores are shallow cuts, 1/4 to 1/2 inch, into

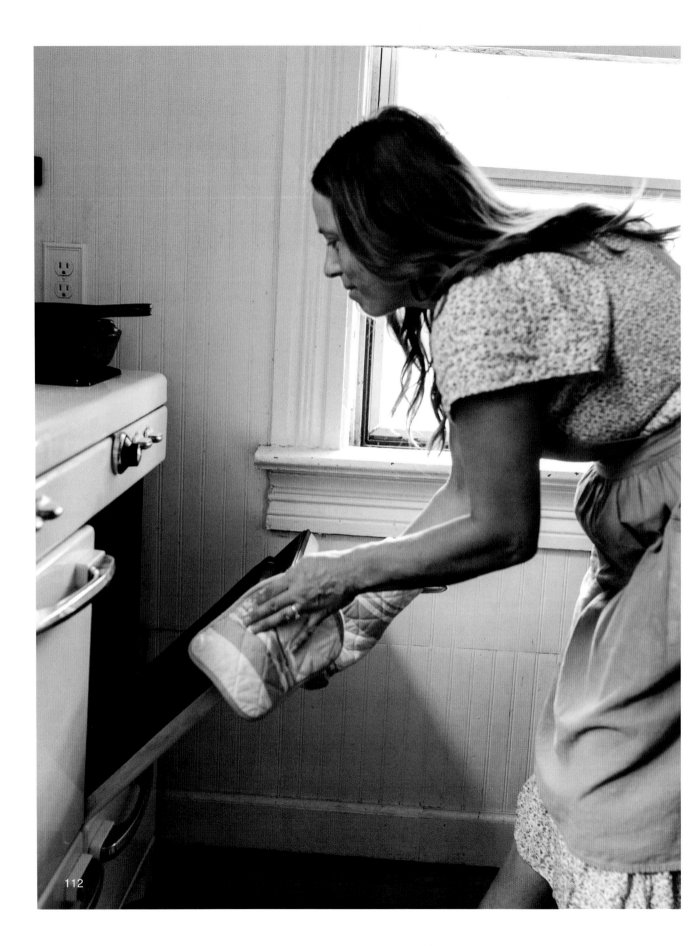

the dough. While they allow the dough to expand a bit, their primary purpose is decorative. Bakers often use both methods together. A popular technique is to use one deep expansion score and a few small artistic scores for appearance.

Bake

High temperatures are essential in producing beautiful bread, especially crusty loaves with airy, open interiors. They also support an even oven spring. The quick expansion of the dough results in light bread with plenty of air pockets.

Many recipes call for turning down the oven temperature after about 20 minutes. This allows for plenty of heat to promote oven spring during the early stages of baking when expansion is the goal. It also prevents overbaking during the later stages, promoting even cooking and browning.

I bake most of my loaves in a Dutch oven, which I preheat in the oven. Baking bread in a Dutch oven captures the steam in the first stage, which ensures a crisp, crackly crust. By contrast, soft-crusted sandwich loaves need lower temperatures and are baked in a loaf pan.

Judging Doneness

You can tell bread is ready by both its color and its temperature. I pull my loaves from the oven when the bread turns golden brown. If you prefer a more precise measurement of doneness, consider taking the temperature of the bread. Artisan-style sourdough is ready when its internal temperature reads 195°F to 210°F. Sandwich breads bake at a lower temperature and are ready when they reach 190°F. Meanwhile, enriched doughs (those made with plenty of added fat) are ready at about 180°F to 190°F.

There's nothing quite so tempting as a fresh loaf straight out of the oven. But resist the urge to slice into a hot (or even warm) loaf and instead let it cool completely. Even though it's out of the oven, several vital processes are taking place. As it cools, the starch begins to harden, and cutting into a loaf too early will result in a gummy crumb. It also results in a rubbery crust.

Storage

Once your bread has cooled completely, you can slice it. Store any leftovers in a paper bag or bread box at room temperature. Avoid storing sourdough in plastic bags or containers, since they can trap moisture. While sourdough is less likely to mold thanks to its high acidity, storing it in plastic can still encourage mold growth. You can also store sourdough sliced-side down on a cutting board or wrapped loosely in a clean tea towel. If you live in a humid climate or want to extend the bread's shelf life, you can store it in the fridge, but this may cause it to turn prematurely stale. For freezing, a ziplock plastic bag is ideal.

Developing a Schedule

Once your starter is happy and bubbling away and you've made a few successful loaves, it's time to develop a routine that works for you. Sourdough needs to fit into your life, not the other way around. But feeding a starter, mixing dough, and letting it rise take time. Fortunately, much of that time is spent waiting. You must wait for the starter to proof and for the dough to ferment. After shaping, you wait again, this time for the dough's final rise. Once it bakes, you must wait for it to cool. Spend these slow hours multitasking. While sometimes there's an entire day between proofing your starter and eating your bread, you need to spend very little time in the kitchen.

Feeding your starter once a week works for most people. Pick a day when you can stick around the house for a bit. If you feed your starter in the early morning, it should be proofed and bubbly sometime around noon. You can make some cookies or muffins with the sourdough discard so that it doesn't go to waste.

Once it's proofed and bubbly, mix up the dough and begin your stretches and folds, if your recipe calls for that technique. Set a timer so that you have a good feel for when you need to check in and tend your dough. Once mixed, most lean dough without much fat will take four to six hours to double. Then, you can shape it and set it in a banneton or proofing basket in the fridge. If you're making a dough with plenty of fat and butter (also called an enriched dough), such as brioche, allow more time—closer to six to eight hours. Added fat slows down fermentation.

The next morning, heat your oven, score the bread, and bake it. This method works well for many home bakers, especially those who bake only once or twice a week. When sorting your schedule, always work backward from the time you'd like your bread to hit the oven, allowing enough time for your dough's final rise, bulk fermentation, mixing, and for your starter to proof.

Navigating the timing of sourdough baking can feel confusing. It's easy to feel overwhelmed. But the process is forgiving—especially when you have a mature starter. Once you're confident, the process gets easier. Soon you might find yourself baking every day.

Sample Schedule

Here are two sample bread baking schedules to give you an idea of how long it will take to make a recipe. Keep in mind that rise times depend greatly on the ambient temperature of your room and that sourdough is forgiving – it's not necessary to be exact with the timing of each step! Feel free to adjust the start times based on when you'd like your bread to hit the oven.

Sample Schedule 1 (Non-enriched Dough)

This sample schedule is for doughs that are not enriched with additional oils or fats, such as No-Knead Sourdough Bread (page 120) or Rosemary Sourdough Bread (page 126).

- 9 am: Feed your sourdough starter. Let it rise for about five hours.

- 2 pm: Make your dough!

- 2 – 5 pm: Stretch and fold your dough. The exact number of stretches and folds and their timing depends on your recipe.

- 5 – 9 pm/bedtime: Allow your dough to rise in a covered bowl on your counter for at least four hours, or until bedtime. This is your bulk fermentation stage.

- 9 pm/bedtime: Shape your dough. Place it in a banneton and put it in the fridge to bake the next morning.

- Next morning: Bake your bread.

Sample Schedule 2 (Enriched Dough)

This sample schedule is for enriched doughs, which are bread doughs made with added fat, such as eggs, butter, or milk. Examples of enriched dough recipes include Sourdough Brioche, Basic Sandwich Bread (page 144) and Cinnamon-Raisin Bread (page 154).

- ◆ 2 pm: Feed your sourdough starter. Let it rise for about five hours.

- ◆ 7pm: Make your dough!

- ◆ 7 pm – 7 am: Allow your dough to rise in a covered bowl on your counter for at least 12 hours. This is your bulk fermentation stage. Do not put your dough in the fridge. (Doing so will halt the bulk fermentation process.)

- ◆ 7 am: Shape your dough and add it to your pan. Allow your dough to rise in the pan at room temperature for two to four hours, or until doubled. This is your second rise.

- ◆ 9 – 11 am: Bake your bread.

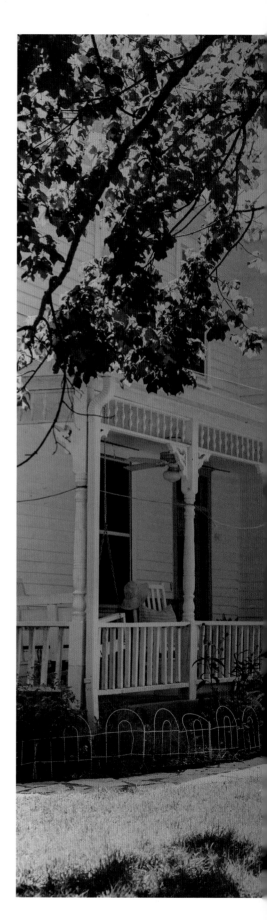

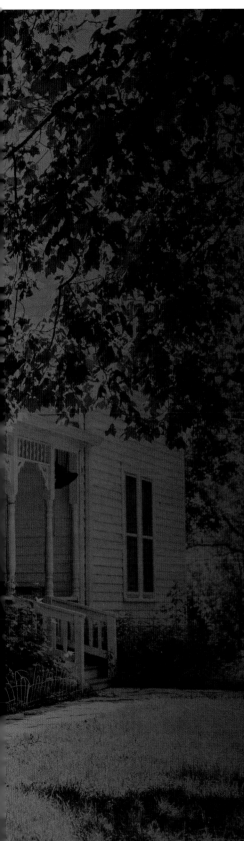

SOURDOUGH AT THE FARMHOUSE

I keep a huge jar of starter since I feed a large family, and fermented grains make an appearance at most of our meals in one way or another. In the morning, I feed the starter until I have at least a full quart. I often don't even bother measuring and add an amount of water and flour that just feels right. While the day goes on, I let that jar sit on the countertop until it's active and bubbly. I'll save some of the sourdough discard for pancakes (page 275), crêpes (page 270), or skillet dinner (page 279).

When the starter is active, I'll work some of it into bread dough before placing the jar in the fridge. Since I come to sourdough hoping to make the most nutritious food for my family, I aim for long-fermented breads. They offer the best flavor anyway. After shaping the dough, I'll drop it in a banneton and tuck it in the fridge so that all that flavor develops slowly overnight.

The next day, I bake. If we're busy, I might just keep the starter in the fridge for a few days. But more often than not, I pull it out and feed it again. On these bulk-prep days, I make plenty of goodies to get us through the week, feeding my starter several cups of flour and water to build up its volume. Perhaps I'll use a cup of starter for bagels, another cup for buns, and yet another for pizza. I let each dough sit at room temperature in separate bowls until bedtime. Then, I put them in the fridge to slow fermentation. This allows me to dirty the mixer bowl only once. Now I have many options in the fridge. I can shape and bake them with little notice.

On my bulk-prep days, I put my starter back in the fridge to rest until the next time. It stays there until I am ready to bulk it back up and use it again. If I feed it several cups of flour and water before my baking day, I still have a few cups in the fridge to pull from. I like to use a refrigerated starter on the fly for the sourdough discard recipes that don't require any waiting.

Same-Day Sourdough Bread

This basic sourdough bread is a staple in our kitchen. It's easy to make, and the ingredients are straightforward and simple. From feeding the starter to baking fresh bread, it's all done in one day. For this reason, it's one of the first recipes I recommend to beginning bakers.

The key to this recipe is an active and bubbly starter. Be sure to feed it first thing in the morning. Allow it to double in volume before mixing up the dough, which takes a few hours. Keep in mind that if your kitchen is cold, it may take more time for the bread to rise. If it is warm, it'll take less, so allow a little flexibility.

1 1/3 cups (315 grams) warm water

1/2 cup (100 grams) active sourdough starter

3 1/3 cups (467 grams) all-purpose flour

1 1/2 teaspoons salt

1 In a large mixing bowl, combine the water, starter, flour, and salt, stirring well until they form a shaggy dough. Cover the bowl, and let the dough rest for 30 minutes, allowing the flour to hydrate fully.

2 Reach underneath one side of the dough and gently pull it up so that it stretches without breaking. Then, fold the dough into the center. Rotate the bowl a quarter turn and repeat the stretch-and-fold process. Repeat twice more until you've gone around the bowl.

3 Cover the bowl and let it rest for 20 minutes. Then, complete another round of stretches and folds. Allow it to rest for 20 minutes more, and then complete one final round of stretches and folds.

4 Let the dough rise in a warm place until it doubles in size, 5 to 8 hours. If your kitchen is cold or your starter is very young, you may need to allow more time.

5 Once the dough has doubled, dust your working surface with a little flour. Gently turn the dough out onto the floured surface. Fold the edges toward the center, and turn it over seam-side down on your counter. Then, carefully cup the dough with both hands and pull it toward you until you feel it release from the countertop. As you work the dough, form it into a ball.

DAILY BREAD

6   Let the dough sit out uncovered for about 15 minutes. Then, transfer the dough to a floured banneton or bowl with a floured tea towel, seam-side up. Cover the dough loosely with a plastic bag or damp kitchen towel and let the dough rise for 1 to 2 hours.

7   An hour before you're ready to bake, place a lidded Dutch oven in your oven and preheat it to 500°F.

8   Gently turn out the dough onto a piece of parchment paper. Dust the top of the dough with flour, and score it by slicing about 1/2 inch deep into the dough at a 45° angle.

9   Grab hold of the edges of the parchment paper, and carefully transfer the dough and the paper to the Dutch oven. Place the lid back on and return the Dutch oven into the oven. Bake for 20 minutes.

10 Remove the lid with oven mitts and turn the oven temperature down to 475°F. Continue baking for about 15 minutes more, or until golden brown.

11 Let the bread cool in the pan for about 5 minutes, and then carefully transfer it to a cooling rack. Allow it to cool completely before slicing and serving.

HOW TO PREVENT YOUR DOUGH FROM STICKING

Use plenty of flour on your tea towel or banneton, or your dough might stick. Err on the side of using too much flour rather than too little. After all, you can dust it off later. Rice flour is an excellent option for flouring your banneton, as it has a coarse texture and tends to stick less.

If it still sticks, your dough may have fermented too long, so keep an eye on your rising times next time you bake.

PREP TIME:
45 MINUTES

BAKE TIME:
45 MINUTES

RISE TIME:
24 TO 28 HOURS

YIELD:
MAKES 2 LOAVES

No-Knead Sourdough Bread

Caring for a family of ten means that my farmhouse kitchen always seems to buzz with activity, so relying on easy recipes is a must. This no-knead sourdough bread is practically effortless. It yields two loaves, so there's always a little extra for the freezer or later in the week.

This recipe takes a little planning, since you mix the dough one day and bake it the next. That extra time allows the bread to develop an even deeper flavor. The crust is crisp, the crumb is soft, and the flavor tastes deliciously tangy.

3 1/2 cups (490 grams) all-purpose flour

1 1/3 cups (186 grams) whole-wheat flour

1 3/4 cups (245 grams) bread flour

2 3/4 cups (650 grams) warm water

1 cup (200 grams) active sourdough starter

4 teaspoons (24 grams) salt

1 In a large bowl, add the all-purpose flour, whole-wheat flour, and bread flour and stir to combine. Then, stir in the water, forming a rough dough. Allow it to rest for 30 minutes to hydrate the flour thoroughly.

2 Pour in the starter. Then, dampen your hands slightly. Work the starter into the flour mixture until well incorporated.

3 Press into the dough about 1/2 inch with the tips of your fingers to give it a dimpled appearance. Then, sprinkle the dough with the salt. Mix the dough with your hands for about 5 minutes, just enough to bring the dough together.

4 Cover the bowl with plastic wrap or a damp towel and let the dough rest for 30 minutes.

5 Reach underneath one side of the dough, gently pull it up, and fold it over the center. Rotate the bowl a quarter turn and repeat the stretch-and-fold process. Repeat twice more until you've gone around the bowl.

6 Cover the bowl and let it rest for 15 minutes. Then, complete another round of stretches and folds. Allow it to rest for 15 minutes more, and then complete a third round of stretches and folds. Let the dough rest for 30 minutes. Then, complete three more rounds of stretches and folds, allowing a 30-minute rest between each round.

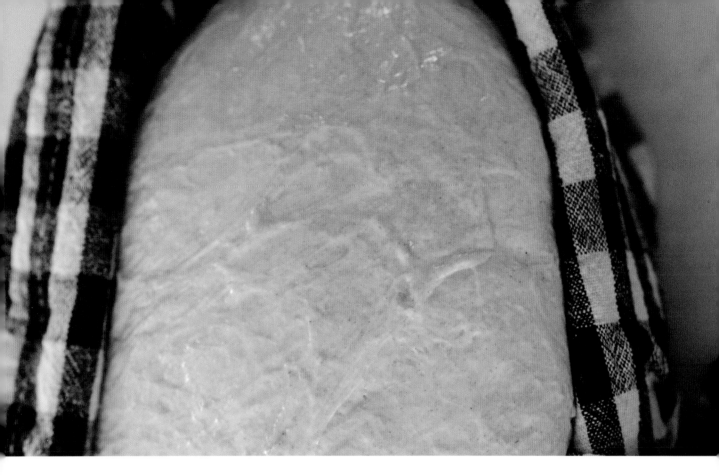

7 Cover the bowl tightly and allow the dough to rise until doubled, about 8 hours.

8 Once the dough has doubled in volume, use a bench scraper to split the dough in half, taking care not to break any of those precious bubbles.

9 Turn the dough out onto a lightly floured working surface. Gently fold the outer edges of the dough toward the center and turn it over so that it rests on the counter seam-side down. Cup the far side of the dough with your hands and gently pull it toward you to shape it into a ball. Let it sit uncovered on your working surface for 15 to 20 minutes.

10 Place the dough seam-side up into a floured banneton or a bowl lined with a floured tea towel. Cover with plastic and transfer it to the fridge for at least 12 and up to 15 hours.

11 The next day, place a Dutch oven in the oven and preheat at 500°F for 1 hour.

12 Gently turn out the dough onto a piece of parchment paper. Dust the top of the dough with flour, and score it by slicing about 1/2 inch deep into the dough at a 45° angle.

13 Grab hold of the edges of the parchment paper, and carefully transfer the dough and the paper to the Dutch oven. Place the lid back on and return the Dutch oven into the oven. Bake for 20 minutes at 500°F with the lid on. Turn the heat down to 475°F and then bake for about 25 minutes more, or until browned on top. Allow it to cool completely before slicing and serving.

Small-Batch Sourdough

Sometimes you need only a little bread—just enough to get by. This recipe makes a smaller loaf with the same deep flavor and crackly crust you get from classic artisan loaves. It's also an excellent jumping-off point for other kinds of bread. You can work chopped fresh herbs, nuts, or other add-ins into the dough for variety. Just sprinkle them over the dough right before you complete the stretches and folds.

The long, slow rise and extra time in the fridge give this artisan-style bread a rich, complex, tangy flavor and crisp, crunchy crust. These techniques also make the bread easier to digest. The good bacteria and yeast in your starter have plenty of time to break down the complex carbohydrates in the flour.

PREP TIME:
45 MINUTES

BAKE TIME:
15 TO 25 MINUTES

RISE TIME:
24 TO 28 HOURS

YIELD:
MAKES 1 LOAF

1 3/4 cup
(245 grams)
all-purpose flour

2/3 cup
(158 grams)
water

1/4 cup
(50 grams)
active
sourdough
starter

1 teaspoon
(6 grams) salt

1 To a large mixing bowl, add the flour, water, starter, and salt. Mix everything together using a dough whisk, wooden spoon, or your hands. It should form a shaggy, rough dough. Cover the bowl tightly and allow the dough to rest for 30 minutes.

2 Reach underneath one side of the dough, gently pull it up, shaking it lightly as you pull, and then fold it over the center. Rotate the bowl a quarter turn, then repeat three more times until you've gone around the bowl. Cover the bowl and let it rest for 30 minutes. Then, complete two more rounds of stretches and folds, allowing a 30-minute rest between each round.

3 After the final stretch and fold, cover the bowl tightly and set it in a warm spot in your kitchen. Let it rise at room temperature for 6 to 12 hours or until doubled. Cover the bowl with a lid, damp kitchen towel, or plastic wrap.

4 Lightly dust your working surface with flour, and then gently tip out the dough. Gently shape it into a ball by pulling it toward you in a circular motion. Let it sit uncovered for at least 15 and up to 20 minutes to help it dry out a bit.

5 Place the dough smooth-side down on your working surface and shape it again. Fold the two sides over to meet in the middle, pinch together, and then repeat on the other two sides.

6 Generously dust a tea towel with flour and set it in a small bowl. Place the dough seam-side up in the prepared bowl and then cover it with a plastic bag. Transfer the dough to the fridge for 12 to 15 hours.

7 An hour before you're ready to bake, place a Dutch oven in a 500°F oven to preheat.

8 Remove the dough right before you plan to bake. Turn it out onto a square of parchment paper. Dust the top with flour and carefully score the dough. Next, lift it by the parchment paper and place it inside the Dutch oven. Bake for 20 minutes with the lid on, then turn the temperature down to 475°F and bake for an additional 15 to 25 minutes, or until golden brown.

WHY DOES SOURDOUGH NEED A LONG RISE TIME?

If you're used to baking bread with commercial yeast, the long, slow rising times required for sourdough baking might surprise you. Sourdough breads often require double the rise time that a similar bread made with commercial yeast might need, so it's wise to plan ahead.

Manufacturers have bred commercial yeast over time to create consistent, quick results. With sourdough baking, you rely on the wild yeast varieties in your starter. Like most wild things, they follow very few rules and seem to do as they please. The wild yeast strains in your starter aren't bred for speed, like baker's yeast, so sourdough tends to take longer to rise.

While sourdough may take more time to rise, that comes with benefits. A lengthier fermentation period allows more time for flavor to develop.

Additionally, those long, slow rises might also make the bread more nutritious. That's because it provides more time to break down phytic acid. Phytic acid is a naturally occurring chemical that binds minerals in grains and makes them hard to absorb. Further, a lengthy fermentation period allows more time for beta-glucan to form. Beta-glucan is a complex carbohydrate associated with cardiovascular health.

Tucking your dough in the fridge allows for even longer rising times. This technique, called retarding the dough, develops flavor without over fermenting. Consider letting the bread rise during the bulk fermentation at room temperature. Shape the loaf. Then, transfer it to the fridge for up to 24 hours before baking. Retarding the dough is an excellent option if you have another time commitment—or if you are just ready to head to bed and don't have time to tend to your dough.

PREP TIME:
45 MINUTES

BAKE TIME:
45 MINUTES

RISE TIME:
24 TO 28 HOURS

YIELD:
MAKES 2 LOAVES

Rosemary Sourdough Bread

This is one of those recipes that makes the home baker look as though they've mastered their craft for years. It's a gorgeous sourdough loaf touched with the aroma of fresh rosemary—all woodsy and warm. It's a delicious partner to an herby tomato soup or a rustic sandwich slathered with a garlicky aioli and stuffed with salami.

If you don't have rosemary, try whatever herbs you have growing in your garden or tucked away in your fridge. I love to work fresh thyme and sliced garlic into this bread, or sprinkle in a spoonful of herbes de Provence.

3 1/2 cups (490 grams) all-purpose flour

1 1/3 cups (186 grams) whole-wheat flour

1 3/4 cups (245 grams) bread flour

2 3/4 cups (650 grams) warm water

1 cup (200 grams) active sourdough starter

4 teaspoons (24 grams) salt

1 tablespoon chopped fresh rosemary

1   In a large mixing bowl, combine the all-purpose flour, whole-wheat flour, bread flour, and the water. Then, add the sourdough starter and salt. Work the ingredients by hand to form a rough dough, then add the chopped rosemary.

2   Reach underneath one side of the dough, gently pull it up, shaking it lightly as you pull, and then fold it over the center. Rotate the bowl a quarter turn, then repeat three more times until you've gone around the bowl.

3   Cover the bowl and let it rest for 15 minutes. Then, complete another round of stretches and folds, working the rosemary into the dough. Allow it to rest for 30 minutes more. Then, complete one final round of stretches and folds.

4   Cover the bowl tightly and allow it to rise until doubled in volume, about 4 hours.

5   Turn the dough out onto a clean working surface and split the dough in half using a bench scraper, taking care not to deflate the dough.

6   Working with half the dough at a time, gently shape it into a ball by pulling it toward you in a circular motion. Let it sit uncovered for at least 15 and up to 20 minutes to help it dry out a bit.

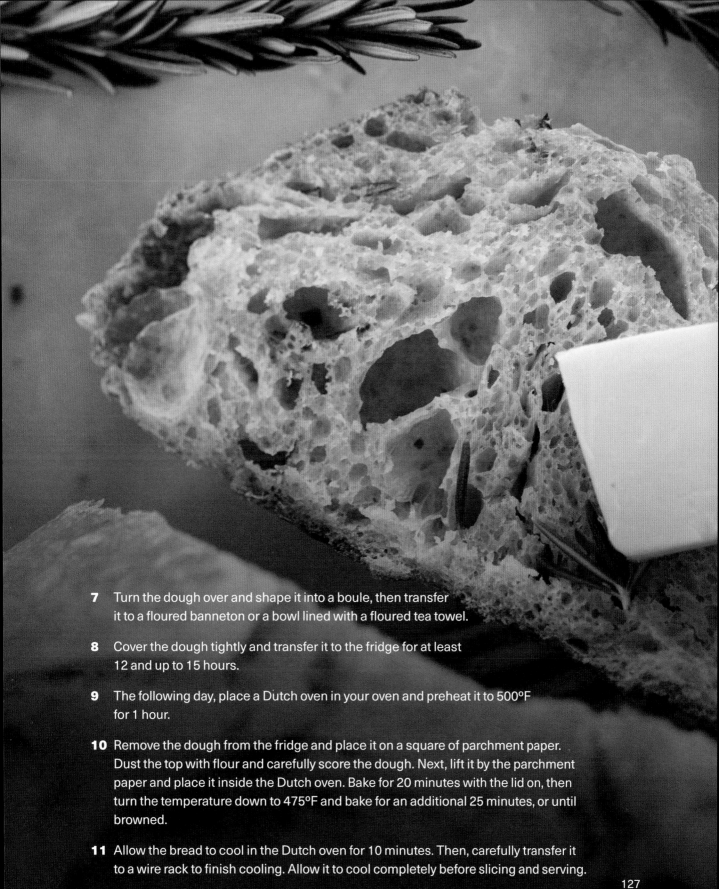

7   Turn the dough over and shape it into a boule, then transfer
    it to a floured banneton or a bowl lined with a floured tea towel.

8   Cover the dough tightly and transfer it to the fridge for at least
    12 and up to 15 hours.

9   The following day, place a Dutch oven in your oven and preheat it to 500°F
    for 1 hour.

10 Remove the dough from the fridge and place it on a square of parchment paper.
    Dust the top with flour and carefully score the dough. Next, lift it by the parchment
    paper and place it inside the Dutch oven. Bake for 20 minutes with the lid on, then
    turn the temperature down to 475°F and bake for an additional 25 minutes, or until
    browned.

11 Allow the bread to cool in the Dutch oven for 10 minutes. Then, carefully transfer it
    to a wire rack to finish cooling. Allow it to cool completely before slicing and serving.

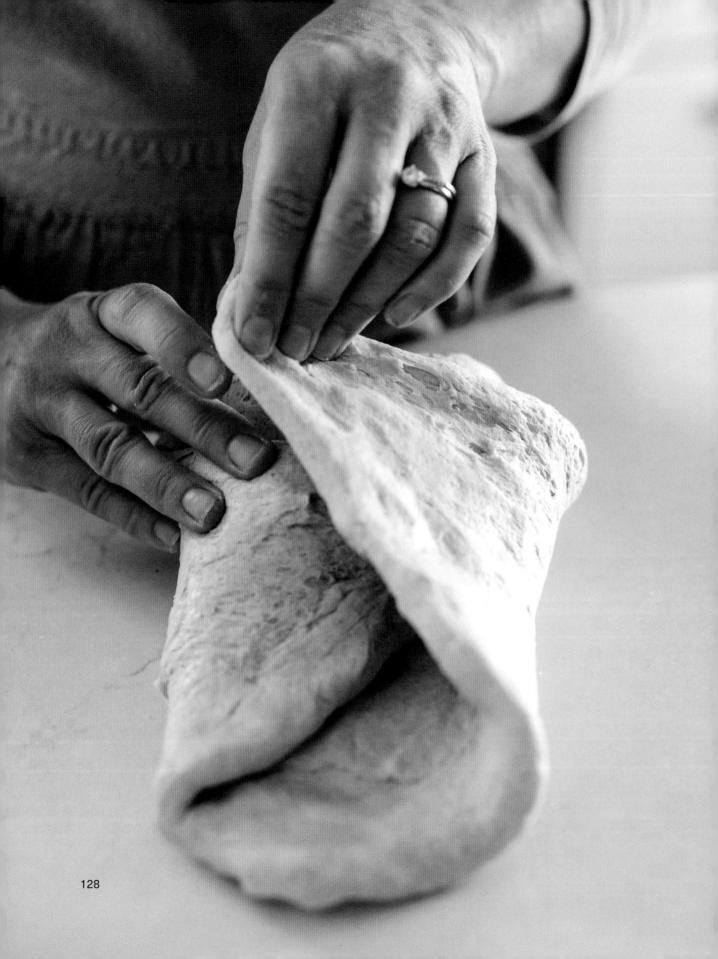

PREP TIME:
5 MINUTES

BAKE TIME:
45 MINUTES

RISE TIME:
24 TO 28 HOURS

YIELD:
MAKES 1 LOAF

Einkorn Sourdough Bread

Einkorn is an ancient wheat that makes a beautiful golden-colored loaf of bread. It also has a rich and complex flavor coupled with a satisfying crisp crust and chewy crumb.

Einkorn is a little tricky to work with. You may find the dough feels stickier and is more challenging to manage than dough made with regular wheat flour. Accordingly, you may need to adjust your technique a little. Don't expect it to pass the windowpane test. Instead of using the stretch-and-fold technique, simply fold the dough onto itself.

3 cups (390 grams) all-purpose einkorn flour

1 cup (140 grams) whole-grain einkorn flour

1 1/4 cups (295 grams) warm water

1 cup (200 grams) active sourdough starter

1 1/2 teaspoons (9 grams) salt

Olive oil, for the bowl

1   In a large mixing bowl, combine the all-purpose einkorn flour, whole-grain einkorn flour, water, starter, and salt. Mix the ingredients by hand until they come together to form a rough, sticky dough.

2   Cover the bowl and let the dough rest for 15 minutes.

3   Tip the dough onto a lightly floured working surface, and pat it down by hand to form a disk about 1 inch thick. Fold the outer edges toward the center, then turn it over and roll the dough into a ball.

4   Drizzle a little olive oil into the bottom of a large bowl, and then place the dough into the bowl and cover it tightly. Allow to rest again for 20 minutes.

5   Repeat the flattening and folding process twice, allowing it to rest for 20 minutes between each round.

6   Shape the dough and cover it with plastic wrap. Allow it to rise until doubled, anywhere from 3 to 12 hours, depending on the warmth of your kitchen and the liveliness of your starter.

(recipe continued on next page)

7 Shape the dough into a boule and place it in a floured banneton. Place the banneton inside a plastic bag and transfer it to the fridge for about 12 to 15 hours.

8 The next day, place a Dutch oven in your oven and preheat it to 450°F.

9 Tip the dough out of the banneton and onto a square of parchment paper. Score the top of the dough, then carefully place the parchment paper and dough into the Dutch oven. Cover with a lid and bake for 30 minutes. Remove the lid and bake for an additional 15 minutes, or until golden brown.

10 Allow the bread to cool in the pan for 10 minutes and then carefully transfer it to a wire rack to cool completely before slicing and serving.

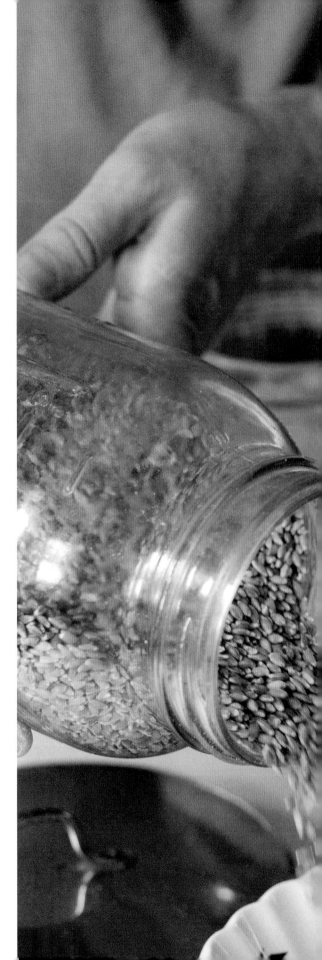

BAKING WITH ANCIENT WHEAT

Einkorn is an ancient variety of wheat, and I often bake with it. Its rich, complex flavor tastes like wheat, only a bit milder and sweeter, with notes of barley and nuts. It also produces beautiful baked goods with a rich golden color thanks to its plentiful beta carotene.

Unlike modern varieties of wheat, einkorn has never been hybridized and has remained in the same form for thousands of years. It's more nutritious, too. Einkorn is richer in protein, B vitamins, and minerals than modern wheat. Researchers have found that sourdough einkorn bread is anti-inflammatory. This is due to both the fermentation process and its particularly abundant antioxidants.

As a distant cousin of wheat, einkorn contains gluten. Its gluten content has a different structure from modern wheat and is also weaker. As a result, some people who experience sensitivities to modern wheat may find einkorn easier to digest—but people with celiac disease should still avoid it.

If you're used to baking only with regular wheat flour, you might find that einkorn behaves differently. It tends to be sticky and absorbs liquid at a slower rate. As a result, einkorn recipes tend to require a little less fat and liquid than you might usually add.

PREP TIME:
45 MINUTES

BAKE TIME:
**40 MINUTES +
1 HOUR TO PREHEAT
THE DUTCH OVEN**

RISE TIME:
24 TO 28 HOURS

YIELD:
MAKES 1 LOAF

Sourdough Rye Bread

The delicious flavor of rye is distinct with notes of molasses and malt. Regular wheat flour, while tasty in its own right, just can't compare. When you add sourdough to the mix, it tastes heavenly. I love the addition of caraway seeds. They bring a vibrant and lively edge to this classic bread. The crumb is chewy but not dense, and it has a rustic edge that I'm sure you'll love.

Try using it as the base for a Reuben sandwich. Toast the bread and slather it with Russian dressing. Then, top it with pastrami, Swiss cheese, and plenty of homemade sauerkraut. It tastes spectacular, I promise.

1 1/4 cup (295 grams) water

1 cup (200 grams) active sourdough starter

2 1/2 cups (350 grams) bread flour

1 cup (140 grams) rye flour

1/2 cup (70 grams) whole-wheat flour

1 1/2 teaspoons (9 grams) salt

1 tablespoon (17 grams) molasses

2 teaspoons (5 grams) caraway seeds

1 In a large mixing bowl, combine the water and starter. Then, mix the bread flour, rye flour, and whole-wheat flour into the starter mixture. Cover the bowl with a damp tea towel and allow the dough to rest for 30 minutes.

2 Reach underneath one side of the dough, gently pull it up, and fold it over the center. Rotate the bowl a quarter turn and repeat the stretch-and-fold process. Repeat twice more until you've gone around the bowl.

3 Cover the bowl and let it rest for 15 minutes. Complete another round of stretches and folds. Allow it to rest for 30 minutes more, and then complete three more rounds of stretches and folds.

4 Cover the bowl tightly and allow it to rise until doubled, 8 to 12 hours.

5 Turn the dough out onto a lightly floured surface. Gently shape the dough into a ball by pulling it toward you in a circular motion. Allow it to rest, uncovered, for 15 to 20 minutes.

6 Turn the dough over, folding the sides of the dough in toward the middle. Place the dough seam-side up in a floured banneton or a bowl lined with a lightly floured tea towel. Cover with a plastic bag and transfer to the fridge for at least 12 and up to 15 hours.

7 Place a Dutch oven in the oven and preheat it at 475°F for 1 hour.

8 Place a square of parchment paper on the counter, and then turn the dough out onto the parchment paper. Dust the top of the dough with flour and then score the bread.

9 Lift the parchment and dough and place them into the preheated Dutch oven, taking care not to burn yourself. Bake the bread with the lid on for 20 minutes. Then, remove the lid and continue baking for 20 minutes more, or until nicely browned.

10 Cool completely before slicing and serving.

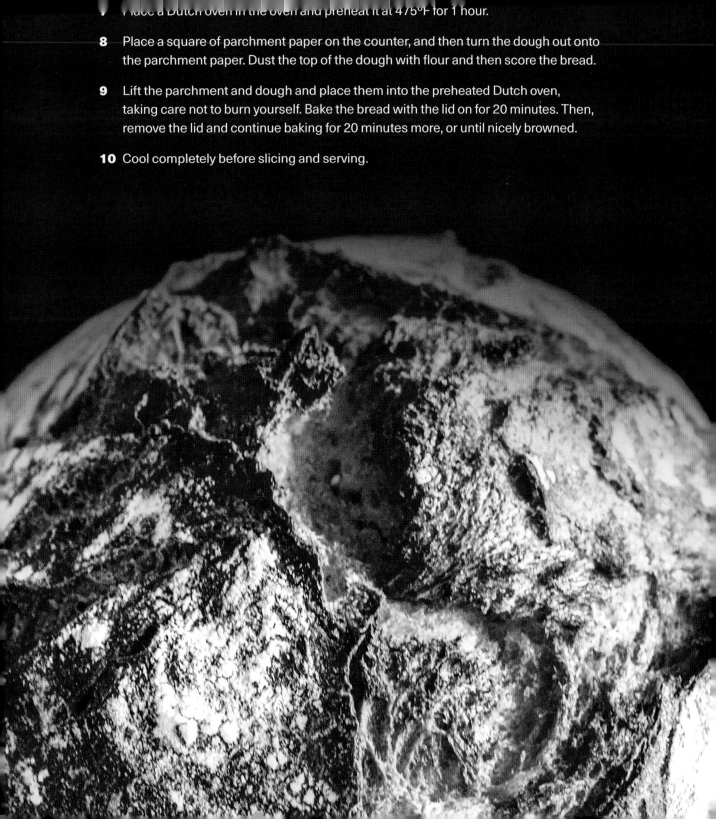

PREP TIME:
45 MINUTES

BAKE TIME:
**45 MINUTES +
1 HOUR TO PREHEAT
THE DUTCH OVEN**

RISE TIME:
24 TO 28 HOURS

YIELD:
MAKES 1 LOAF

Spelt and Walnut Bread

Like einkorn, spelt is an ancient grain related to modern-day wheat. It has a beautiful soft texture and a slightly sweet, nutty flavor. I love to partner it with walnuts, which seem to complement spelt's gorgeous flavor. Spelt gives sourdough bread a tender crumb and hearty texture with tart, slightly earthy undertones.

Spelt has a weaker gluten structure compared to modern wheat, so it's important to use it together with bread flour, which gives the loaf both structure and strength. It's a deliciously wholesome alternative to sourdough breads made entirely with wheat.

1 3/4 cup (245 grams) bread flour

1 1/2 cups (210 grams) white spelt flour

3/4 cup (105 grams) whole-grain spelt flour

1 1/3 cups (314 grams) water

1/2 cup (100 grams) active sourdough starter

2 teaspoons (12 grams) salt

1/2 cup (about 65 grams) coarsely chopped walnuts

1 In a large mixing bowl, whisk together the bread flour, white spelt flour, and whole-grain spelt flour together. Stir in the water, sourdough starter, and salt until it forms a shaggy dough. Cover the bowl tightly and let the dough rest for 30 minutes.

2 Reach underneath one side of the dough, gently pull it up, and fold it over the center. Rotate the bowl a quarter turn and repeat the stretch-and-fold process. Repeat twice more until you've gone around the bowl.

3 Cover the bowl and let it rest for 15 minutes. Then, scatter the walnuts over the dough. Complete another round of stretches and folds, working the nuts into the dough.

4 Allow it to rest for 15 minutes more, and then complete a third round of stretches and folds. Let the dough rest for 30 minutes, then complete three more rounds of stretches and folds, allowing a 30-minute rest between each round.

5 Cover the bowl, and allow it to rise until doubled in volume, 3 to 8 hours.

6 Turn the dough out onto a lightly floured workingsurface. Gently shape the dough by folding it onto itself. Then, turn it seam-side down and gently pull it toward you in a circular motion, creating tension against the working surface. Transfer the dough to a floured banneton, and then cover it with plastic and transfer it to the fridge for at least 12 and up to 15 hours.

7 Place your Dutch oven into your oven, and preheat it to 500°F for at least 1 hour.

8 Remove the dough from the fridge and turn it out onto a square of parchment paper. Dust it with flour and score the loaf. Carefully lift the parchment and dough. Then, place it into the preheated Dutch oven. Bake the bread with the lid on for 20 minutes, then take off the lid and turn down the heat to 475°F. Continue baking for a 25 minutes more, or until golden brown.

9 Let the bread cool in the pan for 10 minutes and then carefully transfer it to a wire rack to cool completely before slicing and serving.

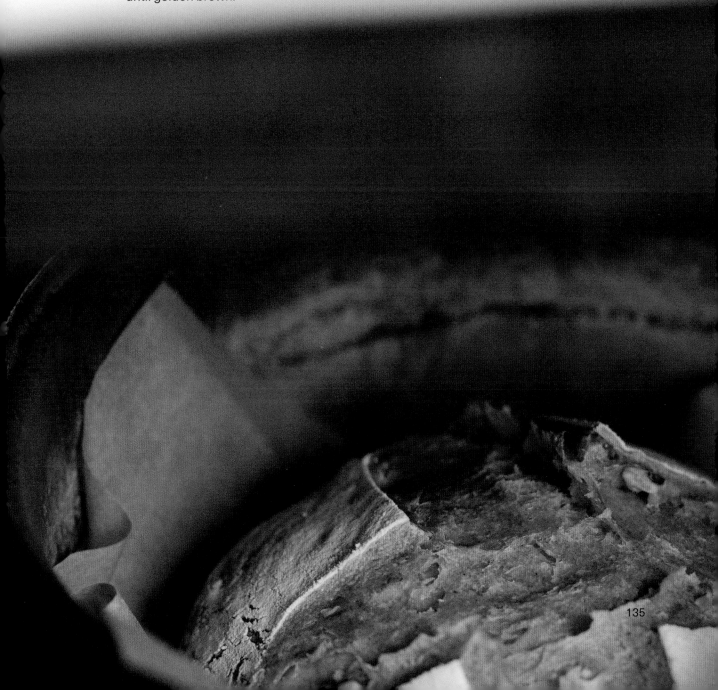

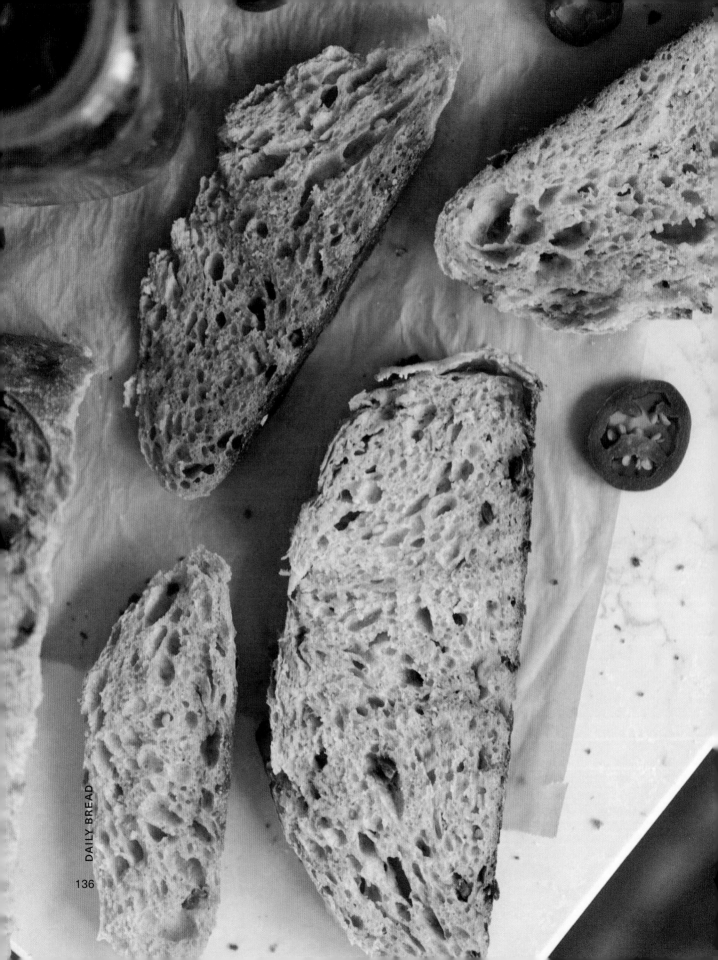

PREP TIME:
2 HOURS

BAKE TIME:
45 MINUTES

RISE TIME:
24 TO 28 HOURS

YIELD:
MAKES 2 LOAVES

Jalapeño-Cheddar Bread

One of the things my kids look forward to the most is a fresh loaf of sourdough bread straight out of the oven. We eat one with dinner nearly every night, but having a little variety is nice. This jalapeño-cheddar bread is a riff on our basic sourdough bread. It's incredibly delicious, with a beautiful crust and a fluffy crumb that's full of cheese with bright pops of heat.

Try it with fresh jalapeños straight from the garden in the summer or pickled jalapeños in the winter. It's tasty either way, especially if you partner it with a meaty chili.

2 3/4 cups (650 grams) warm water

3 1/2 cups (490 grams) all-purpose flour

2 cups (280 grams) bread flour

1 1/3 cups (186 grams) whole-wheat flour

1 cup (200 grams) active sourdough starter

4 teaspoons (24 grams) salt

2 cups (340 grams) shredded cheddar cheese

1/4 cup (64 grams) sliced fresh or pickled jalapeños

1 In a large mixing bowl, combine the water, all-purpose flour, bread flour, and whole-wheat flour by hand until it forms a rough dough. Cover it tightly and let the dough rest for 30 minutes.

2 Pour in the sourdough starter. Then, dampen your hands slightly and work the starter into the flour mixture until well incorporated.

3 Press into the dough about 1/2 inch with the tips of your fingers, giving it a dimpled appearance, and then sprinkle the dough with salt. Mix the dough with your hands for about 5 minutes, just enough to bring the dough together. Cover the bowl and let it rest for 30 minutes.

4 Reach underneath one side of the dough, gently pull it up, and fold it over the center. Rotate the bowl a quarter turn and repeat the stretch-and-fold process. Repeat twice more until you've gone around the bowl.

5 Cover the bowl and let it rest for 15 minutes. Then, scatter the cheddar and jalapeños over the dough. Complete another round of stretches and folds, working the cheese and peppers into the dough. Allow it to rest for 15 minutes more and then complete another round of stretches and folds. Let the dough rest for 30 minutes, then complete three more rounds of stretches and folds, allowing a 30-minute rest between each round.

137

(recipe continued on next page)

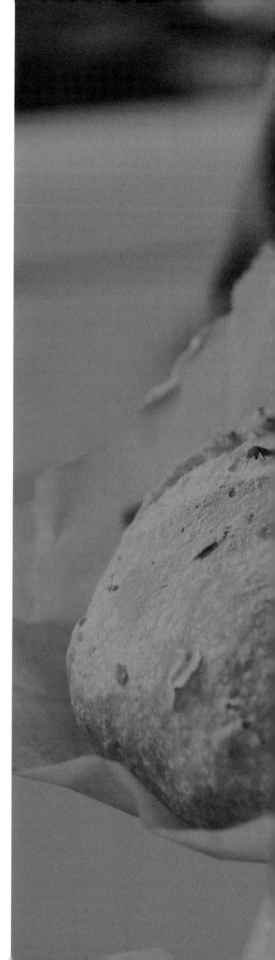

6 Cover the bowl and allow it to rise until doubled in volume, 4 to 6 hours.

7 Turn the dough out onto a lightly floured working surface and then split the dough in half with a bench scraper, taking care not to deflate the dough.

8 Working with one batch of dough at a time, shape the first ball by gently pulling it toward you in a circular motion, creating tension against the working surface. Allow the loaves to rest uncovered for 15 to 20 minutes.

9 Turn them over and shape the dough on a clean working surface by folding the sides of the dough toward the middle. Place the dough seam-side up in a floured banneton or a bowl lined with a lightly floured tea towel. Cover with a plastic bag and transfer to the fridge for at least 12 and up to 15 hours.

10 Place a Dutch oven inside your oven and heat it to 500°F for 1 hour.

11 Remove the dough from the fridge and turn it out onto a square of parchment paper. Dust it with flour and score the loaf. Carefully lift the parchment and dough and place them into the preheated Dutch oven. Bake the bread with the lid on for 20 minutes, then take off the lid and turn down the heat to 475°F. Continue baking for 25 minutes more, or until browned.

12 Let the bread cool in the pan for 10 minutes, and then carefully transfer it to a wire rack to cool completely before slicing and serving.

WORKING WITH HIGH-HYDRATION DOUGHS

Hydration refers to the ratio of water to flour in your dough. High-hydration doughs are wetter and use more liquid. This results in beautiful, airy bread with an open crumb structure. It also makes them more difficult to handle.

Watch your dough closely during bulk fermentation. High-hydration dough tends to ferment faster and needs less time. If you let it ferment too long, it will overproof and turn into a sticky, unworkable mess. Remember dough made with a mature starter ferments faster, and warm kitchens promote fast fermentation, while cold kitchens slow it down.

High-hydration dough requires a gentle hand. Treat it lightly but firmly while it rises, but especially when you shape it. This will make the crumb more open and even. Using a bench scraper helps move your dough efficiently but gently.

If you find the dough too sticky to handle as you stretch and fold it, wet your fingertips with a little water. It will keep the dough from sticking to you.

Additionally, your flour matters. High-hydration recipes benefit the most from wheat flour, especially bread flour. Whole-wheat flour in combination with all-purpose also works. Both the bread and whole-wheat flours have a higher protein content, allowing them to absorb more of the water.

PREP TIME:
15 MINUTES

BAKE TIME:
25 MINUTES

RISE TIME:
15 TO 28 HOURS

YIELD:
MAKES 8 INDIVIDUAL LOAVES

Sourdough Ciabatta Bread

Ciabatta means "slipper" in Italian, so named for the small, slipper-like shape of the loaves. It has a delicately airy crumb and crisp crust, which you achieve by steaming the loaves a little while they bake. Commercial bakeries use special steam-injection ovens to make super-crusty loaves of bread. But you can create the same effect by tucking a cast-iron skillet filled with water into your oven as it preheats. That creates enough steam for beautiful, crisp, golden loaves. They make the best sandwiches thanks to all those air pockets ready to hold on to your sandwich fillings. For a quick lunch, I'll slice the bread through the middle, exposing its gorgeous air bubbles. Then, I'll top it with salami, fresh greens, and cheese.

4 1/2 cups (630 grams) bread flour

2 cups (472 grams) warm water

1 cup (200 grams) active sourdough starter

1 tablespoon (18 grams) salt

1 In a large mixing bowl, combine the flour, water, starter, and salt until it forms a rough dough. Cover the bowl and allow it to rest for 30 minutes.

2 Reach underneath one side of the dough, gently pull it up, and fold it over the center. Rotate the bowl a quarter turn and repeat the stretch-and-fold process. Repeat twice more until you've gone around the bowl.

3 Cover the bowl and let it rest for 30 minutes. Complete two more sets of stretches and folds about 30 minutes apart.

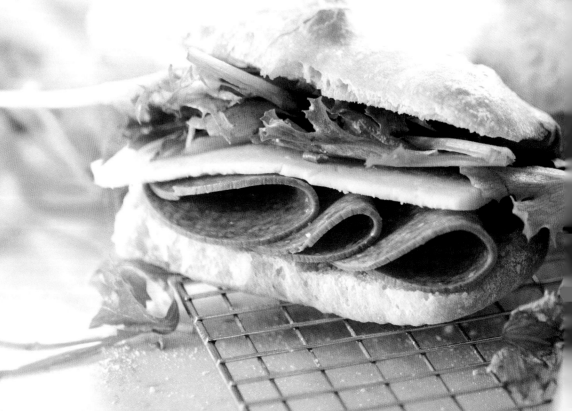

DAILY BREAD

4. Cover the bowl with a damp tea towel and allow the dough to rise until doubled, about 4 hours. Transfer the dough to the fridge and let it ferment for 12 to 24 hours.

5. The next day, dip the dough onto a lightly floured working surface, working gently to keep the bubbles intact. Gently shape the dough into a rectangle, then dust the top with flour.

6. Set aside a rectangular length of parchment paper and dust it with flour. Then, divide the dough into eight equal pieces with a bench scraper. Next, carefully lift the dough one piece at a time using the bench scraper and transfer it to the parchment.

7. Cover the dough with a tea towel and let it rise for 1 to 2 hours, or until puffy.

8. Place a pizza stone on the middle rack of your oven, then place a cast-iron skillet on the lower rack. Pour about 1 cup of water into the skillet. Preheat the oven to 475°F.

9. Carefully lift the parchment paper holding the dough onto the pizza stone, and then bake for about 25 minutes, or until the crust is golden. Transfer to a wire rack to cool completely before serving.

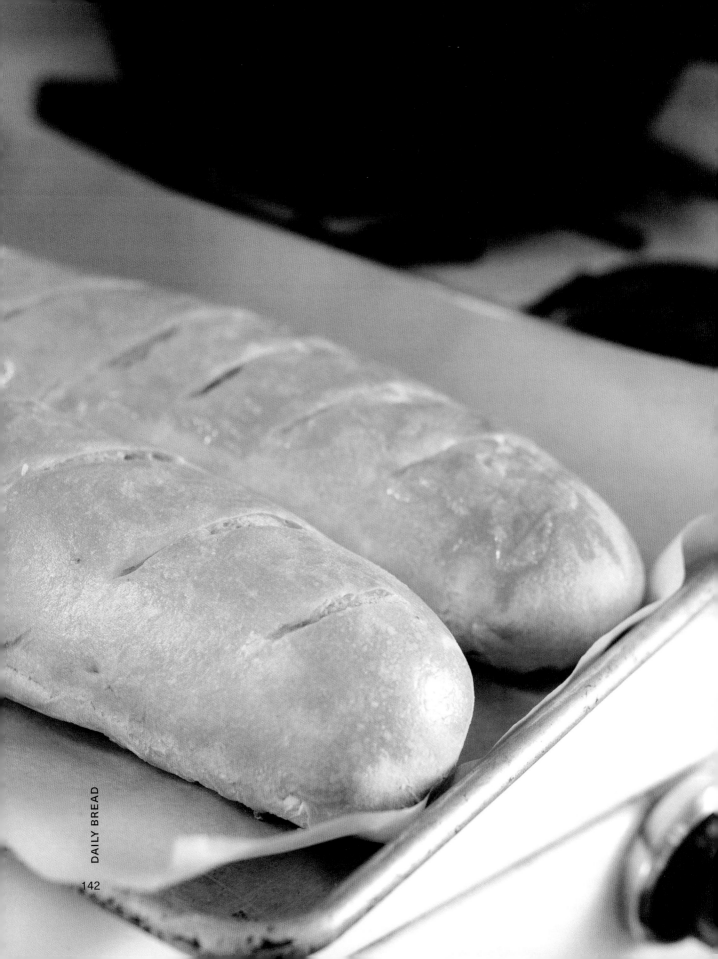

PREP TIME:
15 MINUTES

BAKE TIME:
25 MINUTES

RISE TIME:
11 TO 12 HOURS

YIELD:
MAKES 2 LOAVES

Sourdough French Bread

Every kitchen needs a few stalwart recipes—the workhorses that you make again and again. This sourdough French bread is one of ours. It's a simple, basic, no-frills recipe that I find myself returning to in a million different ways. It makes an excellent table bread and is good for sandwiches. You can also turn it into the most beautiful French Toast Casserole (page 324). Additionally, it's the perfect vehicle for garlic, butter, and cheese. You'll make amazing garlic bread with this as a base.

4 cups (560 grams) all-purpose flour

1 1/4 cups (295 grams) warm water

1 cup (200 grams) active sourdough starter

2 tablespoons (28 grams) olive oil, plus more for the bowl

1 tablespoon (21 grams) honey

2 teaspoons (12 grams) salt

1   In the bowl of a stand mixer equipped with a dough hook, combine the flour, water, starter, olive oil, honey, and salt. Mix on low speed for 8 to 10 minutes, or until the dough turns stretchy and pulls away from the sides of the bowl cleanly.

2   Drizzle a little oil into the bottom of a large mixing bowl, and then transfer the dough from the mixer to your prepared bowl. Cover tightly, then let it rise until doubled or about 8 hours.

3   The next day, punch down the dough and divide it into two equal parts using a bench scraper. Working with half of the dough at a time, shape it by rolling it into a rectangle 1/4 to 1/2 inch thick. Roll it up from the long edge and then pinch the seam closed.

4   Place the loaves onto a parchment-lined baking sheet, then cover them with a tea towel. Allow the dough to rise until doubled, 3 to 4 hours.

5   Preheat the oven to 400°F.

6   Just before baking, score the bread diagonally across by slashing it at a 45° angle. Bake for 25 minutes, or until golden brown and allow to cool completely before slicing.

PREP TIME:
20 MINUTES

BAKE TIME:
45 MINUTES

RISE TIME:
12 TO 14 HOURS

YIELD:
MAKES 2 LOAVES

Basic Sandwich Bread

I will always love those open, airy loaves of artisan sourdough bread. I adore the decorative scoring, the light crumb that soaks up butter, and the crisp, crackling crust. They're a favorite, but sometimes you need something simpler. That's where this sandwich bread hits the mark. It has a tight crumb and a soft, golden-brown crust. Toast it in the morning and slather it with butter and jam. You can also make sandwiches to pack in lunch boxes and picnic baskets.

Keep an eye on your bread. Don't let it overproof, or you'll end up with a wet, sloppy mess.

FOR THE BREAD

8 cups (1,120 grams) all-purpose flour

2 1/2 cups (590 grams) warm water

1 cup (200 grams) active sourdough starter

1/2 cup (113 grams) butter, at room temperature, cut into small pieces, plus more for the pans

2 tablespoons (42 grams) honey

1 tablespoon (18 grams) salt

Oil, for mixing bowl

FOR THE EGG WASH

1 egg yolk

1 tablespoon (15 grams) water

1   **To make the bread:** In the bowl of a stand mixer equipped with a dough hook, combine the flour, water, starter, butter, honey, and salt. Mix on low and allow for 8 to 10 minutes, or until the dough turns stretchy and pulls away from the sides of the bowl cleanly. When the dough is ready, it should pass the windowpane test (see page 13).

2   Drizzle a little oil into the bottom of a large mixing bowl, and then transfer the dough from the mixer to your prepared bowl. Cover tightly, then let it rise in a warm spot in your kitchen until doubled, about 10 hours.

3   Line two loaf pans with parchment paper or grease them with butter. Then, dust your working surface lightly with flour.

4   Tip the dough onto your working surface, then divide it into two equal parts using your bench scraper. Working with one batch of dough at a time, shape it into a rectangle about 1/2 inch thick. Starting at the short end, roll the dough up and then place it in the prepared loaf pan.

5   Cover the dough with a tea towel, then let it rise until it peeks out above the pan and has doubled in volume, anywhere from 2 to 4 hours.

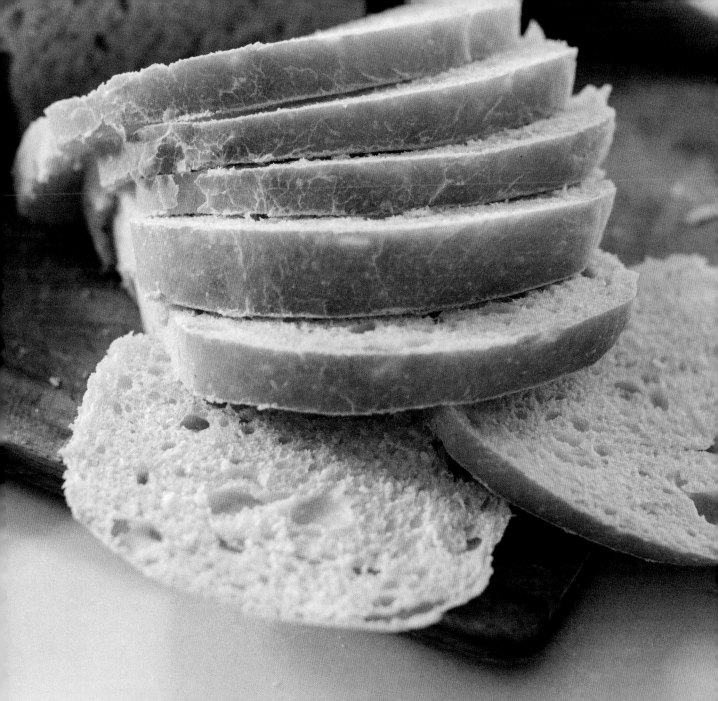

6 About 25 minutes before the bread is ready to bake, preheat the oven to 375°F.

7 **To make the egg wash:** In a small bowl, beat together the egg yolk with the water.

8 Brush the tops of the loaves lightly with egg wash, then transfer them to the oven and bake for 45 minutes, or until the bread is golden brown. Allow the bread to cool in the pans for 10 minutes and then tip the loaves out onto a wire rack to cool completely before slicing. I store leftover slices in a ziplock bag on the counter so it doesn't dry out. You can also throw it in the fridge or freezer for longer storage.

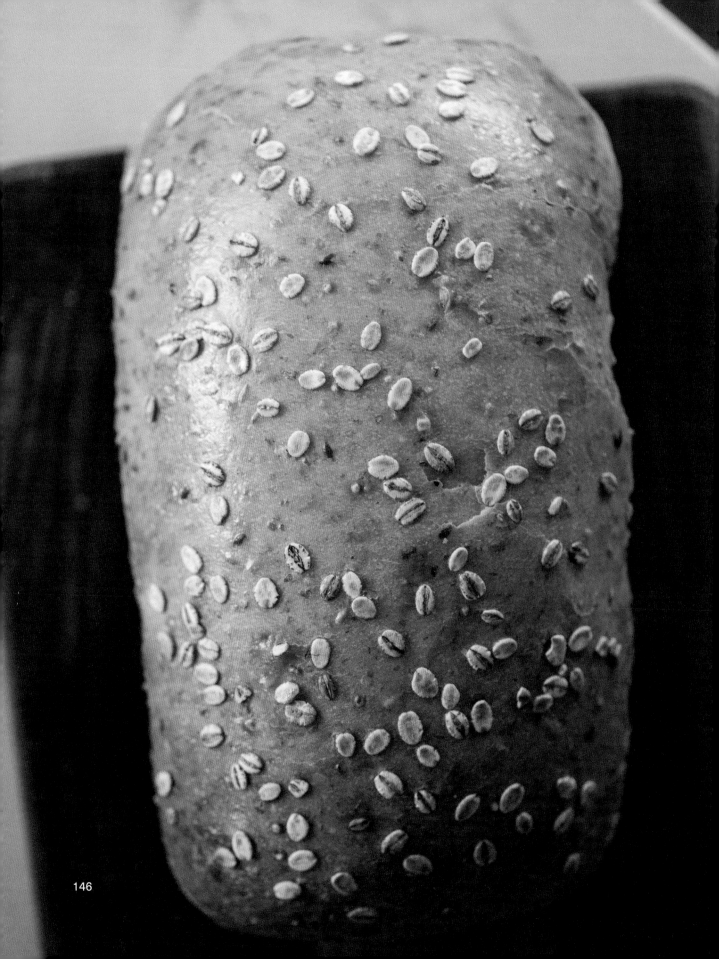

PREP TIME:
20 MINUTES

BAKE TIME:
45 MINUTES

RISE TIME:
6 TO 12 HOURS

YIELD:
MAKES 1 LOAF

Soft Multigrain Bread

Multigrain cereal gives this soft sandwich bread a pleasant, chewy texture and a beautiful flavor with notes of malt. Honey lends a delicate sweetness to the bread. Although it contains plenty of whole grains, you'll find it still has the soft texture of a classic sandwich bread.

Look for a plain cereal (here, cereal means a mix of grains) containing flaked barley, oats, rye, and other grains, but avoid those with added sugar or dried fruit. If you can't find a multigrain cereal mix, you can also use old-fashioned rolled oats in this recipe, too. To prepare the cereal for baking, you must soften it with hot water, ensuring it cools completely before mixing the dough. Hot temperatures can compromise the starter cultures, affecting the bread's rise.

FOR THE BREAD

3 tablespoons (42 grams) butter, plus more for the pan

1/2 cup (40 grams) multigrain cereal

1 1/2 cups (354 grams) boiling water

3 1/2 (490 grams) cups all-purpose flour

1 cup (200 grams) active sourdough starter

3 tablespoons (63 grams) honey

1 1/2 teaspoon (9 grams) salt

FOR THE EGG WASH

1 egg yolk

1 tablespoon (15 grams) water

1 **To make the bread:** In a small saucepan, melt the butter, then set it aside and allow it to cool to room temperature.

2 In the bowl of a stand mixer equipped with a dough hook, place the multigrain cereal. Add the water and let the mixture cool for about 1 hour, or until it reaches room temperature.

3 Add the melted butter, flour, sourdough starter, honey, and salt to the mixer. Mix on low speed for 10 to 12 minutes, or until it pulls away from the sides of the bowl, becoming smooth and glossy.

4 Cover the bowl and let it rise for 10 to 12 hours, or until doubled.

5 Butter a 9-by-5-inch loaf pan or line it with parchment paper.

(recipe continued on next page)

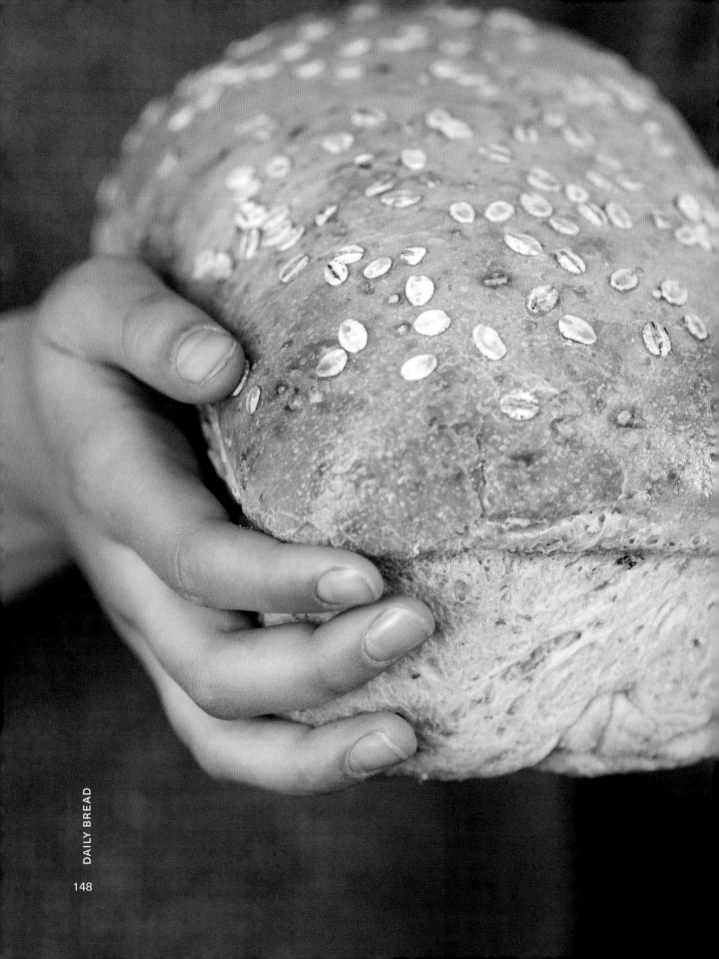

6   Shape the dough by rolling it flat into a rectangle, then roll it up from the short end into a log. Place the dough in the prepared loaf pan. Cover the dough with a towel or plastic wrap and let it rise for 2 to 4 hours at room temperature, or until doubled.

7   Preheat the oven to 375°F.

8   **To make the egg wash:** In a small bowl, beat the egg yolk with the water.

9   Brush the tops of the loaves lightly with egg wash. Transfer them to the oven and bake for 45 minutes, or until the bread is golden brown. Allow the bread to cool in the pan for 10 minutes. Then, tip the loaves out of their pans and let them cool on a wire rack completely before slicing.

PREP TIME:
30 MINUTES

BAKE TIME:
25 MINUTES

RISE TIME:
12 TO 16 HOURS, PLUS OVERNIGHT CHILL

YIELD:
MAKES 2 LOAVES

Sourdough Brioche

Brioche is a French-style of bread that's delightfully soft and airy. The kids love it for its delicate texture and rich flavor, and I find myself making it time and time again. Sometimes, I'll work a few tablespoons of chopped fresh rosemary into the dough. It gives it a woodsy aroma that reminds me of Christmas. Leftovers make the most delicious bread pudding, too.

Like most fortified breads, brioche gets its tender crumb and rich flavor from plenty of butter, eggs, and milk. They work together to enrich the dough, lending a decadent quality to the bread. However, they can make the bulk fermentation take a little longer. Using bread flour in combination with all-purpose helps strengthen the dough.

This recipe produces a wet dough that seems as though it couldn't possibly come together. Then, as if by magic, the dough turns smooth and glossy. If you find yourself tempted to add more flour, resist the urge. Instead, give the ingredients a little more time in the mixer.

FOR THE BREAD

1 cup (200 grams) active sourdough starter

1/2 cup (122 grams) milk

3 cups (420 grams) bread flour

1/2 cup (70 grams) all-purpose flour

1 cup (226 grams) butter, at room temperature, plus more for the pans

1/4 cup (48 grams) sugar

4 eggs

1 1/2 teaspoons (9 grams) salt

FOR THE EGG WASH

1 egg yolk

1 tablespoon (15 grams) water

1 **To make the bread:** In the bowl of a stand mixer equipped with a dough hook, combine the sourdough starter, milk, bread flour, all-purpose flour, butter, sugar, eggs, and salt. Knead for about 15 minutes on low speed, or until the dough pulls away from the sides of the bowl and turns smooth and glossy.

2 Cover the bowl tightly and place it in a warm spot for 6 to 8 hours, or until doubled. Transfer to the fridge, and let it chill overnight.

3 The next day, lightly flour your working surface. Then, butter two loaf pans or line them with parchment paper.

4 Tip the dough onto your working surface, then divide it into sixteen equal portions.

5 Working one at a time, roll the individual pieces of dough into balls and then place eight balls into each loaf pan. Cover and allow to rise for 6 to 8 hours, or until doubled.

6 Preheat the oven to 425°F.

7 **To make the egg wash:** In a small bowl, beat the egg yolk with the water and then brush it over the loaves of bread.

8 Bake for 25 minutes, or until the brioche starts to turn golden. Let the bread cool in its pan for 5 minutes, then turn it onto a wire rack to finish cooling before slicing.

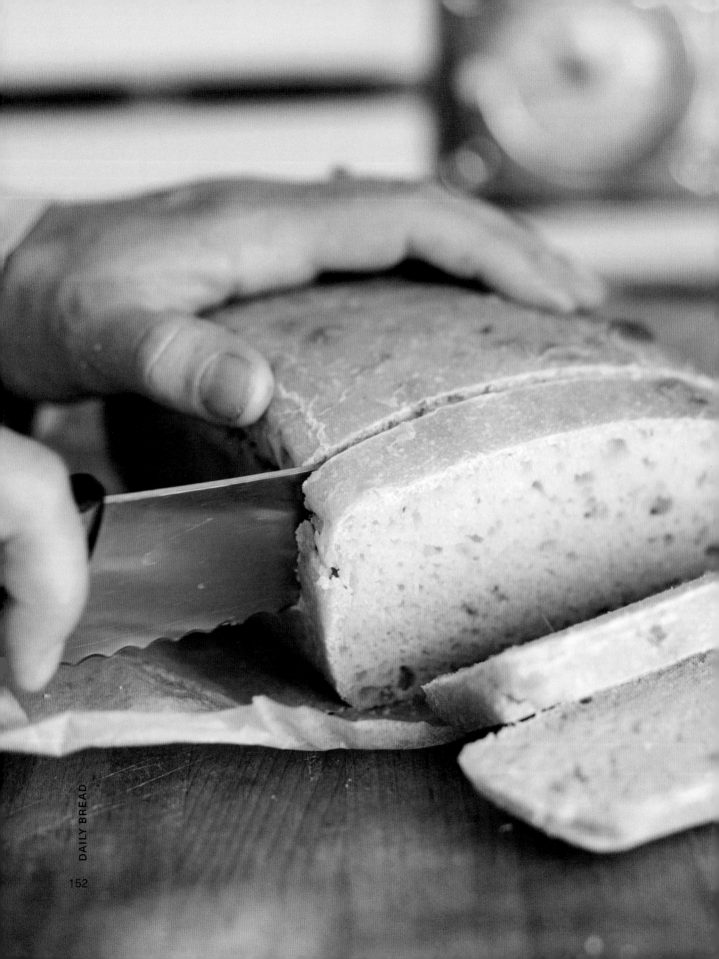

PREP TIME:
20 MINUTES

BAKE TIME:
45 MINUTES

RISE TIME:
10 TO 12 HOURS

YIELD:
MAKES 2 LOAVES

Rosemary-Garlic Potato Bread

If you're ever stuck with leftover mashed potatoes, make this bread. The potatoes give it a delicious sweetness and their starch content makes the loaves utterly tender and fluffy. They also provide a good boost of nutrition, adding more fiber, potassium, and B6. If you don't have leftover mashed potatoes, peel, boil, and mash a medium Russet potato and add it to the dough.

1 cup (210 grams) mashed potatoes

8 medium garlic cloves, finely chopped

1 tablespoon finely chopped fresh rosemary

1 cup (200 grams) active sourdough starter

2 cups (488 grams) milk

1/4 cup (57 grams) butter, at room temperature, plus more for the pans

5 1/2 cups (770 grams) all-purpose flour

1/4 cup (48 grams) sugar

2 teaspoons (12 grams) salt

1   In a small bowl, stir together the mashed potatoes, garlic, and rosemary until well incorporated.

2   In a stand mixer equipped with a dough hook, combine the mashed potato mixture with the milk, butter, flour, sugar, and salt. Knead the dough on low speed for 10 to 15 minutes, until it becomes smooth and elastic and pulls away from the sides of the bowl.

3   Transfer the dough to a greased bowl, covering it tightly. Allow the dough to rise in a warm spot in your kitchen for about 8 hours, or until it doubles.

4   After the bulk rise, divide the dough into two equal-sized portions and shape each into a ball.

5   Grease two loaf pans or line them with parchment paper and place the shaped dough into the pans. Cover the pans tightly and let the dough rise again for 2 to 4 hours, or until it doubles in size.

6   Preheat the oven to 350°F.

7   Bake the loaves for 45 minutes, or until the crust is golden brown. Let the bread cool in its pan for 5 minutes, then turn it onto a wire rack to cool before slicing.

PREP TIME:
15 MINUTES

BAKE TIME:
35 MINUTES

RISE TIME:
10 TO 12 HOURS

YIELD:
MAKES 2 LOAVES

Cinnamon-Raisin Bread

This sweet bread is brimming with cinnamon-dusted raisins—so many that the dough can hardly contain them all. We like to slice it thickly and toast it before slathering it with heaps of rich, golden butter. It's a treat just as much as it's bread. You start the process the night before you plan to bake. The starter does its work as you sleep, leavening the dough. In the morning, you shape it and let it rise. By late afternoon, it's ready to bake.

1 cup (200 grams) active sourdough starter

1 1/2 cups (354 grams) room-temperature water

1/2 cup (113 grams) melted coconut oil, plus more for the bowl

1/2 cup (168 grams) honey

6 cups (840 grams) all-purpose flour

1 tablespoon (18 grams) salt

2 cups (340 grams) raisins

1 cup (236 grams) hot water

1/2 cup (100 grams) brown sugar

3 tablespoons (24 grams) cinnamon

1 In the bowl of a stand mixer equipped with a dough hook, combine the starter, room-temperature water, coconut oil, and honey. Add the flour and salt and mix the dough on low speed for 10 to 15 minutes, or until stretchy and pliable.

2 Lightly grease two mixing bowls with coconut oil. Then, divide the dough into two equal portions. Place each in a prepared bowl. Cover the bowls tightly and let the bread rise overnight, about 8 hours.

3 In a medium mixing bowl, add the raisins and cover them with hot water. Place a lid on the bowl or cover it with a tea towel to keep out debris and let them soak overnight.

4 The next day, lightly dust your working surface with flour. Working with one portion of dough at a time, tip your dough out onto the prepared working surface. Gently press it down with your fingertips and then roll it into a large rectangle about 1/2 inch thick.

5 Drain the raisins, discarding their soaking liquid, and return them to their bowl. Stir in the brown sugar and cinnamon until the raisins are lightly coated.

6 Sprinkle the raisin mixture evenly over the two portions of rolled dough. Then, starting from the short side, roll the dough up tightly, pinching it closed at the ends. Place the dough into loaf pans and cover them lightly with a tea towel. Allow them to rise for 2 to 4 hours, or until doubled in size.

7 Preheat the oven to 400°F.

8 When the oven comes to temperature, bake the bread for about 35 minutes, or until browned on top. Allow the bread to cool for 5 minutes in its pans, and then transfer it to a wire rack to cool completely before slicing and serving. I store leftover slices in a ziplock bag on the counter so it doesn't dry out. You can also throw it in the fridge or freezer for longer storage.

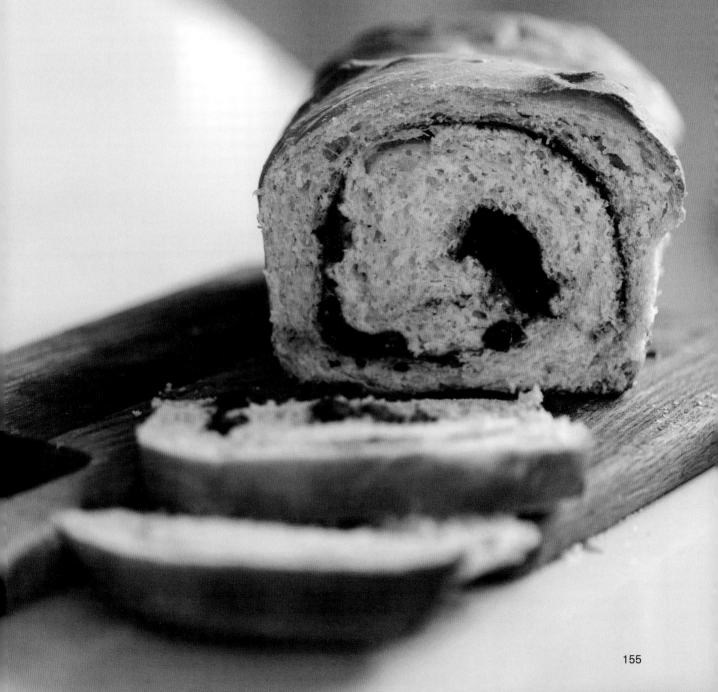

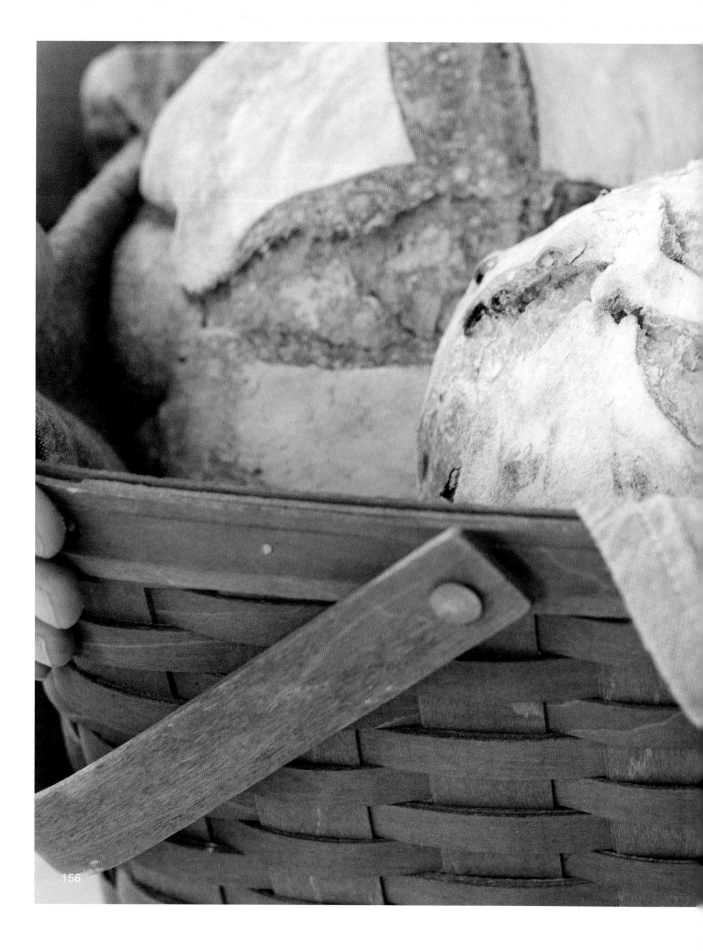

CHAPTER 5

Beyond the Loaf

I LOVE AIRY-CRUMBED, crisp-crusted sourdough boules and buttery loaves of sandwich bread. But it's fun to use sourdough for other types of bread, too. Just about any bread that is leavened with baker's yeast can be made even better with a sourdough starter. Sourdough gives the same breads their rise and loft, but it also yields a beautiful, rich, tangy flavor.

With a little know-how, you can use sourdough to make bagels, dinner rolls, pizza, pretzels, and much more. As with baking artisan-style bread, sourdough versions of specialty breads take more time. So plan ahead. While sourdough is a slow process, its slowness is part of its charm. That's where the magic happens. Long, slow rises mean big flavor and deep satisfaction.

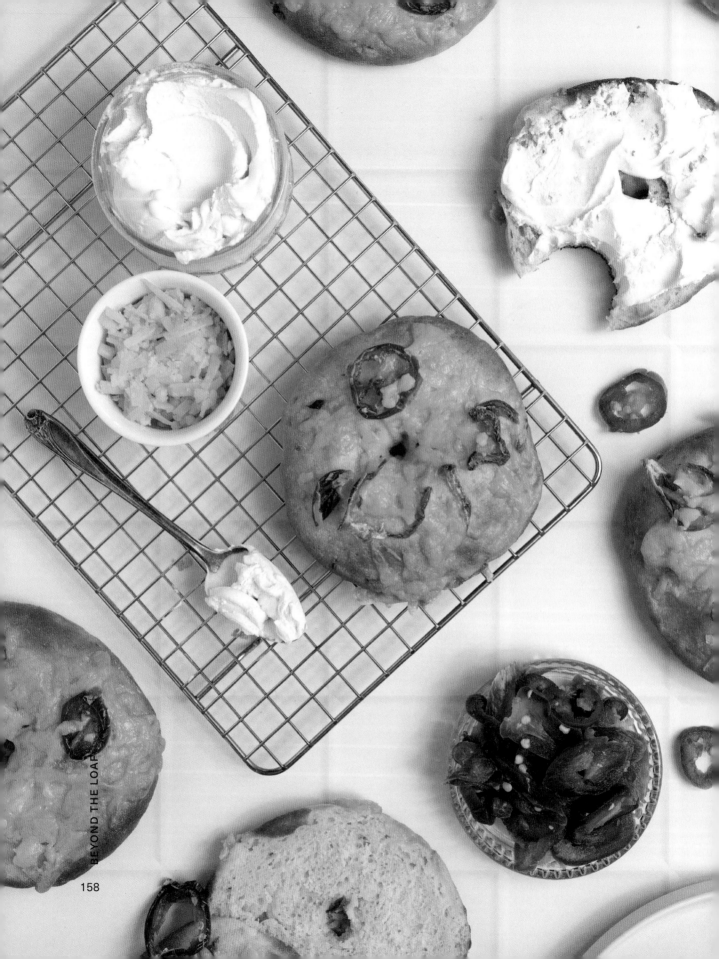

Jalapeño-Cheddar Bagels

Sourdough bagels are a favorite in our house. They're easy to grab on the go. Toast them in the morning for breakfast and schmear them with cream cheese. For lunch, stuff them with fresh veggies and deli meats. While plain bagels get the job done, I find that a little shredded cheddar cheese and some diced jalapeños bring out the flavor. They transform bagels into something special.

I'm partial to pickled jalapeños in this recipe because they add a nice acidity. However, if your garden is brimming with fresh peppers, use those instead. If you're looking for a simpler option, you can make plain bagels by skipping the cheese and jalapeños. They'll still be delicious.

FOR THE DOUGH

1/2 cup (100 grams) active sourdough starter

1 cup (236 grams) water

2 tablespoons (42 grams) honey

2 teaspoons (12 grams) salt

4 cups (560 grams) all-purpose flour, divided

1/2 cup (85 grams) shredded cheddar cheese

1/4 cup diced (64 grams) pickled jalapeños

FOR THE BATH

8 cups (1,888 grams) water

1 tablespoon (14 grams) baking soda

1 tablespoon (12 grams) sugar

FOR TOPPING THE BAGELS

1/2 cup (85 grams) shredded cheddar cheese

1/4 cup (64 grams) thinly sliced pickled jalapeños

1   **To make the dough:** In the bowl of a stand mixer equipped with a dough hook, combine the starter, water, and honey. Add 2 cups (280 grams) of the flour and salt and mix on low speed for about 10 minutes, or until they come together to make a stiff dough. Gradually add the remaining 2 cups (280 grams) of flour, the cheddar, and jalapeños and continue mixing until the dough becomes smooth and pliable.

2   Cover the bowl tightly and allow it to ferment for 8 to 12 hours or until doubled in a warm spot in your kitchen.

3   The next day, divide the dough into eight equal pieces. Roll each piece into a ball, slightly flatten it, and then poke a hole in the middle of the dough with your finger. Stretch the hole a bit to widen it. Place on parchment-lined backing sheet and cover the shaped dough with a tea towel and let it rise in a warm spot for 2 to 4 hours, or until puffy.

(recipe continued on next page)

4   Preheat the oven to 425°F and line a baking sheet with parchment paper.

5   **To make the bath:** In a large pot, bring the water to a boil, then stir in the baking soda and sugar. Using a slotted spoon, gently place the bagels in the boiling water one or two at a time to prevent overcrowding. Boil them for about 1 minute, then flip them and boil them for 1 minute more.

6   **To top the bagels:** Gently lift the bagels out of the pot with a slotted spoon. Shake off any excess water and place them onto your prepared baking sheet. Sprinkle them evenly with extra shredded cheese and jalapeños.

7   Bake for 20 to 25 minutes, or until the bagels are golden brown and the cheese is melted and crisp on top. You can store any remaining bagels in a ziplock bag in the fridge or freezer. I like to pre-slice them before freezing so that it's easy to reheat them by popping them into a toaster on a low setting.

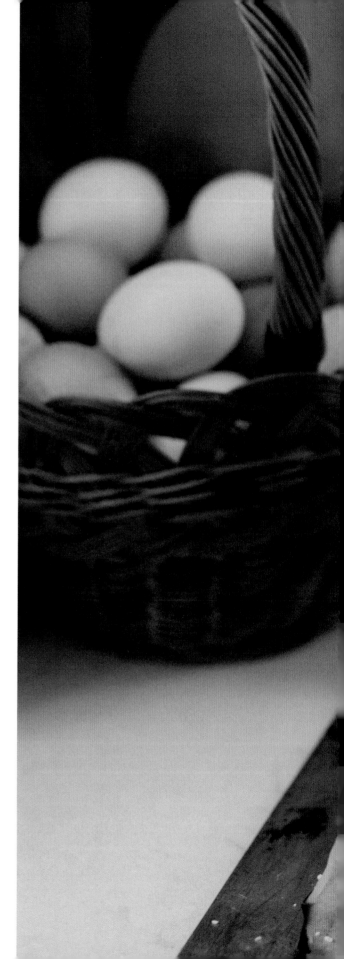

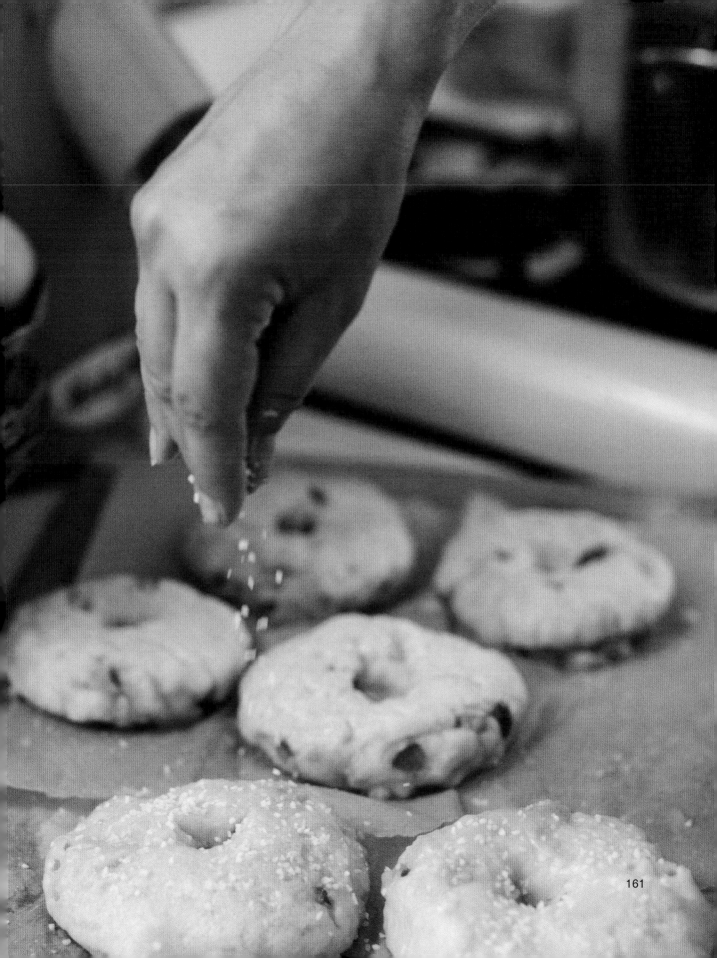

PREP TIME:
20 MINUTES

BAKE TIME:
20 MINUTES

RISE TIME:
10 TO 16 HOURS

YIELD:
MAKES 15 PRETZELS

Soft Sourdough Pretzels

When my kids are looking for a snack, I love to pull out a batch of these soft, chewy pretzels. They're fun to make together—rolling the dough into ropes and twisting them to form the classic pretzel shape. We love to serve them with a coarse, German-style mustard or a cheese sauce. For variety, consider skipping the salt topping. Instead, dust them with grated parmesan cheese, cinnamon and sugar, or even everything-bagel seasoning.

Just before you bake the pretzels, you need to tuck them into an alkaline bath. This technique gives them a beautiful brown color and chewy texture. Traditionally, bakers boil them in lye water. But I've found that a combination of baking soda and brown sugar works just as well, with no need for specialized ingredients.

FOR THE DOUGH

1/2 cup (100 grams) active sourdough starter

1 cup (236 grams) water

2 tablespoons (42 grams) honey

3 cups (420 grams) all-purpose flour

1 1/2 teaspoons (9 grams) salt

FOR THE WATER BATH

9 cups (2,124 grams) water

2 tablespoons (28 grams) baking soda

2 tablespoons (24 grams) brown sugar

FOR THE EGG WASH AND TOPPING

1 egg yolk

1 tablespoon (15 grams) water

1 tablespoon (about 13 grams) coarse sea salt

(recipe continued on next page)

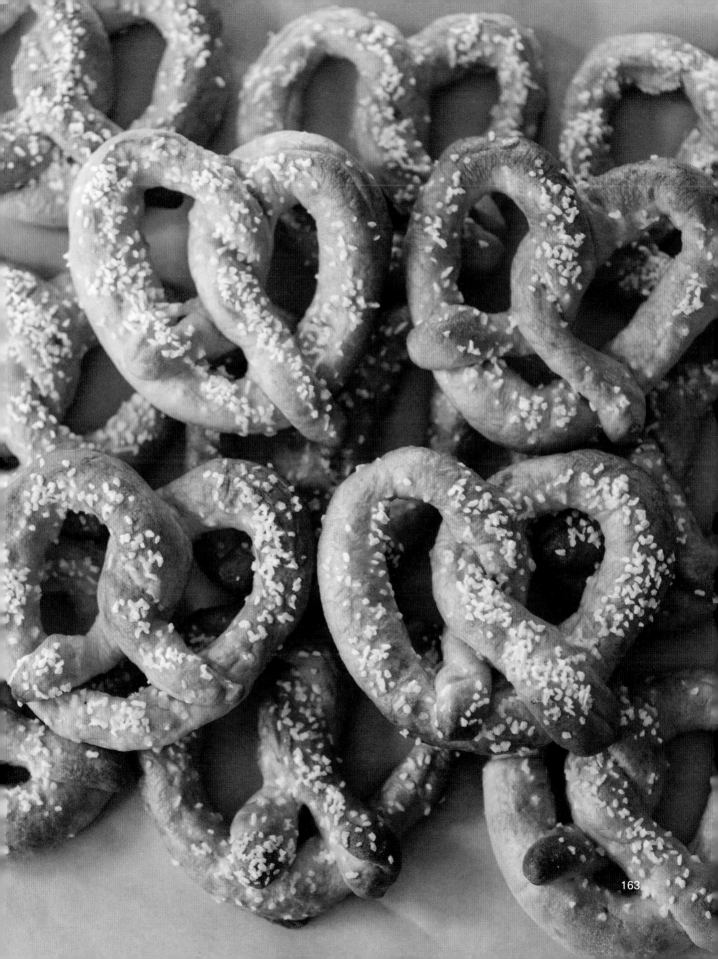

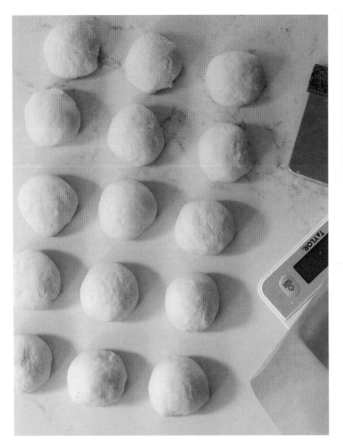

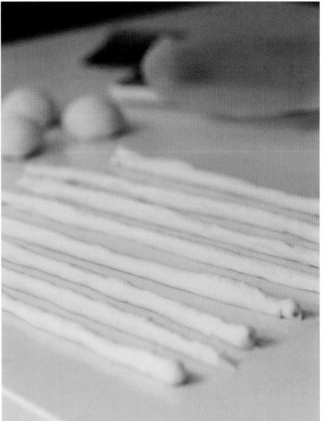

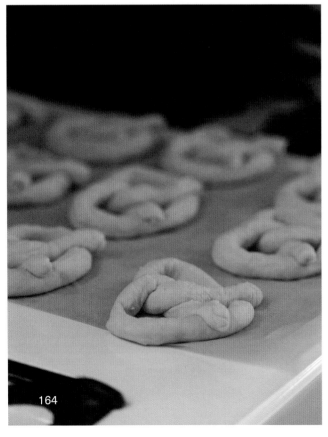

164

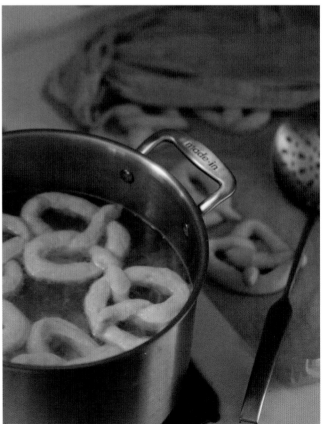

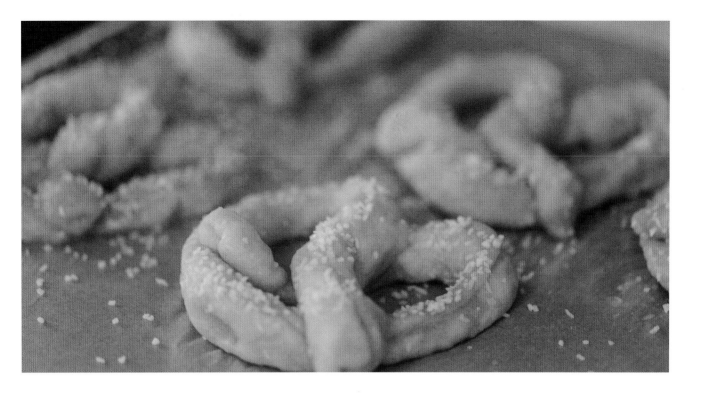

1 **To make the dough:** In the bowl of a stand mixer equipped with a dough hook, combine the starter, water, and honey. Add the flour and salt and mix on the lowest speed for about 10 minutes, or until the ingredients form a smooth, pliable dough that pulls away from the sides of the bowl. Cover the bowl tightly and let the dough rise at room temperature for 8 to 12 hours, or until doubled.

2 The next day, divide the dough into fifteen equal pieces. Roll each piece into an 18-inch rope and curving it into a *U* shape. Twist the ends of the rope around each other twice and press into the bottom of the *U* shape. Cover the shaped dough and allow it to rise for about 2 to 4 hours, or until slightly puffy.

3 Preheat the oven to 425°F and line a baking sheet with parchment paper.

4 **To make the water bath:** In a large stock pot, bring the water, baking soda, and brown sugar to a boil. Working in batches of one or two, boil the pretzels for 30 seconds on each side. Then, gently lift them from the pot with a slotted spoon, shaking off any excess water, and place them on the prepared baking sheet.

5 **To make the egg wash and top the pretzels:** In a small bowl, whisk the egg yolk and water together to form a uniform slurry. Brush each pretzel with egg wash, then sprinkle it with coarse salt.

6 Bake for 15 minutes, or until the pretzels are amber brown. Let them cool for about 10 minutes before serving. Store leftovers in an airtight container at room temperature for up to 3 days.

PREP TIME:
20 MINUTES

BAKE TIME:
25 MINUTES

RISE TIME:
9 TO 10 HOURS

YIELD:
MAKES 8 ROLLS

Basic Dinner Rolls

These fluffy, buttery rolls are delicious with just about any meal. They're perfect for sopping up leftover stew or gravy and help fill out lighter meals such as soups and salads. The trick is to start the rolls the night before, and then they'll be ready for dinner the next day. All that extra time allows the rolls to develop that rich, tangy sourdough flavor.

You can bake these rolls in either a spacious 9-by-13-inch dish, which allows some separation between them. Or bake them in a dish as small as 8 by 8 inches, which knits the rolls more closely together so that you can pull them apart.

FOR THE DOUGH

1/2 cup (100 grams) active sourdough starter

3/4 cup (177 grams) warm water

1/4 cup (57 grams) melted butter, plus more for the bowl and baking dish

2 cups (280 grams) all-purpose flour

1/4 cup (48 grams) sugar

1/2 teaspoon salt

FOR THE EGG WASH

1 egg yolk

1 tablespoon (15 grams) water

1 **To make the dough:** In the bowl of a stand mixer equipped with a dough hook, combine the starter, water, and butter. Add the flour, sugar, and salt and knead the mixture on low speed for 10 to 15 minutes, or until the dough becomes smooth and elastic.

2 Drizzle a little melted butter into a large mixing bowl. Transfer the dough to the prepared bowl and cover it. Allow it to rise overnight, about 8 hours, or until doubled.

3 The next day, lightly butter a 9-by-13-inch or 8-by-8-inch baking dish or line it with parchment paper.

4 Divide the dough into eight equal portions and place them in the prepared pan. Cover with a tea towel and let them rise for about 2 to 4 hours, or until doubled.

5 Preheat the oven to 375°F.

6 **To make the egg wash:** In a small bowl, beat the egg yolk with the water, then brush it lightly over the dough.

7 Transfer the rolls to the oven and bake for 25 to 30 minutes, or until golden brown. Serve immediately with butter.

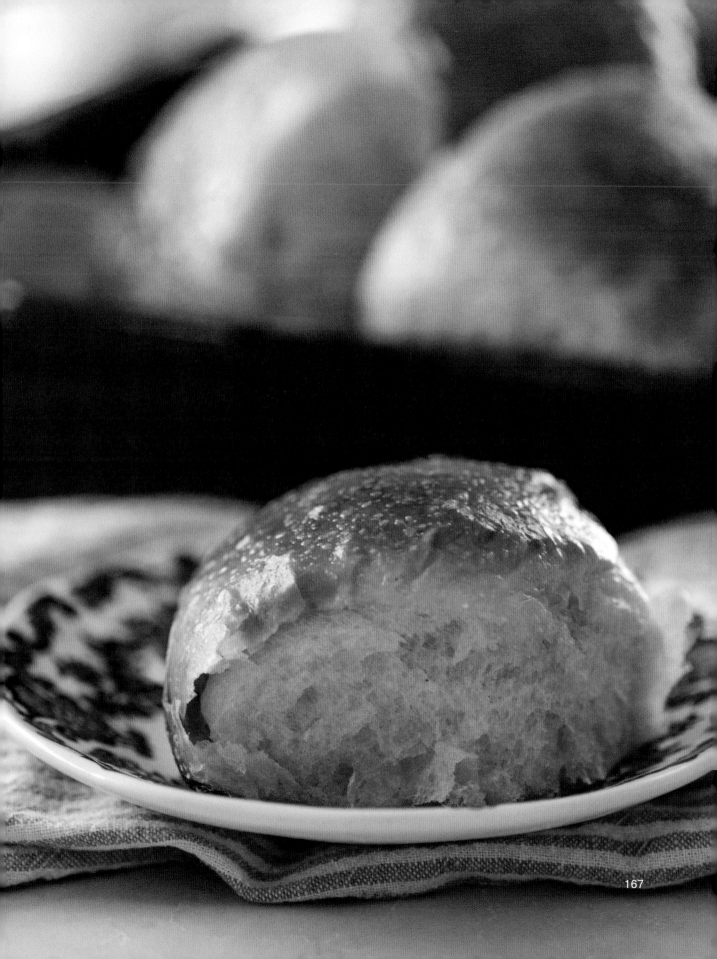

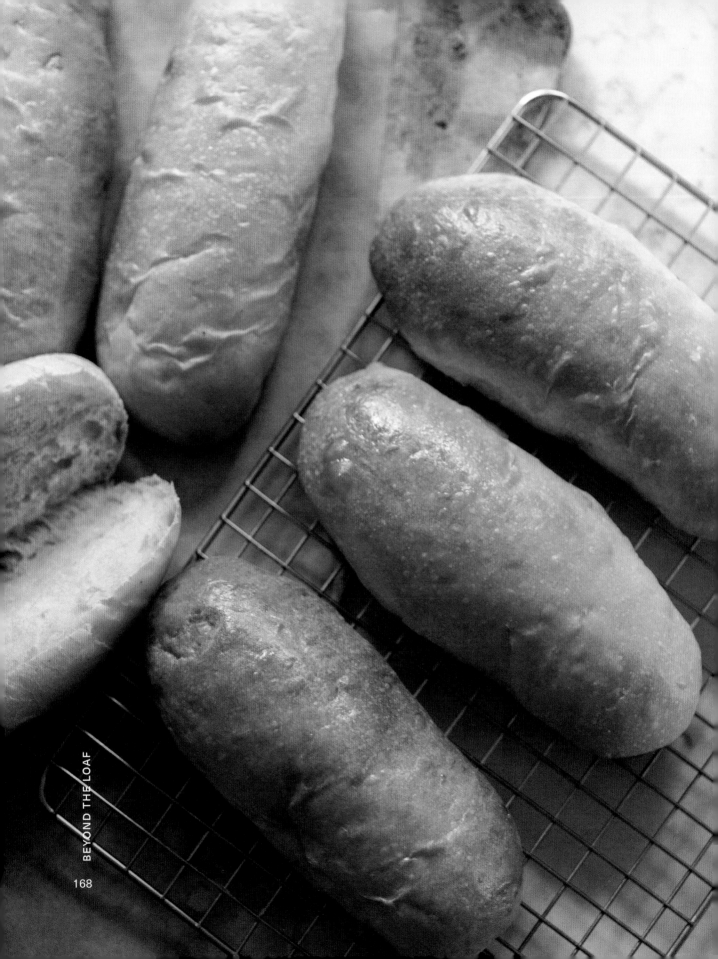

PREP TIME:
15 MINUTES

BAKE TIME:
30 MINUTES

RISE TIME:
10 TO 16 HOURS

YIELD:
**MAKES 8 HAMBURGER BUNS
OR 10 HOT DOG BUNS**

Hamburger and Hot Dog Buns

In the summer, the garden at my farmhouse brims over with fresh vegetables. Heirloom tomatoes tumble from vines. Crisp lettuce grows from dark, rich soil. Cucumbers arrive practically begging for the pickle jar. Celebrating that abundance is part of our family's summer traditions.

One of our favorite ways to celebrate is to host a backyard barbecue. There's something so wholesome and satisfying about grilling up burgers that are truly made from scratch—from the homegrown vegetables to the soft, sesame-topped bun. It'll be the best burger you ever make. Don't worry—if your little ones prefer hot dogs, this same dough works equally well for hot dog buns, too.

FOR THE BUNS

1/2 cup (100 grams) active sourdough
  starter

3/4 cup (177 grams) warm water

1/4 cup (57 grams) melted butter, plus more
  for the bowl

3 tablespoons (63 grams) honey

1 egg

3 cups (420 grams) all-purpose flour

1 teaspoon (6 grams) salt

FOR THE EGG WASH AND TOPPING

1 egg yolk

1 tablespoon (15 grams) water

2 tablespoons (18 grams) sesame seeds,
  optional

(recipe continued on next page)

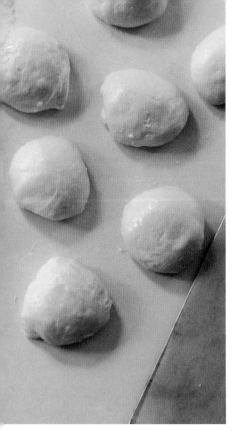
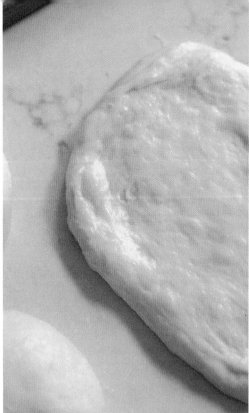
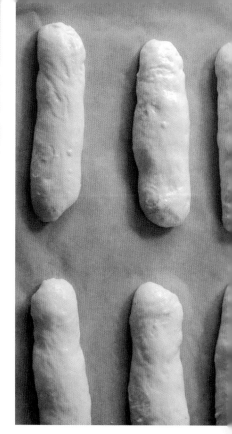

1. **To make the buns:** In the bowl of a stand mixer equipped with a dough hook, combine the starter, water, butter, honey, and egg. Add the flour and salt and knead the mixture on low speed for about 10 minutes, or until the dough becomes smooth and elastic.

2. Tip a little butter into a bowl, then transfer the dough to the prepared bowl. Cover it tightly, and allow it to rest for 8 hours, or until doubled. Then, transfer the bowl to the fridge and let it chill overnight for 8 to 12 hours.

3. The next day, divide the dough into eight equal pieces for hamburger buns and ten equal pieces for hot dog buns.

4. For hamburger buns, form the dough into balls and then press them down to create a flat surface on top, tucking any remaining dough underneath.

5. For hot dog buns, roll the dough out to form a 6-by-4-inch rectangle, then roll them up starting from the long edge.

6. Cover the shaped buns with plastic wrap or a damp tea towel and let them rise 2 to 4 hours or until doubled.

7. Preheat the oven to 350°F.

8. **To make the egg wash and top the buns:** In a small bowl, whisk the egg yolk and water together. Brush the egg wash over the buns and sprinkle them with sesame seeds, if you like.

9. Bake the buns for 25 to 30 minutes, or until golden brown. Allow to cool before serving. Store in a glass container with an airtight lid or a ziplock bag so they don't dry out.

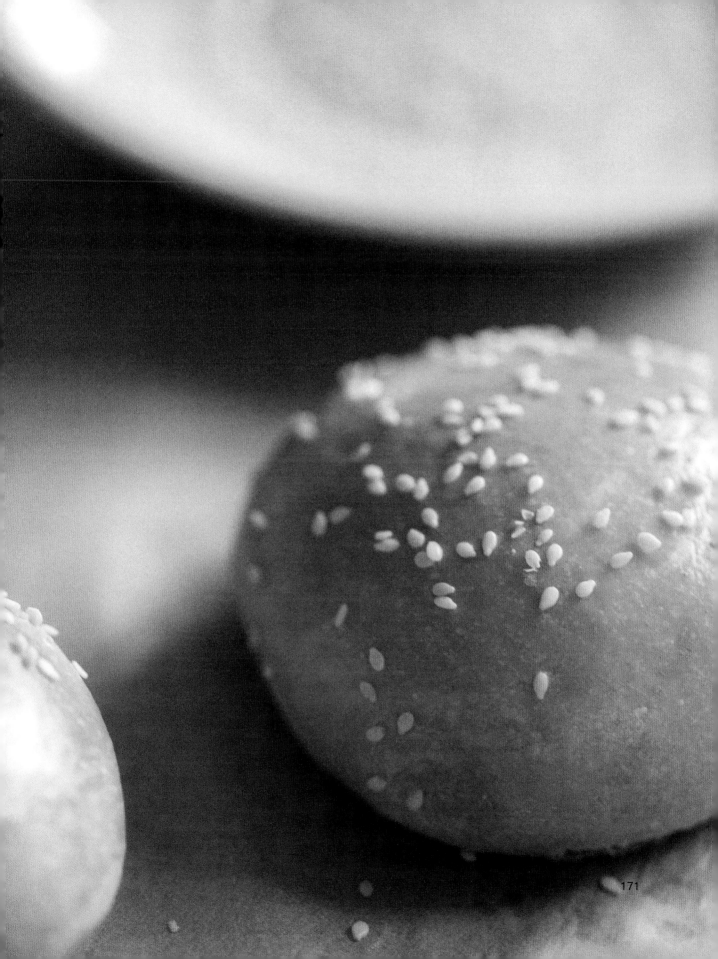

PREP TIME:
20 MINUTES

BAKE TIME:
25 MINUTES

RISE TIME:
10 TO 12 HOURS

YIELD:
MAKES 8 ROLLS

Rosemary-Garlic Dinner Rolls

While a crusty loaf of bread is nice at the dinner table, my family always enjoys a basketful of dinner rolls. They're soft and delicate, infused with fresh rosemary and a touch of garlic. You can easily substitute other herbs, if you prefer. Thyme is delicious, and oregano is lovely, especially if you top the rolls with a dusting of parmesan cheese as they bake.

FOR THE DOUGH

1/2 cup (100 grams) active sourdough starter

3/4 cup (177 grams) warm water

1/4 cup (57 grams) melted butter

2 1/2 cups (350 grams) all-purpose flour

1/4 cup (48 grams) sugar

1/2 teaspoon salt

2 teaspoons finely chopped fresh rosemary

3 medium garlic cloves, finely chopped

Olive oil, for the bowl

FOR THE EGG WASH

1 egg yolk

1 tablespoon (15 grams) water

1 **To make the dough:** In the bowl of a stand mixer equipped with a dough hook, combine the sourdough starter, water, and butter. Add the flour, sugar, salt, rosemary, and garlic and knead on low speed for 10 to 15 minutes, or until the dough turns smooth and pliable.

2 Drizzle a little olive oil in a large mixing bowl, and then scoop the dough into the prepared bowl. Cover the bowl tightly, and let the dough rise overnight, about 8 hours or until doubled.

3 The next day, grease a 9-by-13-inch baking dish. Then, turn the dough out onto a floured surface and divide into eight equal portions with a bench scraper. Form the dough into small, round balls and then place them in the prepared baking dish. Cover the dish with a damp tea towel, and then let the dough rise for 2 to 4 hours, or until doubled.

4 Preheat the oven to 375°F.

5 **To make the egg wash:** In a small bowl, whisk together the egg yolk and water. Gently brush the egg wash over the rolls and then transfer them to the oven and bake for 25 to 30 minutes, or until fragrant and golden brown. Allow them to cool before serving.

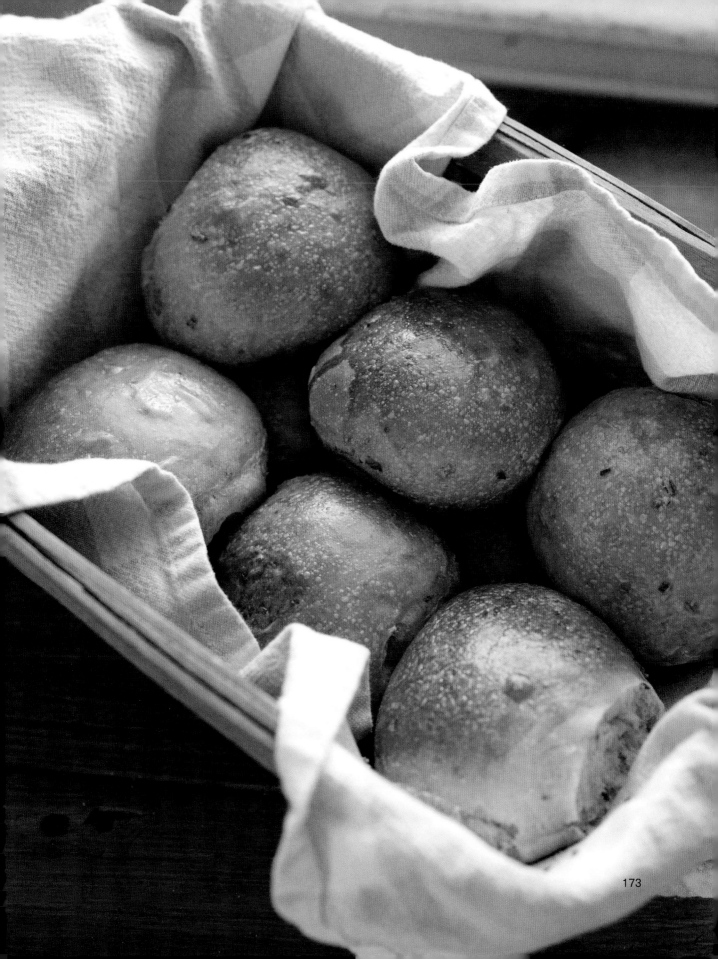

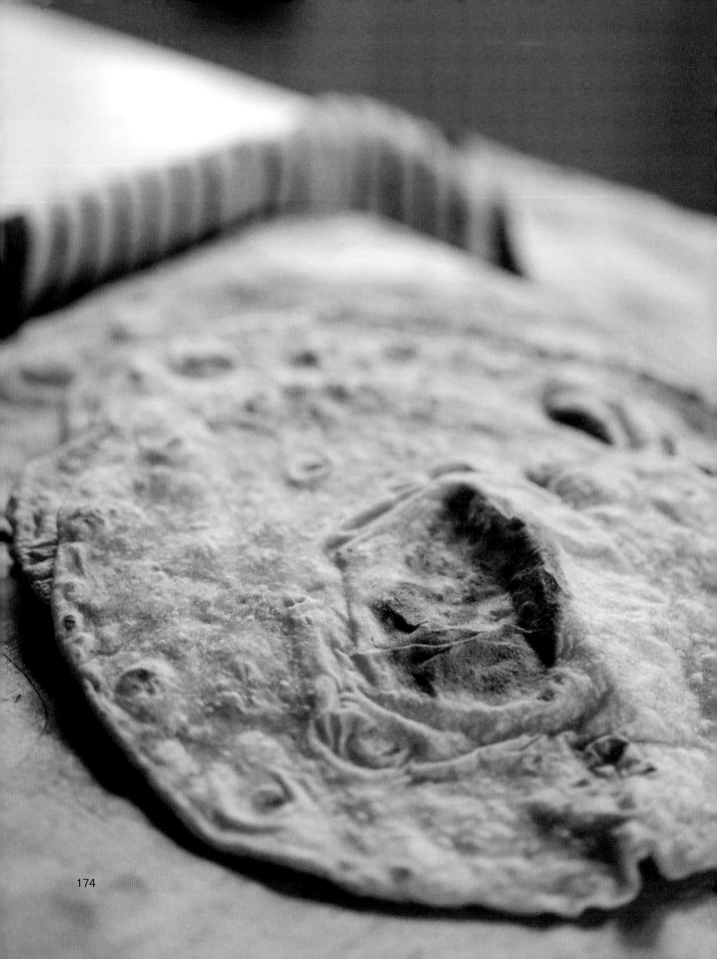

PREP TIME:
10 MINUTES

COOK TIME:
20 MINUTES

RISE TIME:
12 HOURS

YIELD:
**MAKES
12 TORTILLAS**

Tortillas

Tortillas are a lifesaver in our house. You can turn them into easy, well-loved meals. Everyone seems to love breakfast tacos, burritos for lunch, and quesadillas for a snack. With just five basic ingredients (sourdough starter, flour, water, oil, and salt), these tortillas are perfect for a quick summer wrap or your favorite tacos. You can use an active sourdough starter or sourdough discard. Either works!

To make cooking these tortillas fast and easy, I love getting four cast-iron skillets going at one time. And there's no need for a tortilla press. You can easily just roll these out with a rolling pin.

3 cups (420 grams)
  unbleached all-purpose flour

1 cup (200 grams)
  active sourdough starter

3/4 cup (177 grams)
  filtered water

1/4 cup (56 grams)
  extra-virgin olive oil

1 1/2 teaspoons (9 grams) salt

Coconut oil, for cooking

1 In the bowl of a stand mixer equipped with a dough hook, combine the flour, sourdough starter or discard, water, olive oil, and salt. Mix on low speed for about 3 minutes, or until the dough is thoroughly combined and slightly elastic.

2 Drizzle a little olive oil in a large bowl, and then scoop the dough into the prepared bowl. Cover tightly and allow it to sit at room temperature until slightly puffy, about 12 hours.

3 Dust your working surface lightly with flour, and then tip the dough out onto it. Divide it into twelve equal portions and form them into balls. Roll out each ball of dough into an 8-inch circle.

4 Heat a cast-iron skillet over medium heat for about 3 minutes and melt a little coconut oil in the pan. Working one at a time, place a tortilla into the pan and cook for 1 minute on each side. Transfer to a plate and continue cooking all the tortillas.

5 Serve immediately or store them in an airtight container at room temperature for up to 3 days.

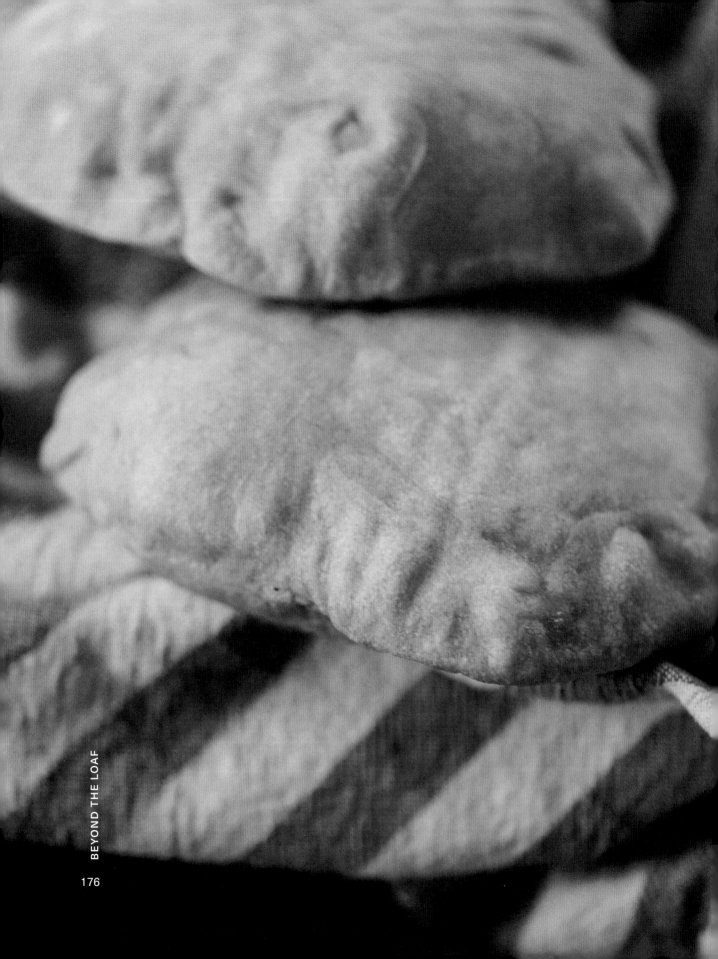

176

PREP TIME:
10 MINUTES

BAKE TIME:
5 MINUTES

RISE TIME:
8 1/2 TO 9 HOURS

YIELD:
MAKES 8 PITAS

Pita Bread

I love making these easy pita breads throughout the year. In the wintertime, we serve them with hearty soups or as a vessel for pocket sandwiches stuffed with all sorts of delicious things. When summer finally peeks its head up, I pack them with ripe tomatoes, leafy greens, cucumbers, and other seasonal vegetables.

You make them the same way you might make tortillas or flatbread—rolling out small portions of dough into circles. With pita, you'll allow them to rise and puff up just a bit. That creates a beautiful pocket of air that expands as the pitas bake, and the result is light and delicious.

1/2 cup (100 grams) active sourdough starter

1 cup (236 grams) water

2 tablespoons (113 grams) olive oil, plus more for the bowl

2 cups (280 grams) all-purpose flour

1/2 cup (70 grams) whole-wheat flour

1 tablespoon (12 grams) sugar

1 teaspoon (6 grams) salt

1. In the bowl of a stand mixer equipped with a dough hook, combine the starter, water, olive oil, all-purpose flour, whole-wheat flour, sugar, and salt. Knead the mixture on low speed for 10 minutes, or until the dough becomes stretchy and smooth.

2. Drizzle a little olive oil into a large mixing bowl, place the dough in it, and cover with a lid or plastic wrap. Allow the dough to rise for 8 hours at room temperature or up to 12 hours in the fridge, or until it doubles in size.

3. Lightly flour your working surface, then divide the dough into eight equal portions. Shape them into small balls, then let them rest for about 15 minutes.

4. Roll each ball into a thin 6-inch circle with a rolling pin, ensuring it is no more than 1/4 inch thick, and then cover them with a damp tea towel. Allow the circles of dough to rise for 30 minutes to 1 hour, or until they become puffy.

5. While the pitas are undergoing their last rise, place a pizza stone in your oven and preheat it to 500ºF.

6. Arrange the dough onto the hot baking surface and bake for approximately 5 minutes, or until the pitas puff up nicely. Transfer them to a wire rack to cool completely before serving. Store any leftovers in an airtight container or a ziplock bag so they don't dry out.

177

PREP TIME:
10 MINUTES

BAKE TIME:
10 MINUTES

RISE TIME:
2 TO 12 HOURS

YIELD:
MAKES ABOUT 8 FLATBREADS

Sourdough Flatbread

In the whirlwind of our bustling homestead, a quick and reliable recipe is a game changer. This sourdough flatbread has become my go-to. It saves the day when time is scarce and your patience wears thin. While other sourdough recipes often demand planning, this flatbread recipe fits seamlessly into the ebb and flow of the day. It's perfect for those chaotic days when you need to fill bellies, but nothing seems to follow a schedule.

You can mix a handful of ingredients together at breakfast time. By lunch, the flatbreads are ready to roll into neat little circles that you toss in a hot pan for a few minutes. Fill them with beans, rice, and cheese for homemade burritos. They're also a delicious way to transform leftovers. I often tuck leftover chicken and roast vegetables into these flatbreads. It's such an easy lunch.

The dough is ready in just a few hours. If the clock insists on ticking faster than anticipated and you find the day has gotten away from you, simply tuck the dough into the fridge overnight. It will rest leisurely in the cold, developing flavor at its own pace. By the next morning, it will still be there, patiently waiting for you.

1 cup (200 grams) active sourdough starter

1/2 cup (122 grams) milk

2 cups (280 grams) all-purpose flour

1 teaspoon (6 grams) salt

Olive oil, for cooking

1   In a large mixing bowl, combine the starter, milk, flour, and salt to form a rough dough. Knead the dough for a few minutes.

2   Cover the dough and allow it to rise for 2 to 4 hours or until puffy. For a longer fermentation, you can transfer the bowl to the fridge and allow it to rise overnight, 8 to 12 hours or until puffy.

3   The next day, lightly dust your working surface with flour. Then, turn the dough out onto it and divide it into eight equal pieces. Roll each piece to about 1/4-inch thickness.

4   Heat a cast-iron skillet over medium heat. Drizzle a little olive oil onto the hot pan, and then, working with one flatbread at a time, drop it into the skillet. Cook the flatbreads on each side for 1 or 2 minutes, or until they puff a bit and begin to brown in spots.

5   Serve warm or store in an airtight container for a few days or up to 1 week.

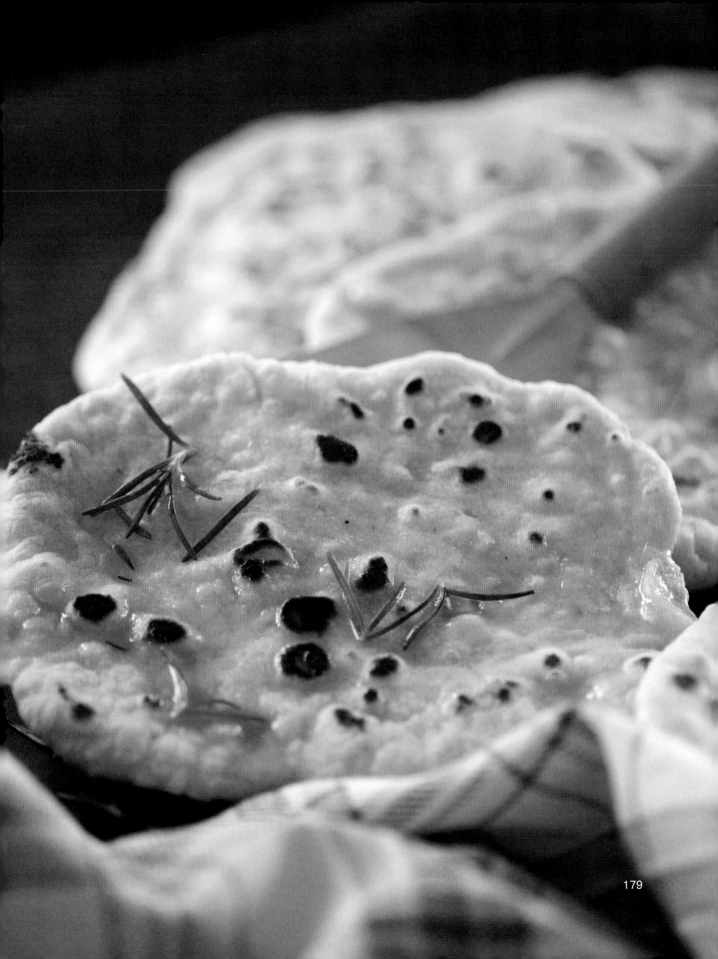

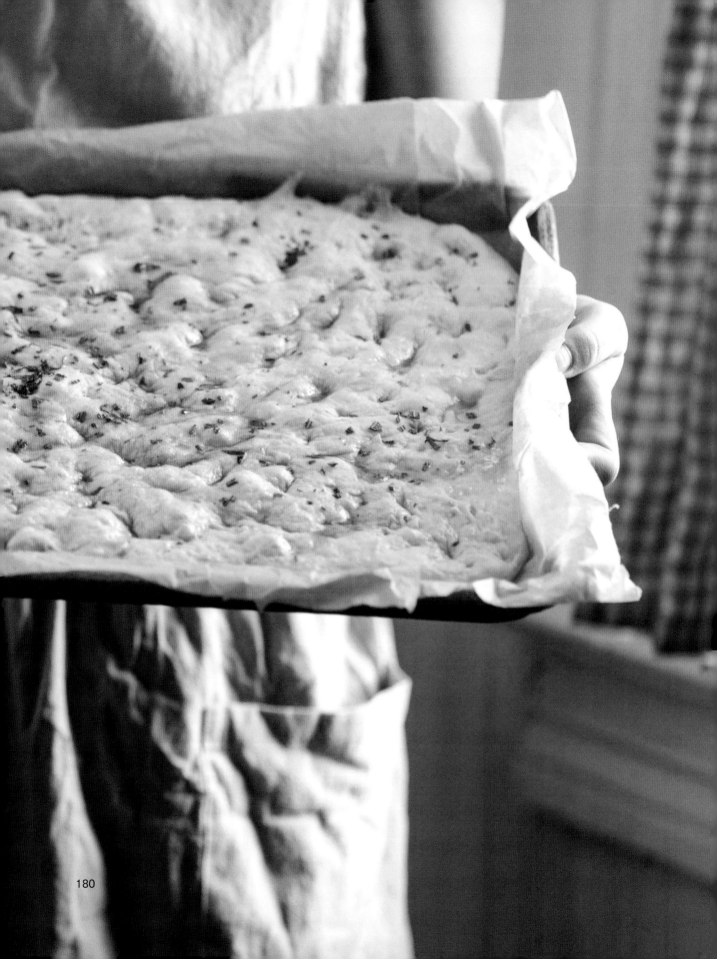

PREP TIME:
20 MINUTES

BAKE TIME:
20 MINUTES

RISE TIME:
10 TO 14 HOURS

YIELD:
SERVES ABOUT 12

Rosemary Focaccia

Fragrant with rosemary and extra-virgin olive oil, this delicious focaccia fills the house with its fantastic aroma as it bakes. I also like its versatility. In the summer months, we'll top it with fresh cherry tomatoes. In autumn and winter, you can top it with delicata squash, garlic, and sage. If you're craving something more robust, top it with mozzarella and sausage. You can also substitute the all-purpose flour with Khorasan wheat flour in the exact same quantity for a richer dough flavor.

1 cup (200 grams) active sourdough starter

1 1/2 cups (354 grams) warm water

1/2 cup (113 grams) extra-virgin olive oil, divided, plus more for the bowl and for drizzing

1 tablespoon (21 grams) honey

2 teaspoons (12 grams) salt

4 cups (560 grams) all-purpose flour

2 sprigs fresh rosemary, chopped

1 teaspoon garlic powder

1 In the bowl of a stand mixer equipped with a dough hook, combine the starter, water, 1/4 cup (57 grams) of the olive oil, the honey, and salt. Gradually add the flour, about 1/2 cup (70 grams) at a time, continuing to mix for about 10 minutes, or until the dough is smooth and elastic and begins pulling away from the sides of the bowl.

2 Drizzle a little olive oil into a large mixing bowl, then scoop the dough into the prepared bowl. Cover the bowl tightly and allow the dough to rise at room temperature for about 8 hours, or until doubled.

3 The next day, line a rimmed baking sheet with parchment paper, then pour the remaining 1/4 cup (57 grams) of olive oil into the bottom.

4 Tip the dough onto the prepared baking sheet, then press it down carefully with your fingertips. Cover the dough, then allow it to rise for 2 to 4 hours, or until puffy.

5 Preheat your oven to 400°F.

6 Drizzle olive oil over the dough and sprinkle it with chopped rosemary and garlic powder. Bake for 20 minutes, or until the bread turns golden brown and the rosemary releases its fragrance. Store in an airtight container or a ziplock bag so it doesn't dry out.

PREP TIME:
20 MINUTES

BAKE TIME:
13 MINUTES

RISE TIME:
8 1/4 HOURS

YIELD:
**MAKES ABOUT
4 MEDIUM PIZZA CRUSTS**

Basic Sourdough Pizza

Pizza is a standby in a house full of hungry children, and our farmhouse is no different. Sure, everyone loves the classic combination of cheese and pepperoni, but sometimes I like to get creative and top our pizzas with pesto cream sauce and walnuts. Another favorite is fig jam with goat cheese, prosciutto, and arugula. I'll even serve pizza for breakfast, topped with tomatoes, cheese, crispy bacon, and eggs.

You can start the dough in the morning, and it will be ready by dinner. Then, add your favorite toppings and bake. A pizza stone helps ensure a beautiful, evenly cooked crust. It's worth the investment. You can also bake the pizzas in a pizza pan or on a baking sheet lined with parchment paper.

1/2 cup (100 grams) active sourdough starter

1 1/2 cups (354 grams) water

2 tablespoons (28 grams) olive oil, plus more for the bowl

4 cups (560 grams) all-purpose flour

2 teaspoons (12 grams) salt

Pizza sauce and toppings of your choice

1. In the bowl of a stand mixer equipped with a dough hook, combine the starter, water, and olive oil. Add the flour and salt and mix the dough on medium speed for about 10 minutes, or until the dough is smooth and elastic.

2. Drizzle a little olive oil into a large mixing bowl. Then, scoop the dough into the oiled bowl and cover it tightly. Allow it to rest at room temperature for about 8 hours, or until doubled.

3. Place a pizza stone in the oven and preheat it to 475°F.

4. Lightly dust your working surface with flour, then gently tip out the dough. Divide it into four equal sections, and let them rest for about 15 minutes.

5. Roll out one portion of dough at a time to about 1/4-inch thickness, creating a slight ridge around its perimeter. Next, spread pizza sauce evenly over the dough and top it with your favorite ingredients.

6. Transfer the pizzas to the hot baking surface and bake them for 13 to 15 minutes, or until the crust is browned and the cheese has melted. Turn the oven to broil, and broil for 3 to 4 minutes more, or until the toppings begin to caramelize. Serve immediately.

7. You can freeze the uncooked dough for up to three months, or store in a Ziplock bag or airtight container for up to a week.

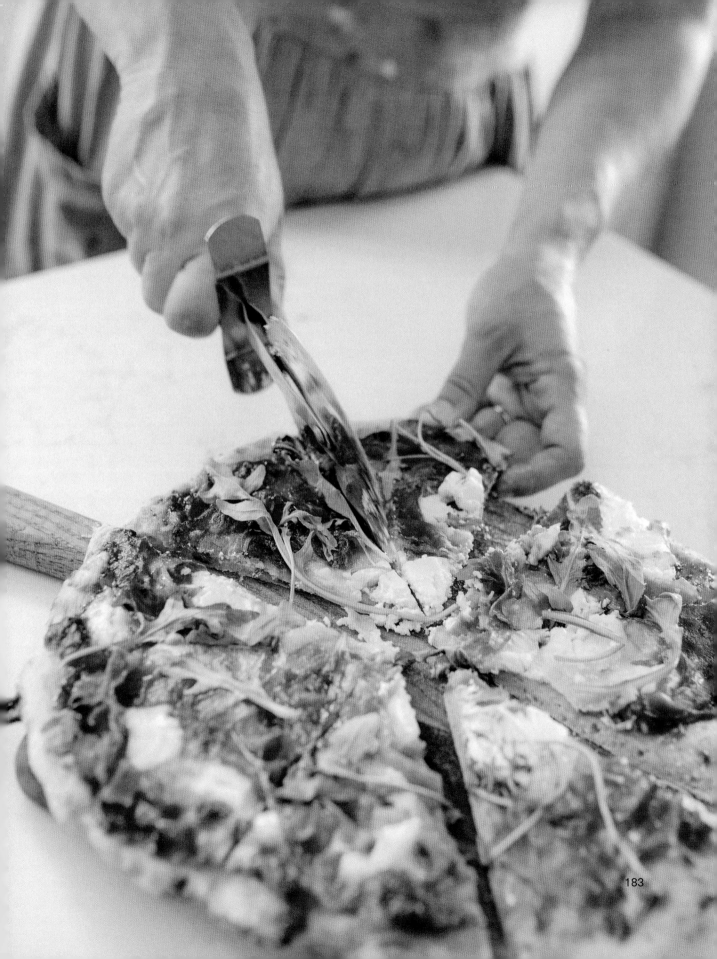

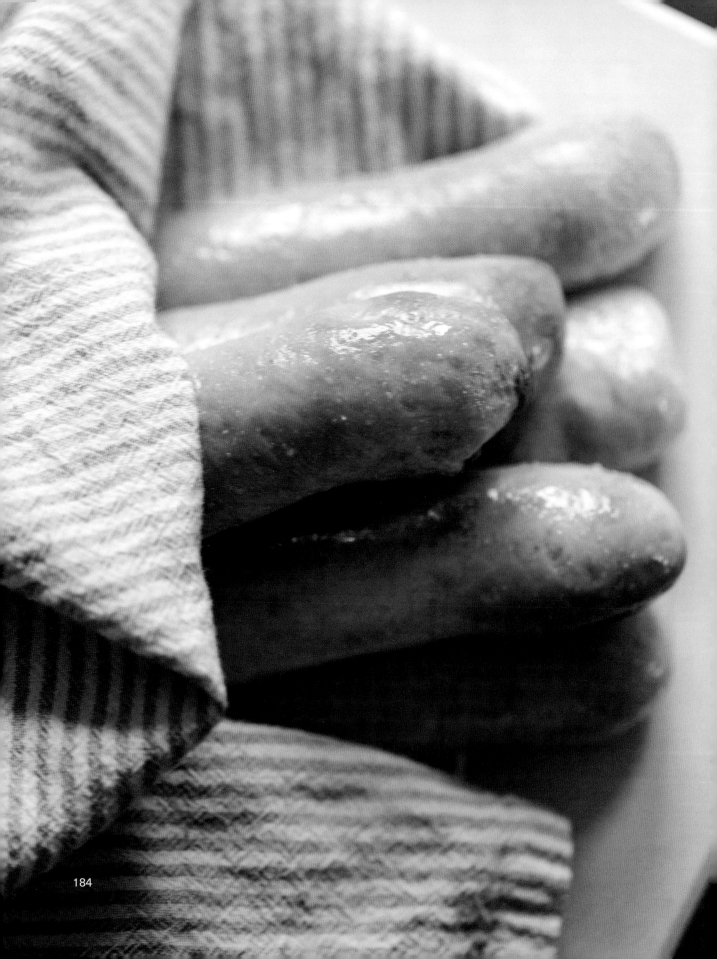

PREP TIME:
20 MINUTES
BAKE TIME:
20 MINUTES
RISE TIME:
9 TO 10 HOURS
YIELD:
MAKES ABOUT 12 BREADSTICKS

Parmesan-Herb Breadsticks

I absolutely adore baking big, lofty loaves of bread for my family, and luckily, they're just as enthusiastic about devouring them. However, there are times when we could all use a little variety—something that's both new and familiar all at once. That's where these buttery, herby breadsticks come into play. They're a tasty riff on the classic, only upgraded with parmesan cheese and garlic.

Since they're individually portioned, they make lunchtime a breeze. You can tuck them neatly into lunch boxes or serve them in a big communal breadbasket for family dinners. They're a natural match for a hearty bowl of pasta Bolognese and equally delicious partnered with a comforting soup brimming with garden vegetables.

FOR THE DOUGH

1/2 cup (100 grams) active sourdough starter

1 cup (236 grams) water

3 tablespoons (42 grams) butter, melted

2 3/4 cups (385 grams) bread flour

1/4 cup (about 25 grams) finely grated parmesan cheese

2 tablespoons (24 grams) sugar

1 1/2 teaspoons (9 grams) salt

FOR THE TOPPING

3 tablespoons (42 grams) butter

1/4 teaspoon salt

1/4 teaspoon garlic powder

1 teaspoon Italian herb blend

(recipe continued on next page)

1. **To make the dough:** In a stand mixer equipped with a dough hook, combine the starter, water, and butter. Add the flour, cheese, sugar, and salt and knead the dough on medium-low speed for about 10 minutes, or until you achieve a soft, smooth dough that is glossy and elastic.

2. Cover the bowl tightly and place it in a warm spot in your kitchen. Let the dough rise for 8 hours, or until it doubles in size.

3. Dust your working surface with flour, and then tip out the dough. Divide it into twelve evenly sized balls using a bench scraper. Roll each piece of dough into a log about 8 inches long.

4. Line a baking sheet with parchment paper. Carefully place the pieces of dough a few inches apart on the prepared sheet. Cover with a towel and allow the breadsticks to rise for 1 to 2 hours, or until they become puffy and double in size.

5. Preheat the oven to 400°F.

6. Transfer the baking sheet to the oven and bake the breadsticks for 20 minutes or until they turn golden brown on top.

7. **To make the topping:** While the breadsticks bake, melt the butter in a small saucepan and stir in the salt and garlic powder.

8. When the breadsticks have finished baking and are still hot, brush them with the butter mixture, then sprinkle them with the herbs. Let them cool before serving. Store in airtight container or a ziplock bag so they don't dry out.

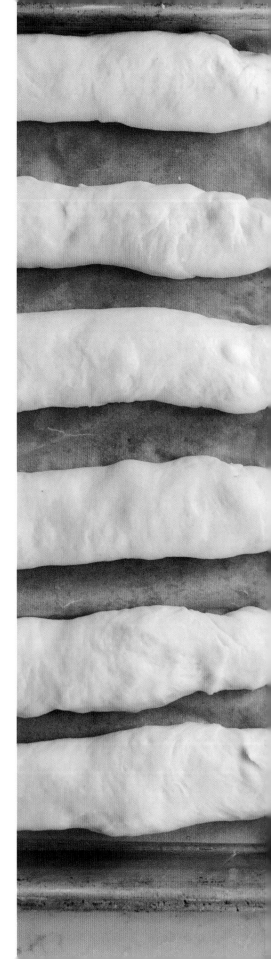

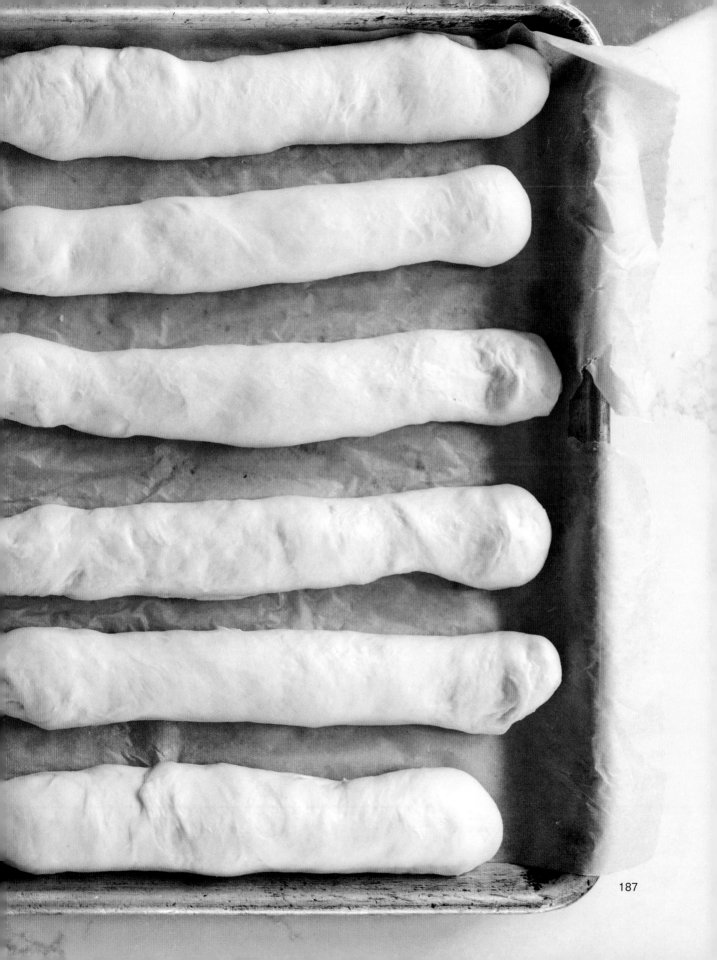

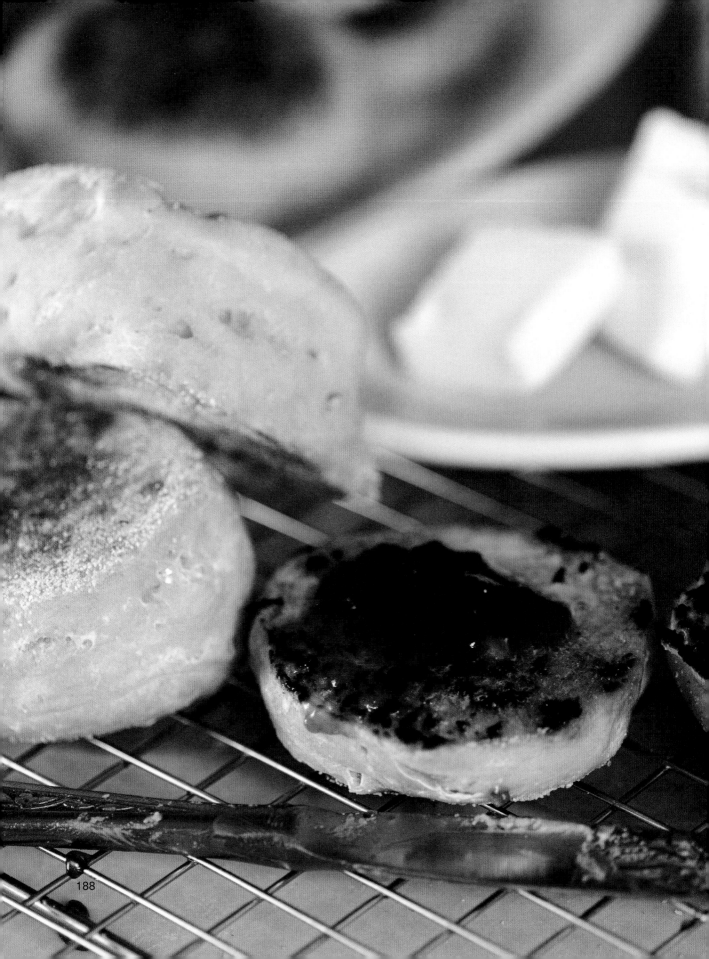

PREP TIME:
15 MINUTES

COOK TIME:
N/A

RISE TIME:
12 TO 24 HOURS

YIELD:
MAKES 12 MUFFINS

English Muffins

These English muffins have earned a permanent spot on our breakfast table. Pop them in the toaster and slather on some butter and jam. Or get creative by turning them into breakfast sandwiches topped with eggs, ham, cheese, and sliced tomatoes or a sprinkle of fresh herbs.

Making these English muffins is a process that requires some time and a touch of patience, but it's absolutely worth it. You can start them the night before, and then finish the batter at breakfast time. If the batter seems a little runny, add a touch more flour. Monitor the temperature carefully as you work to prevent the outside from scorching and to ensure they cook all the way through. My favorite trick is to transfer individual portions of dough one by one to a warm oven as I work. That way, they stay nice and warm and are sure to cook through.

1/2 cup (100 grams) active sourdough starter

1 cup (236 grams) water

2 1/2 cups (600 grams) all-purpose flour

1 tablespoon (21 grams) honey

1 teaspoon (6 grams) salt

1 teaspoon baking soda

Coconut oil, for the skillet

1 In a large glass mixing bowl, combine the starter and water. Add the flour and mix until a rough dough forms. Cover the bowl with a towel and let it sit at room temperature for 12 to 24 hours.

2 Once the dough has risen, beat in the honey, salt, and baking soda until fully incorporated.

3 Line a rimmed baking sheet with parchment paper and place it in the oven, then preheat the oven to 300°F.

4 Heat a cast-iron skillet on high heat. Drop a little coconut oil into the pan and let it melt.

5 Divide the dough into twelve equal parts. Working one at a time, drop each portion into the hot skillet. Turn the heat down to low and let cook for about 10 minutes, or until the dough puffs and doubles in size.

6 Turn the heat up to medium-low and continue cooking 3-5 minutes until the bottoms are slightly browned. Flip once; wait until the muffin releases easily from the pan. Transfer the muffin to the oven and then continue working through the remaining portions of dough.

7 Serve warm. Store any leftovers in an airtight container at room temperature for up to 5 days.

PREP TIME:
15 MINUTES

BAKE TIME:
35 MINUTES

RISE TIME:
9 TO 10 HOURS

YIELD:
MAKES 12 BUNS

Spiced Buns with Raisins

I love to serve these buns on cozy mornings. There's nothing like opening a bun and slathering it with butter, which melts into all the nooks and crannies of the sweet, spiced crumb. Pops of raisins give the buns a sweet edge that's hard to resist, especially if you serve them with a steaming-hot mug of coffee touched with a spoonful of fresh cream.

FOR THE DOUGH

2 cups (280 grams) all-purpose flour

1 1/2 cups (210 grams) bread flour

1/2 cup (96 grams) cup sugar

1 teaspoon (6 grams) salt

1 teaspoon cinnamon

1/2 teaspoon allspice

1/4 teaspoon nutmeg

1 cup (244 grams) milk

1/2 cup (100 grams) active sourdough starter

6 tablespoons (84 grams) butter, at room temperature, plus more for the baking dish

2 teaspoons (10 grams) vanilla extract

1 egg, beaten

2/3 cup (120 grams) raisins

FOR THE EGG WASH

1 egg yolk

1 tablespoon (15 grams) water

1 **To make the dough:** In a large mixing bowl, mix together the all-purpose flour, bread flour, sugar, salt, cinnamon, allspice, and nutmeg. Stir in the milk, starter, butter, vanilla, and egg until well combined. Allow the dough to rest for 10 minutes.

2 Sprinkle the raisins over the dough. Then, reach underneath one side of the dough, gently pull it up, and fold it over the center. Rotate the bowl a quarter turn and repeat the stretch-and-fold process. Repeat twice more until you've gone around the bowl.

3 Cover the bowl and let it rest for 15 minutes. Then, complete two more rounds of stretches and folds. Cover the bowl tightly, and allow the dough to rise for about 8 hours, or until doubled.

4 Lightly dust your working surface with flour, and then divide the dough into twelve equal portions. Shape each portion of dough into a ball, pulling against the work surface to create some surface tension.

5   Rub a little butter inside a 9-by-13-inch baking dish, and then place the buns into the dish. Cover them with a tea towel or a piece of plastic wrap. Allow them to rise at room temperature for about 2 to 4 hours, or until doubled.

6   Preheat the oven to 350ºF.

7   **To make the egg wash:** In a small bowl, whisk together the egg yolk and water. Then, brush it over the buns.

8   Transfer the buns to the oven and bake for about 35 minutes, or until golden brown. Allow them to cool completely before serving. Store in airtight containeror a ziplock bag so they don't dry out.

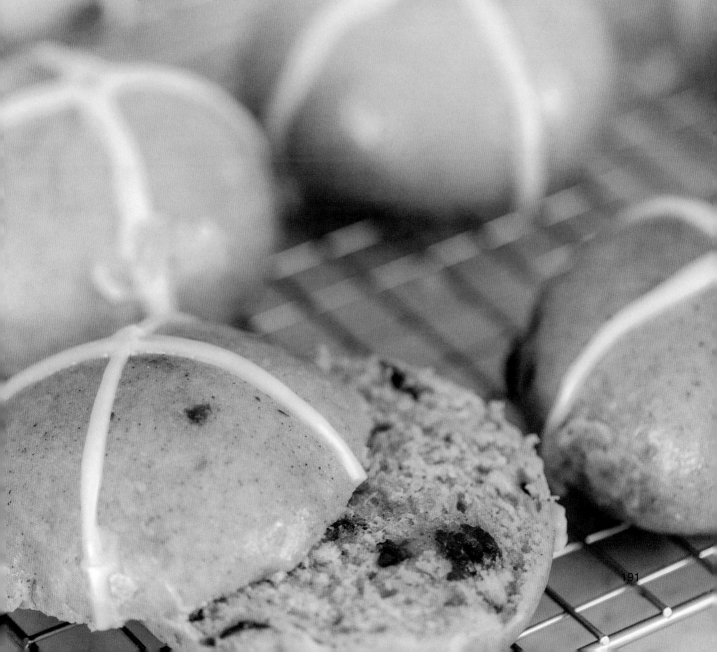

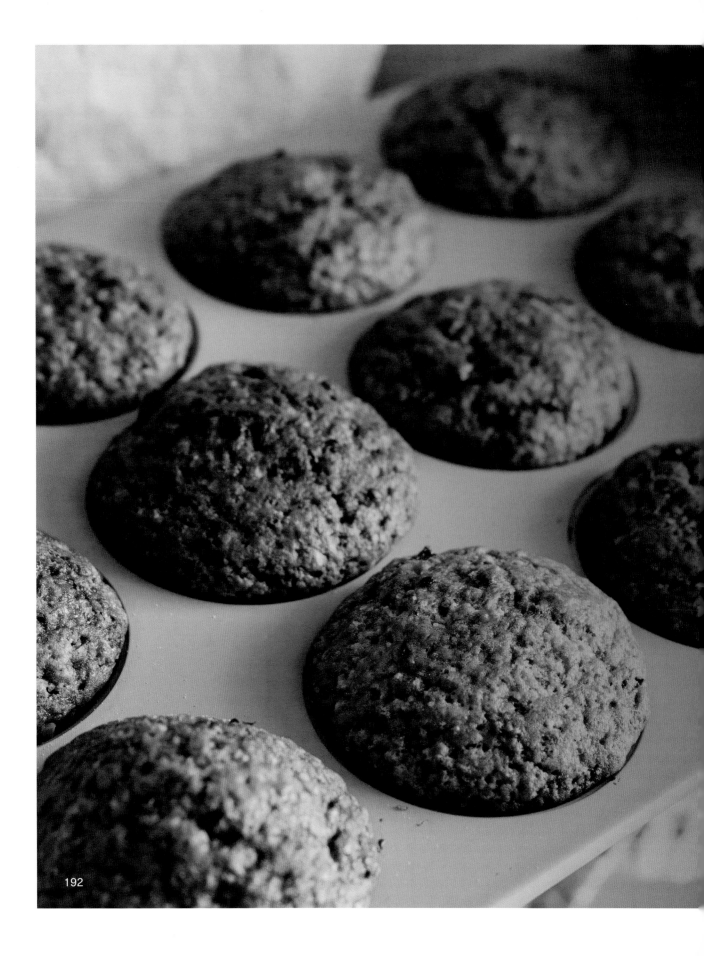

CHAPTER 6

Pastries and Quick Breads

ON MANY MORNINGS, the aroma of freshly baked muffins or scones fills the kitchen, mingling with the perfume of hot coffee. It's hard to resist. It feels like home when the kitchen is bustling and warm from the oven's heat. The kids sit at the table, slathering muffins with fresh, golden-yellow butter before they head out to play. It's a wonderful way to start the day.

From time to time, the homey scones and muffins make way for fancier pastries—treats that need a touch more effort and practice. These we save for special occasions such as holidays or family visits. Then, it's time for little fruit-topped tarts or sweet rolls.

When I first started baking, I soon realized I had more sourdough starter than I could manage. Or, at least, it felt that way. Instead of simply baking bread, I realized that you can just as easily convert quick breads and pastries to sourdough, too. It lends a richer, more complex flavor to muffins and quick breads, and I like them better.

Yeast gives traditional loaves of bread their rise. In contrast, quick breads rely on a chemical reaction between acidic ingredients, such as buttermilk, and alkaline ingredients, such as baking soda. Sourdough starter is naturally acidic. It combines beautifully with baking soda to make soft-crumbed quick breads, muffins, biscuits, and scones with deep and rich flavor.

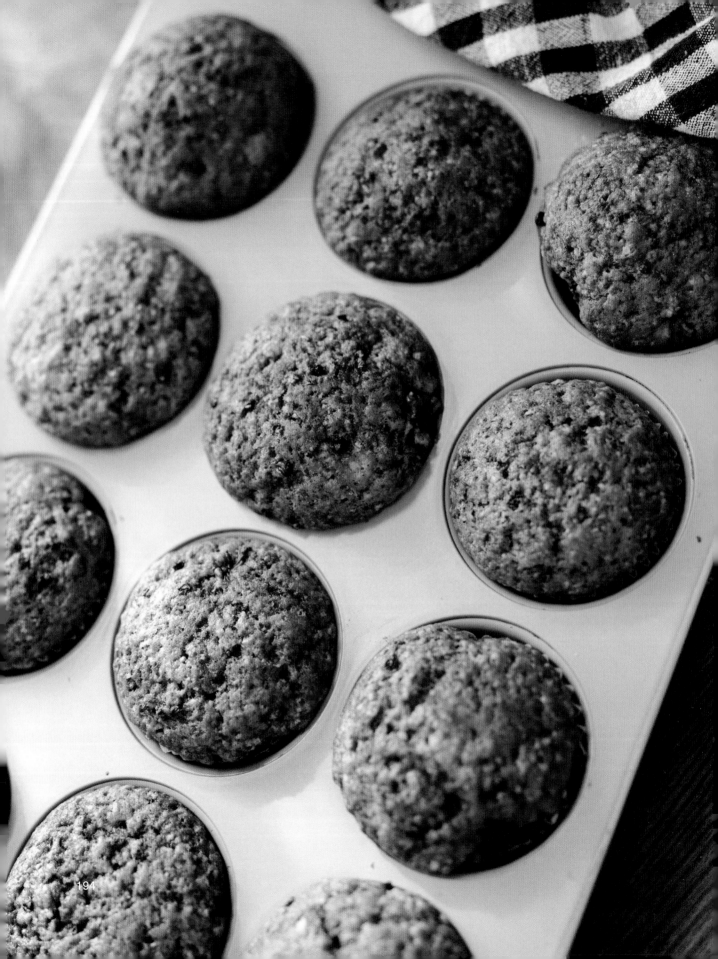

Blackberry Muffins

In the summer, blackberry bushes come alive with little white star-shaped flowers. By early fall, these flowers form plump, ripe berries. If you're lucky enough to live near a berry farm or grow them yourself, you can pick baskets of them. Enjoy plenty fresh by the handful and reserve the rest for this easy muffin recipe.

If fresh berries are a little harder to come by in your community, you can always make this recipe with frozen berries instead. Dust the berries with a little flour before folding them into the batter to prevent them from sinking to the bottom of the muffins as they bake.

2 cups (280 grams) all-purpose flour

2 teaspoons (10 grams) baking powder

1/2 teaspoon baking soda

1 teaspoon cinnamon

1/2 teaspoon salt

1/2 cup (125 grams) sourdough discard

1/2 cup (113 grams) butter, melted

1 teaspoon (5 grams) vanilla

1 cup (192 grams) sugar

2 eggs, at room temperature

1 cup (170 grams) fresh or frozen blackberries

1 Preheat the oven to 425°F and and arrange paper liners in a muffin tin.

2 In a medium bowl, whisk together the flour, baking powder, baking soda, cinnamon, and salt.

3 In a large mixing bowl, whisk together the sourdough discard, butter, vanilla, and sugar. Beat the eggs into the batter one at a time until thoroughly incorporated.

4 Gradually add the flour mixture to the egg mixture, stirring until just combined. Gently fold the blackberries into the batter.

5 Spoon the batter into the prepared muffin tin, filling the cups three-quarters full. Bake for 6 minutes at 425°F, then decrease oven temperature to 350°F. Continue baking for 13 to 15 minutes more, or until golden brown on top and a toothpick inserted into the center of the muffins comes out clean.

6 Transfer the muffins to a wire rack and allow them to cool completely before serving. Store in an airtight container or a ziplock bag so they don't dry out.

PREP TIME:
10 MINUTES

BAKE TIME:
20 MINUTES

RISE TIME:
0 MINUTES

YIELD:
MAKES 12 MUFFINS

Lemon Poppy Seed Muffins

These muffins are easy to pack for snacks or breakfast on the go. They're bursting with the vibrant flavor of lemon, which you incorporate both into the glaze and the muffins themselves.

FOR THE MUFFINS

2 cups (280 grams) all-purpose flour

1 cup (192 grams) sugar

2 tablespoons (18 grams) poppy seeds

2 teaspoons (10 grams) baking powder

1/2 teaspoon baking soda

1/2 teaspoon salt

1/2 cup (125 grams) sourdough discard

1 cup (244 grams) milk

1/2 cup (113 grams) butter, melted

2 large eggs, at room temperature

1 tablespoon (15 grams) lemon juice

1 teaspoon (5 grams) vanilla extract

FOR THE GLAZE

1 cup (113 grams) powdered sugar

2 tablespoons (30 grams) lemon juice

1 Preheat your oven to 400°F and arrange paper liners in a muffin tin.

2 **To make the muffins:** In a large mixing bowl, combine the flour, sugar, poppy seeds, baking powder, baking soda, and salt.

3 In a separate large mixing bowl, whisk the sourdough discard, milk, butter, eggs, lemon juice, and vanilla until they form a smooth, uniform batter. Slowly beat the dry ingredients into the wet ingredients, taking care not to overmix.

4 Spoon the batter into the prepared muffin tins.

5 Bake for 20 minutes, or until a toothpick inserted in the middle of the muffins comes out clean and the edges of the muffins turn golden brown.

6 Transfer the muffins to a wire rack and allow them to cool completely while you prepare the glaze.

7 **To make the glaze:** In a small bowl, whisk the powdered sugar and lemon juice until combined. Drizzle the glaze over the muffins and then serve. Store in an airtight container or a ziplock bag so they don't dry out.

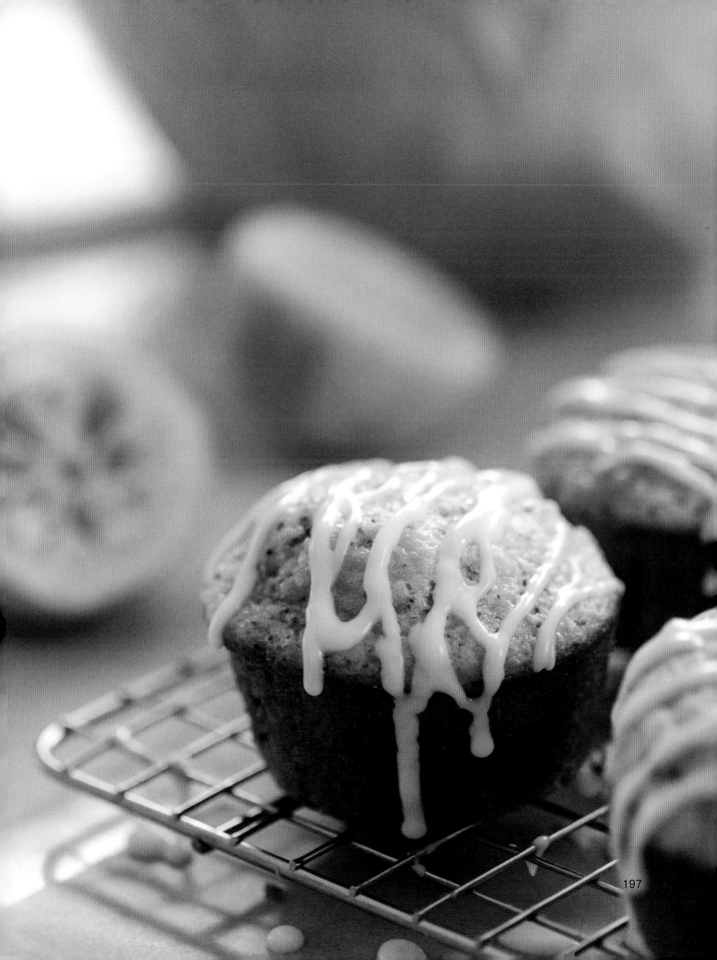

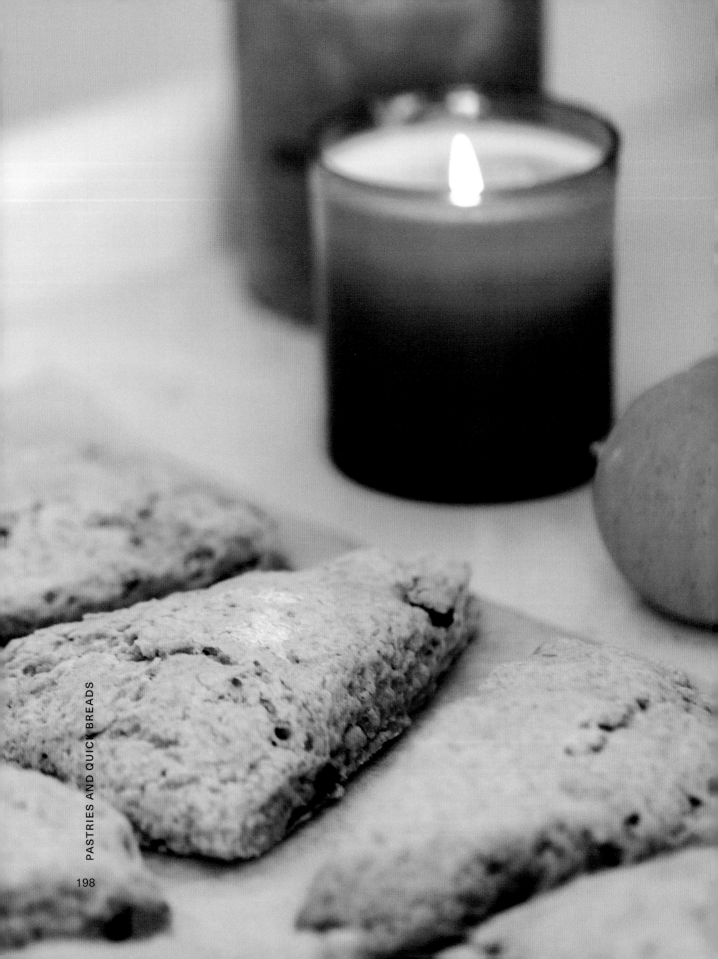

PREP TIME:
**15 MINUTES +
10 MINUTES CHILL TIME**

BAKE TIME:
20 MINUTES

RISE TIME:
0 MINUTES

YIELD:
MAKES 8 SCONES

Pumpkin Scones

I love keeping a garden. One of my favorite vegetables to grow is winter squash—especially the giant Jarrahdale pumpkins. With their pale, soft sage-green outsides and vibrant orange flesh, they're beautiful and look picture-perfect sitting on your porch. They also taste delicious and make an absolutely gorgeous pumpkin purée. You can certainly use canned pumpkin purée if you don't grow your own.

These scones tend to spread, so there's a bit of a trick to this recipe. The key is to keep them very cold before you bake them. Using frozen butter and popping them in the freezer for 10 minutes before baking keeps them nice and cold.

2 1/2 cups (350 grams) all-purpose flour

1/2 cup (96 grams) coconut sugar

1 tablespoon (14 grams) baking powder

1 tablespoon (8 grams) pumpkin pie spice

1/2 teaspoon salt

1/2 cup (113 grams) butter, cubed, frozen

1 cup (142 grams) semi-sweet chocolate chunks

1/2 cup (125 grams) sourdough discard

1/2 cup (120 grams) pumpkin purée

1/4 cup (60 grams) heavy cream

1 egg

1 teaspoon (5 grams) vanilla extract

1 Preheat your oven to 400°F and line a baking sheet with parchment paper.

2 In a large bowl, mix together the flour, sugar, baking powder, pumpkin pie spice, and salt. Cut in the cubed butter using a fork or pastry blender. Stir in the chocolate chunks.

3 In a separate large bowl, beat the sourdough discard, pumpkin purée, heavy cream, egg, and vanilla. Stir the wet ingredients into the flour mixture until well combined, taking care not to overmix.

4 Lightly flour your working surface. Tip out your dough onto it. Shape the dough into a 12-inch circle, and cut it into eight equal wedges.

5 Transfer the scones to the prepared baking sheet and place them in the freezer for 10 minutes.

6 Bake for 20 minutes, or until the edges start to turn golden and a toothpick inserted into the center of the scones comes out clean.

7 Transfer the scones to a wire rack and allow them to cool for 10 minutes before serving. Store in an airtight container or a ziplock bag so they don't dry out.

PREP TIME:
15 MINUTES

BAKE TIME:
20 MINUTES

RISE TIME:
0 MINUTES

YIELD:
MAKES 8 SCONES

Chocolate-Coconut Scones

These scones remind me a bit of old-fashioned German chocolate cake. The combination of chocolate and coconut is unforgettable—and almost decadent, especially at breakfast. I like to use dark maple syrup in this recipe as a sweetener, as it lends a delicious robust sweetness that marries well with dark chocolate.

FOR THE SCONES

3 3/4 cups (525 grams) all-purpose flour

1 cup (226 grams) cold butter, diced

1/2 cup (45 grams) unsweetened shredded coconut

2 tablespoons (28 grams) baking powder

1 tablespoon (18 grams) salt

1/2 cup (125 grams) sourdough discard

1 cup (240 grams) heavy cream

4 eggs

3 tablespoons (60 grams) maple syrup

8 ounces (228 grams) semi-sweet chocolate chunks

FOR THE EGG WASH

1 egg yolk

1 tablespoon (15 grams) water

2 tablespoons (25 grams) sugar

1 Preheat the oven to 400°F and line two baking sheets with parchment paper.

2 **To make the scones:** In the bowl of a stand mixer equipped with a paddle attachment, add the flour, butter, coconut, baking powder, and salt. Mix at low speed until the butter is broken down to the size of peas, but no smaller. Take care not to overmix.

3 In a medium bowl, whisk together the sourdough discard, heavy cream, eggs, and maple syrup. Pour the wet ingredients into the dry ingredients and mix on low speed until just combined. Fold in the chocolate chunks.

4 Dust your working surface with flour and then roll out the dough until it's 1 inch thick. Cut the scones into rounds about 3 inches across with a biscuit cutter. Arrange the scones on the prepared baking sheets.

5 **To make the egg wash:** In a small bowl, whisk together the egg yolk and water and brush it lightly over the scones, then sprinkle them with sugar.

6 Bake for 20 to 22 minutes, or until evenly brown.

7 Transfer the scones to a wire rack to cool before serving. Store any leftovers in an airtight container at room temperature for up to 3 days.

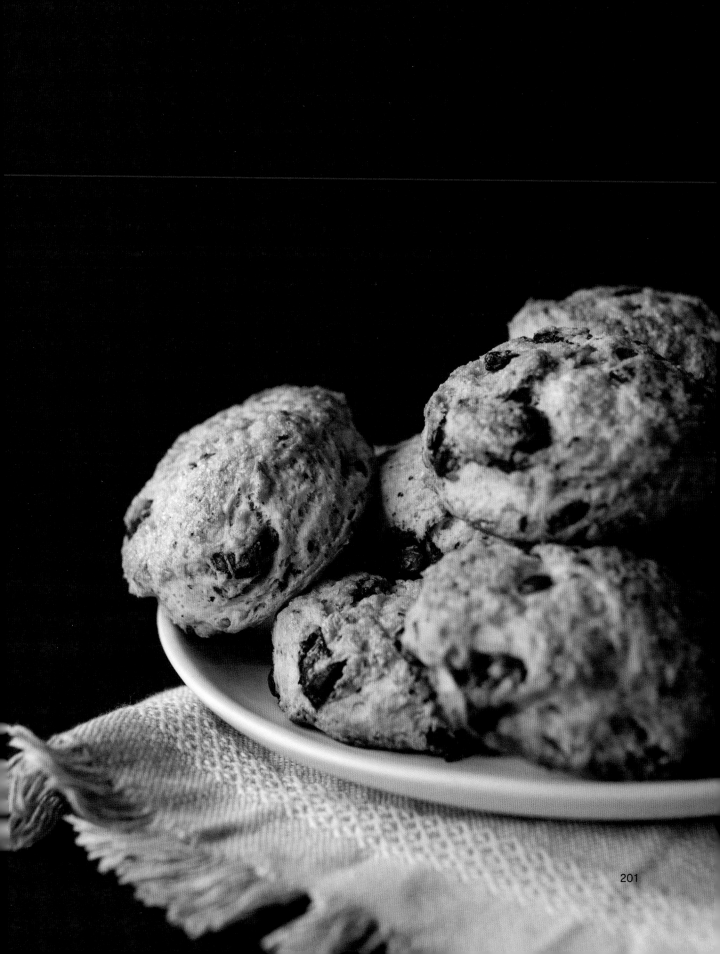

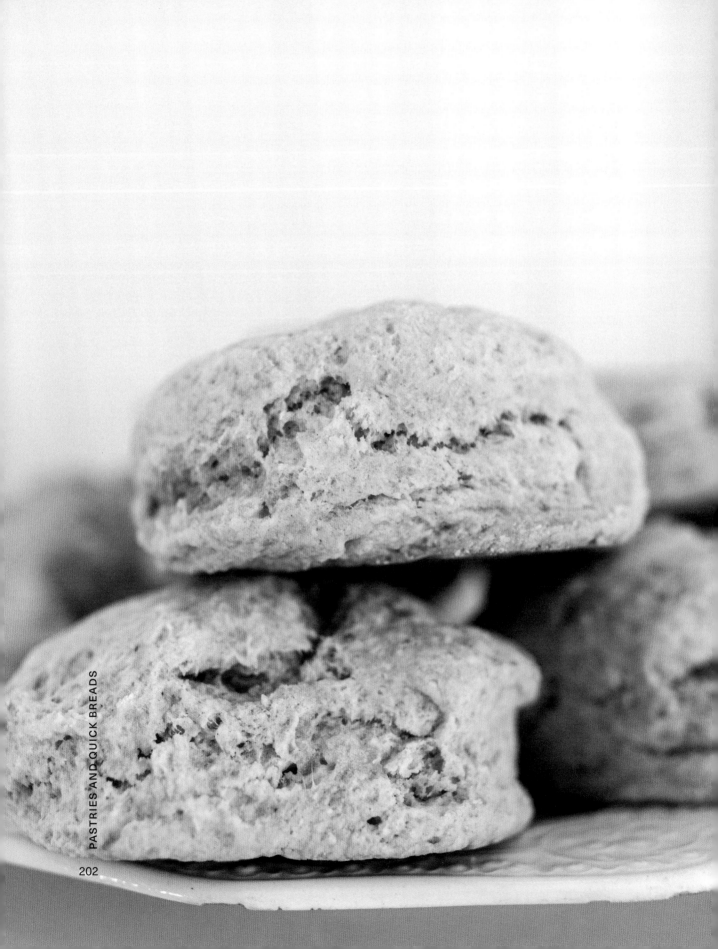

PREP TIME:
10 MINUTES

BAKE TIME:
20 MINUTES

RISE TIME:
10 TO 12 HOURS

YIELD:
MAKES ABOUT 12 BISCUITS

Sourdough Biscuits

I love to serve these biscuits straight out of the oven, drenched in butter with plenty of homemade jam or a spoonful of raw wildflower honey. Sourdough discard gives them a tart, slightly tangy edge that tastes incredibly delicious.

There's a lot of flexibility in this recipe. Preparing the dough in advance and allowing it to soak at room temperature for a few hours produces a wonderfully tender biscuit with a complex flavor. It also makes the biscuits a little easier to digest. You can make the dough up to a day in advance, which is great if you're running behind schedule. For people who have a tough time digesting grains, longer fermentation periods can often make them a little easier on your stomach.

2 cups (280 grams) all-purpose flour

1/2 cup (113 grams) cold butter, cut into chunks

1 cup (250 grams) sourdough discard

1/2 cup (122 grams) milk

1 tablespoon (12 grams) granulated sugar

2 teaspoons (10 grams) baking powder

1 teaspoon (5 grams) baking soda

3/4 teaspoon salt

1. To a large mixing bowl, add the flour and then toss in the cold butter. Work the butter into the flour with a fork or pastry blender until it comes together. Add the sourdough discard, milk, and sugar to the bowl and stir until well combined.

2. Cover the bowl and let it rest at room temperature for 10 to 12 hours.

3. Add the baking powder, baking soda, and salt to the dough. Mix everything together well to form a uniform and pliable dough.

4. Preheat the oven to 400°F, then line a baking sheet with parchment paper and lightly dust your working surface with flour.

5. Turn the dough onto your working surface, then pat it into a rectangle about 3/4 inch thick. Dip a 3- to 4-inch-diameter biscuit cutter in flour, and then cut out the biscuits. Transfer them to the baking sheet, keeping the biscuits about 2 inches apart.

6. Bake for 14 to 20 minutes, or until golden brown. Store in an airtight container or a ziplock bag so they don't dry out. You can also throw them in the freezer for longer storage.

203

PREP TIME:
15 MINUTES

BAKE TIME:
50 MINUTES

RISE TIME:
0 MINUTES

YIELD:
MAKES 1 LOAF

Banana Bread

Whenever you have bananas just teetering on the edge of being overripe, make this banana bread. It's a delicious treat that comes together in about an hour (with only 10 minutes of active time). Plus it packs well, so you can wrap it neatly in some parchment paper and kitchen twine. Then, take it to a friend's home as a little gift, or bring it to a potluck.

While this recipe is just about as basic as you can get, a big spoonful of sourdough discard does a lot of the heavy lifting. It brings a rich complexity to such a staple baked good. You can also add in chopped dark chocolate chunks, toasted walnuts, or even flaked coconut if you want to take the treat to the next level. Just fold them into the batter right before you pour it into the loaf pan.

2 cups (280 grams) all-purpose flour

2 teaspoons (10 grams) baking powder

1 teaspoon (5 grams) baking soda

1 teaspoon (6 grams) salt

1 cup (200 grams) dark brown sugar

1/2 cup (114 grams) melted butter, plus more for the pan

3 ripe bananas (about 350 grams), mashed

1/2 cup (125 grams) sourdough discard

2 large eggs

1 teaspoon (5 grams) vanilla extract

1   Preheat the oven to 350°F and lightly grease a 9-by-5-inch loaf pan with butter.

2   In a medium mixing bowl, whisk together the flour, baking powder, baking soda, and salt. Set aside.

3   In the bowl of a stand mixer equipped with a paddle attachment, add the brown sugar and butter and mix on medium speed until light and fluffy. Beat in the bananas, sourdough discard, eggs, and vanilla until they form a uniform batter.

4   Pour the batter into the prepared loaf pan. Transfer to the oven and bake for 50 to 60 minutes, or until a toothpick inserted into the center of the bread comes out clean. Allow the bread to cool in the pan for 1 hour, then slice and serve. Store any leftovers in an airtight container at room temperature for up to 4 days.

PASTRIES AND QUICK BREADS

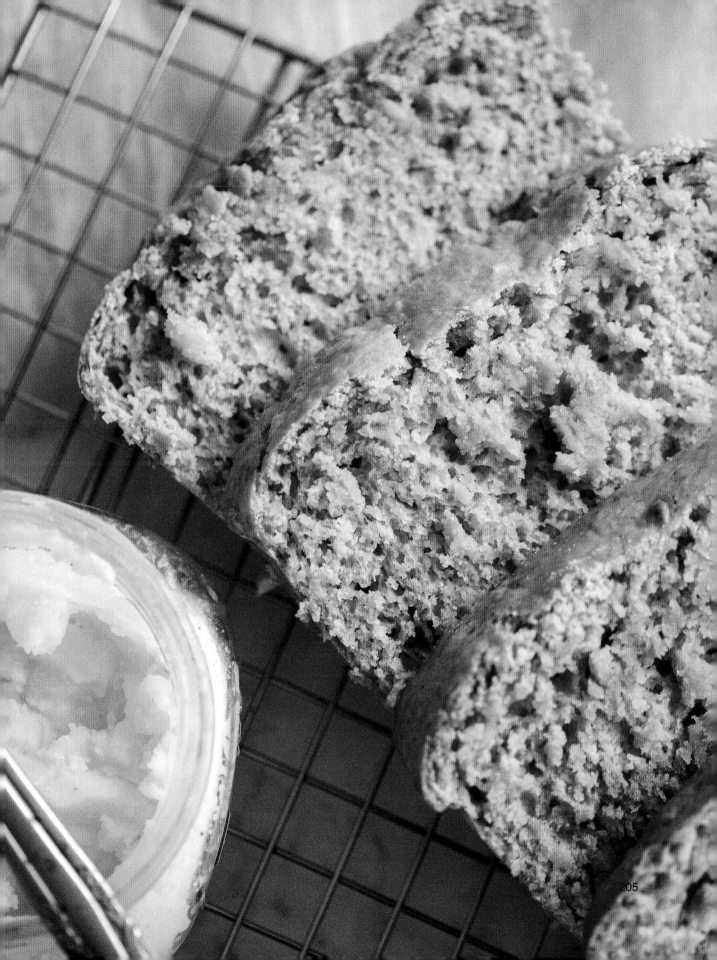

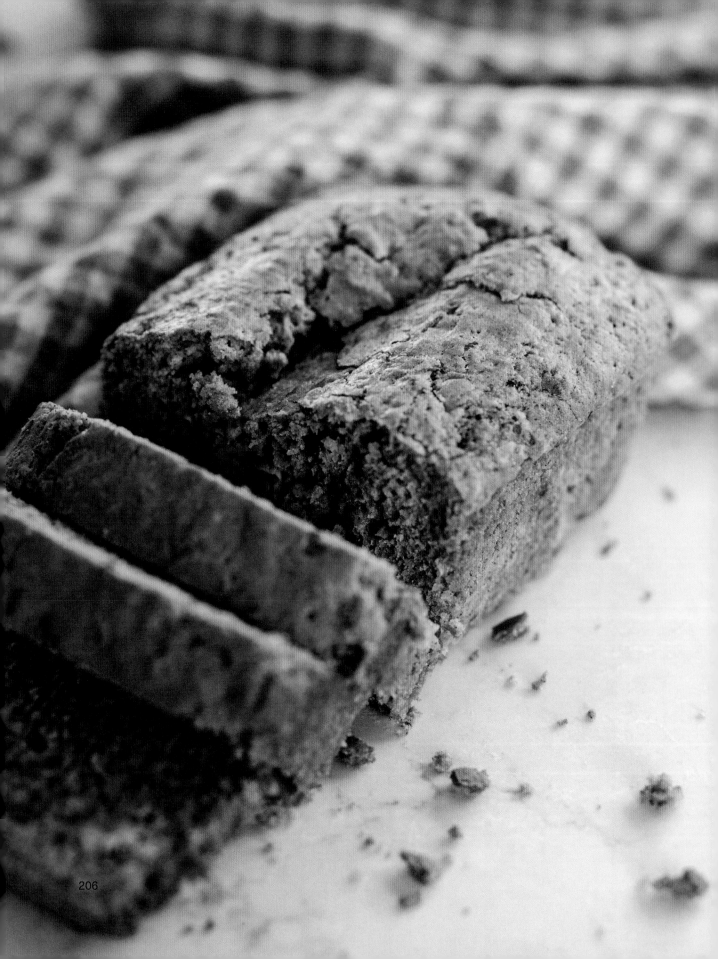

PREP TIME:
15 MINUTES

BAKE TIME:
1 HOUR

RISE TIME:
0 MINUTES

YIELD:
MAKES 1 LOAF

Zucchini Bread

In late summer, zucchini takes over my garden. No matter how many my children pick, there always seems to be more. We can never seem to eat it all, so I set to work grating it to make loaf after loaf of this easy zucchini bread. Serve it with plenty of butter for breakfast or a glass of milk for a snack.

The best part is that it freezes easily; just wrap it tightly first. You can pull it out in the depths of winter while your garden sleeps. Even on those dark cold days, you can still enjoy the bounty of homegrown food.

2 cups (280 grams) all-purpose flour

2 teaspoons (6 grams) cinnamon

2 teaspoons (10 grams) baking powder

1 teaspoon (5 grams) baking soda

1 teaspoon (6 grams) salt

1 1/4 cup (250 grams) brown sugar

1/2 cup (114 grams) unsalted, melted butter, plus more for the pan

1/2 cup (125 grams) sourdough discard

2 eggs

1 teaspoon (5 grams) vanilla

2 cups (about 225 grams) grated zucchini

1　Preheat the oven to 350ºF and lightly grease a 9-by-5-inch loaf pan with butter.

2　In a medium bowl, whisk together the flour, cinnamon, baking powder, baking soda, and. Set aside.

3　In a large bowl, beat together the brown sugar and butter for about 5 minutes, or until light and fluffy. Beat in the sourdough discard, eggs, and vanilla. Then, fold in the zucchini.

4　Stir the flour mixture into the wet ingredients a little at a time until just incorporated.

5　Pour the batter into the prepared loaf pan and bake for 50 to 60 minutes, or until a toothpick inserted in the center comes out clean.

6　Allow the bread to cool in the pan for 1 hour before slicing. To store, cover with foil or place inside an airtight container.

PREP TIME:
15 MINUTES

COOK TIME:
12 TO 18 MINUTES

RISE TIME:
14 TO 16 HOURS

YIELD:
MAKES 16 DONUTS

Cinnamon-Sugar Donuts

Richly indulgent, these donuts will become a favorite treat in your home—especially when you serve them with a big mug of coffee. The subtle addition of cinnamon to the dough, followed by gentle dredging in cinnamon sugar, adds an extra layer of flavor to a morning favorite.

Allowing the dough to rest in the fridge develops an optimal flavor and texture. This step prevents overfermentation, so make sure to plan ahead. While the process requires some patience, the resulting donuts strike a perfect balance of softness and depth. They capture the essence of thoughtful, unhurried baking.

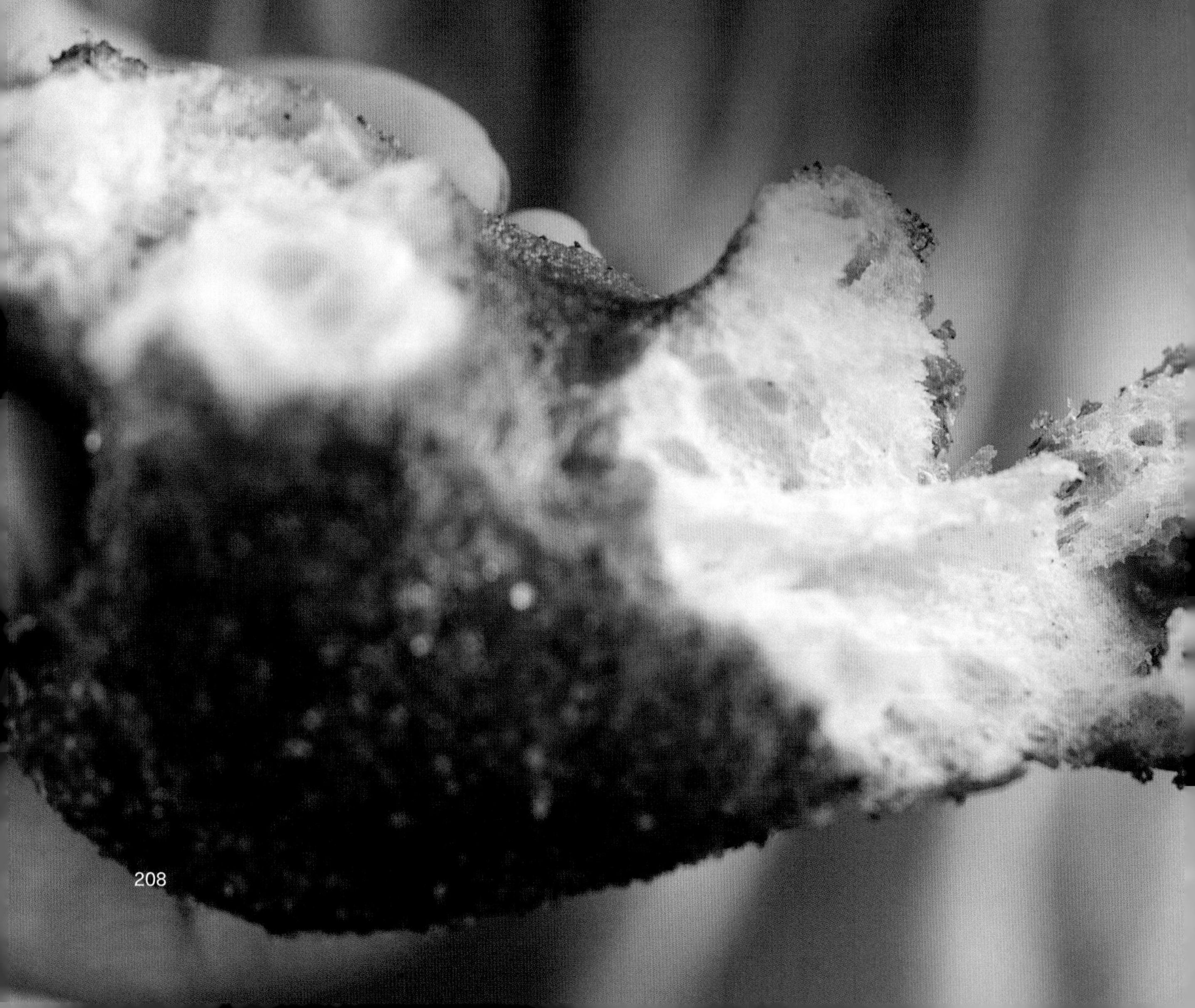

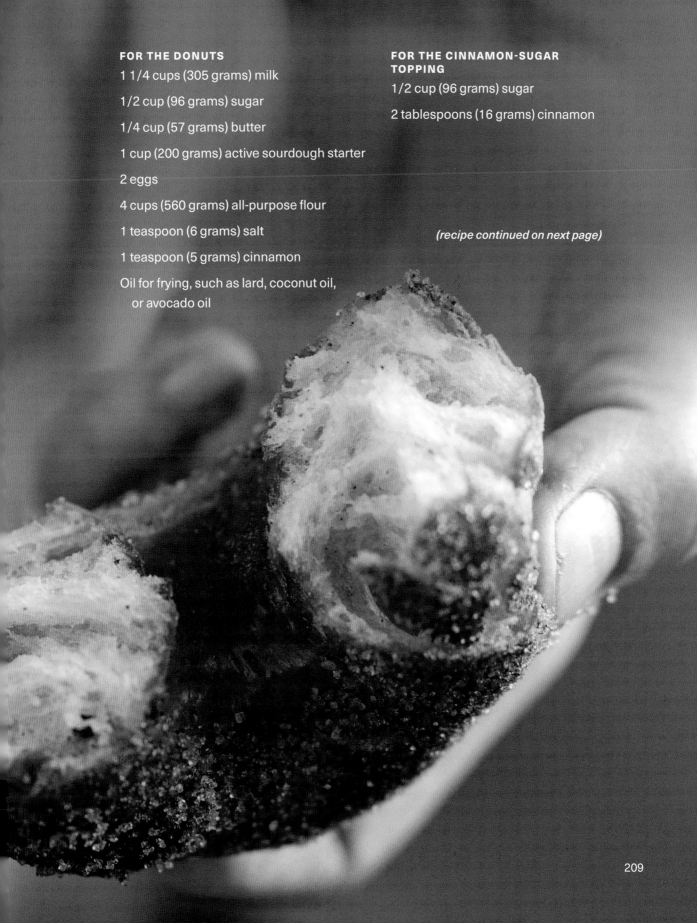

FOR THE DONUTS

1 1/4 cups (305 grams) milk

1/2 cup (96 grams) sugar

1/4 cup (57 grams) butter

1 cup (200 grams) active sourdough starter

2 eggs

4 cups (560 grams) all-purpose flour

1 teaspoon (6 grams) salt

1 teaspoon (5 grams) cinnamon

Oil for frying, such as lard, coconut oil,
   or avocado oil

**FOR THE CINNAMON-SUGAR
TOPPING**

1/2 cup (96 grams) sugar

2 tablespoons (16 grams) cinnamon

(recipe continued on next page)

209

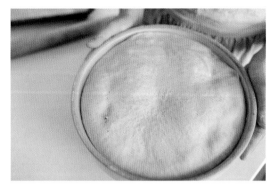

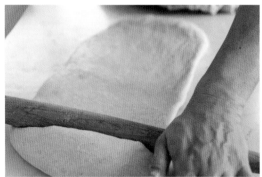

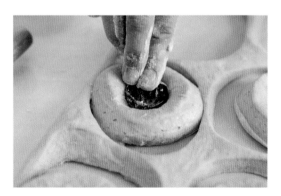

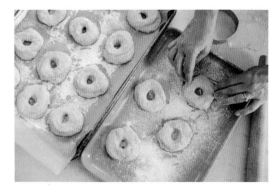

1 **To make the donuts:** In a small saucepan over low heat, combine the milk, sugar, and butter and mix until the sugar dissolves. Transfer the mixture to the bowl of a stand mixer equipped with a dough hook and allow it to cool to room temperature.

2 Beat in the starter and eggs. Add the flour, salt, and cinnamon and knead on low speed for about 10 minutes, or until the dough becomes elastic and pulls away from the sides of the bowl.

3 Cover the mixing bowl tightly, and leave it in a warm place to rise for 5 to 6 hours, or until doubled in bulk. Then, transfer it to the fridge and let it chill overnight, at least 8 hours.

4 To make the topping: The following day, in a small bowl, whisk together the sugar and cinnamon and set aside.

5 Dust your working surface lightly with flour. Turn out the dough and then roll it into a rectangle about 1/2 inch thick.

6 Cut out the donuts using a biscuit cutter or a mason jar, then cut the interior hole using a small lid from an olive, avocado, or other oil jar. Place your donuts on a baking sheet. Cover them with a damp tea towel or plastic wrap for 1 1/2 to 2 hours and allow them to rise.

7 Add about 1/2 inch of oil to a cast-iron skillet over medium heat. When the oil reaches 375ºF on a cooking thermometer, or when a small piece of dough sizzles when you add it to the pan, you are ready to fry your donuts.

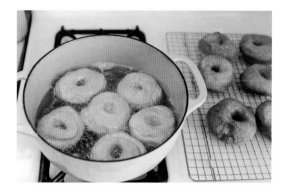

8 Place a square of parchment paper on your counter for easier cleanup and then place a wire cooling rack over it.

9 Fry the donuts in small batches for 2 to 3 minutes or until golden on one side. Then flip them and fry for another 2 to 3 minutes on the other side, or until they puff and turn golden. Be careful not to crowd the pan. Transfer the donuts to the wire rack. Allow them to cool for about 30 seconds. Then, dip them in the cinnamon sugar and return them to the rack to cool completely.

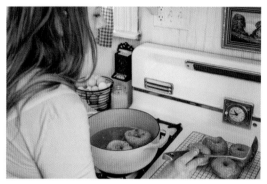

10 Store any leftovers in an airtight container at room temperature for up to 2 days.

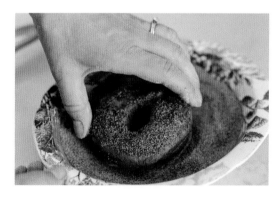

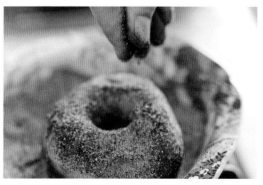

Strawberry Brioche Tarts

In early summer, the garden bursts with vivid pops of red strawberries nestled among their dark green vines. I gather what I can and make these delightful handheld tarts. Sun-kissed and perfectly ripe, the berries mingle with vanilla-scented cream cheese for a luscious tart filling. It captures the essence of summer—sweet, bright, and playful. Instead of a stiff crust, I opt for a tender and flaky brioche-style dough made golden-rich with plenty of butter and fresh eggs. The result is a lovely little tart that packs easily for a picnic and won't crumble on your plate.

Versatility is the hallmark of this recipe, and let the seasonal changes guide you. In late summer, you can substitute fresh blueberries. As autumn approaches, you might try blackberries with just a hint of cardamom to bring out their flavor.

FOR THE DOUGH

1 cup (200 grams) active sourdough starter

4 eggs

1/2 cup (122 grams) milk

3 cups (420 grams) bread flour

1/2 cup (70 grams) all-purpose flour

1 cup (226 grams) butter, at room temperature

1/4 cup (48 grams) sugar

1 1/2 teaspoons (9 grams) salt

FOR THE CUSTARD

1 egg

8 ounces (226 grams) cream cheese, at room temperature

1/4 cup (48 grams) sugar

1 teaspoon (5 grams) vanilla extract

FOR THE STRAWBERRY TOPPING

1 cup (about 150 grams) diced strawberries

1 tablespoon (12 grams) sugar

FOR THE EGG WASH

1 egg white reserved from the custard

1 tablespoon (15 grams) water

1. **To make the dough:** In the bowl of a stand mixer equipped with a dough hook, combine the starter, eggs, and milk. Add the bread flour, all-purpose flour, butter, sugar, and salt and knead on low speed for about 15 minutes, or until the dough is smooth and glossy and pulls away from the sides of the bowl.

2. Cover the bowl tightly and place it in a warm spot for 6 to 8 hours, or until doubled. Transfer to the fridge, and let it chill overnight.

3. Lightly flour your working surface, and then tip out the dough. Divide it into twelve equal portions using a bench scraper and shape them into balls. Cover them with a towel and allow them to rise again, about 2 hours, until puffed up.

4. To make the custard: While the dough rises, separate the egg white and add the yolk to a medium bowl, reserving the egg white for the egg wash. Beat in the cream cheese, sugar, and vanilla.

5. **To make the strawberry topping:** In a medium bowl, toss the strawberries with the sugar.

6. **To make the egg wash:** In a small bowl, whisk the reserved egg white with the water.

7. When the dough is ready, preheat the oven to 350°F and line a baking sheet with parchment paper.

8. Gently place the dough balls on the baking sheet. Flatten them down with the palm of your hand, then press down in their centers to form a divot. Fill with the custard and sprinkle with the strawberry topping. Brush the pastries with the egg wash, then bake for 20 minutes, or until cooked through and golden brown.

9. Allow the tarts to cool completely on a wire rack before you serve them. Store in an airtight container or a ziplock bag so they don't dry out, in the refrigerator.

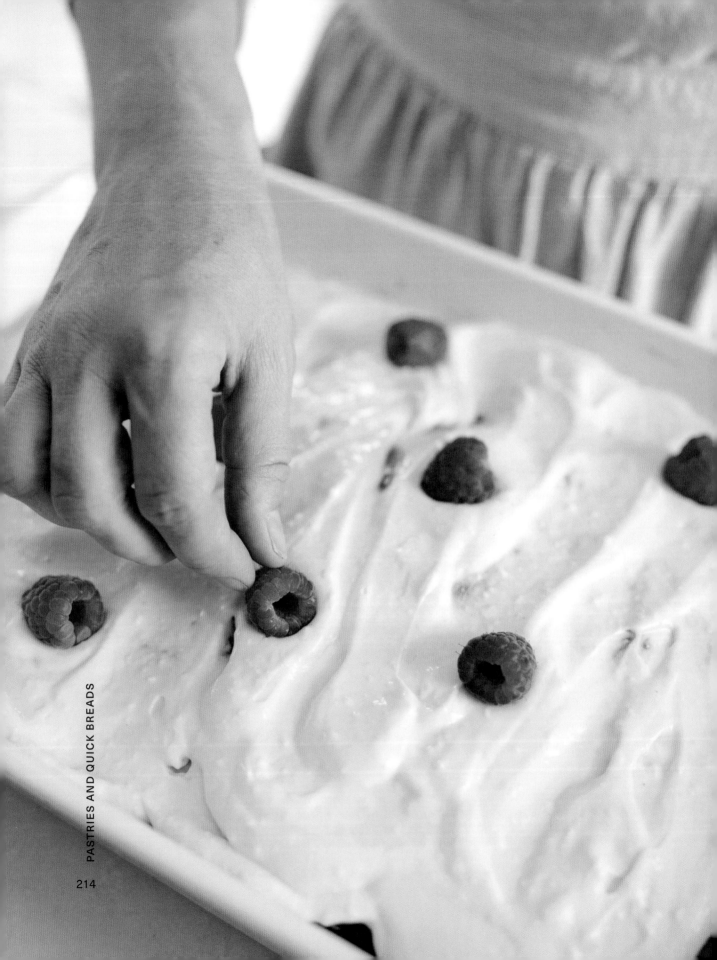

214

PREP TIME:
30 MINUTES

BAKE TIME:
25 MINUTES

RISE TIME:
8 HOURS

YIELD:
MAKES 12 ROLLS

Raspberry Sweet Rolls

Few things rival the comforting charm of classic cinnamon rolls, except, perhaps, these raspberry-filled sweet rolls. A butter-infused dough envelops vibrant, sweet-tart berries to make gorgeous sweet rolls. Then, you slather them in a simple honey-vanilla cream-cheese frosting touched by the lightest slip of lemon.

Preparing the dough takes a little time, so plan to start the night before. I'm sure you'll find it's worth the effort.

FOR THE DOUGH

1/2 cup (100 grams) active sourdough starter

1/2 cup (118 grams) water

1/2 cup (113 grams) melted coconut oil, plus more for the bowl

1/2 cup (168 grams) honey

2 eggs

4 cups (560 grams) all-purpose flour

1 teaspoon (5 grams) baking soda

1 teaspoon (5 grams) baking powder

1/2 teaspoon salt

FOR THE FILLING

3 cups (420 grams) fresh or frozen raspberries

1/3 cup (64 grams) granulated sugar

3 teaspoons (9 grams) cornstarch

1/2 cup (113 grams) butter, at room temperature

1/2 cup (100 grams) light brown sugar

FOR THE FROSTING

6 ounces (170 grams) cream cheese, softened

1/2 cup (120 grams) heavy cream

1/2 cup (168 grams) honey

2 teaspoons (10 grams) vanilla extract

1 teaspoon (5 grams) lemon juice

(recipe continued on next page)

1. **To make the dough:** In the bowl of a stand mixer equipped with a dough hook, combine the starter, water, coconut oil, honey, and eggs. Add the all-purpose flour and mix on low speed for about 10 minutes, or until the dough is smooth, glossy, and pulls away from the sides of the bowl. It should pass the windowpane test (see page 13). If it doesn't, continue mixing for a few minutes further.

2. Lightly grease a large mixing bowl with coconut oil, then place the dough in the bowl. Cover it tightly and let it rest in a warm spot in your kitchen for at least 8 hours, or until doubled.

3. Preheat the oven to 375°F.

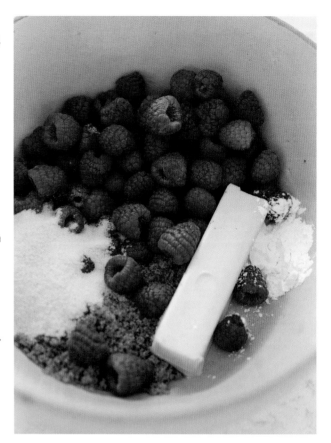

4. Return the dough to the bowl of the stand mixer and add the baking soda, baking powder, and salt. Mix on medium speed for about 5 minutes, or until the baking powder, baking soda, and salt are incorporated.

5. Lightly dust your working surface with flour and then tip the dough out onto it. Roll it into a rectangle about 1/4 inch thick.

6. **To make the filling:** In a small bowl, stir together the raspberries, granulated sugar, cornstarch, butter, and light brown sugar, then spoon it evenly over the dough.

7. Working from the long side, roll the dough up tightly. When you reach the end, pinch the edge closed. Slice the rolled dough into twelve even rolls.

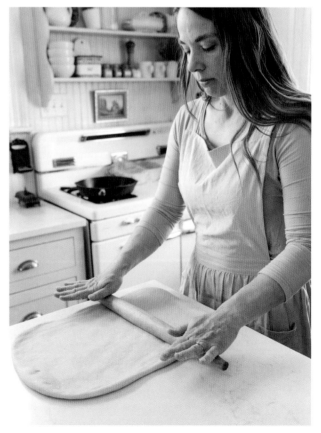

8. Place the rolls into a well-seasoned 14-inch cast-iron skillet or baking dish. Bake for 20 to 25 minutes, or until the rolls are lightly browned and the dough is cooked through. Allow them to cool for 10 minutes while you prepare the frosting.

9. **To make the frosting:** In a medium mixing bowl, beat the cream cheese, heavy cream, honey, vanilla, and lemon juice to form a smooth frosting. Spread the frosting over the rolls and serve. To store, cover with foil or place inside an airtight container and keep refrigerated up to a week.

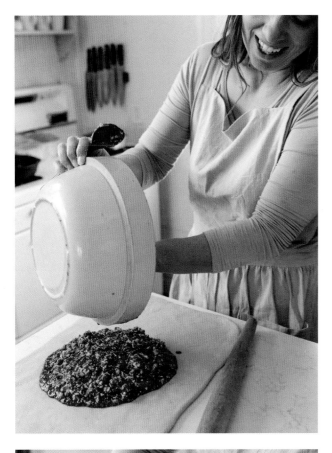

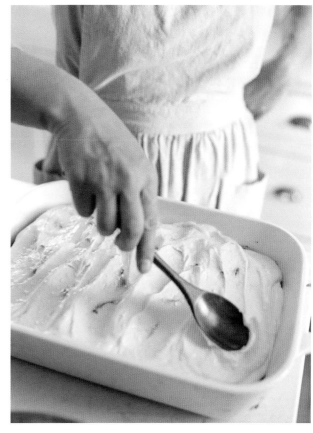

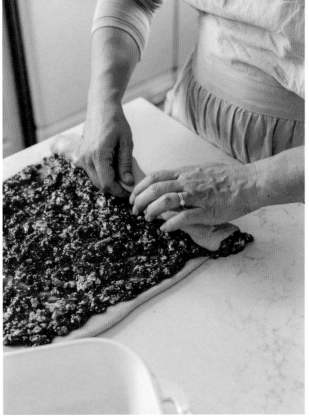

HOW TO SLICE SWEET ROLLS

When slicing sweet rolls and sticky buns, it makes sense to cut them with a sharp knife just as you would anything else. But the pressure applied as you slice through the dough with a knife can leave rough, jagged cuts. As a result, the buns and sweet rolls may not expand quite as evenly in the oven as you had hoped. Instead, slide a 12-inch length of string or dental floss underneath the dough. Bring it up over the dough, crossing the two ends at the top. Then, pull firmly on the ends of the string. It'll slice straight through the dough cleanly. That means fewer utensils to wash, cleaner cuts, and better expansion as the rolls bake.

PREP TIME:
30 MINUTES

BAKE TIME:
25 MINUTES

RISE TIME:
8 HOURS

YIELD:
MAKES 12 BUNS

Sticky Buns

Rising early in the morning in our bustling farmhouse gives me a moment of peace before the frenzy of the day begins. I pour myself a mug from our French press and top it with fresh cream. The smell of fresh coffee fills the air. It's a simple pleasure, fortifying and energizing me for the day ahead. Breakfast is on my mind. Feeding eight children is no small task. But when I can, I love taking time for something memorable.

In those quiet morning hours, I pull out the dough I made the night before. I roll it out and dress it with brown sugar, honey, and pecans before tucking the buns into the oven. Their sweet aroma fills the air in no time, and the children come down hungry and ready to eat. Sitting down to eat together, I'm reminded of the richness in the simplicity of a home-made life.

FOR THE DOUGH

1/2 cup (100 grams) active sourdough
  starter

1/2 cup (118 grams) lukewarm water

4 cups (560 grams) all-purpose flour

1/2 cup (112 grams) butter, melted,
  plus more for the bowl

1/2 cup (168 grams) honey

2 eggs

1 teaspoon (5 grams) baking soda

1 teaspoon (5 grams) baking powder

1/2 teaspoon salt

FOR THE FILLING

1/4 cup (57 grams) butter,
  at room temperature

1/2 cup (100 grams) light brown sugar

1 tablespoon (8 grams) cinnamon

FOR THE TOPPING

3/4 cup (150 grams) firmly packed light
  brown sugar

6 tablespoons (84 grams) butter

1/4 cup (85 grams) honey

1/2 teaspoon salt

1 1/2 cups (170 grams) coarsely chopped
  pecans

PASTRIES AND QUICK BREADS

218

(recipe continued on next page)

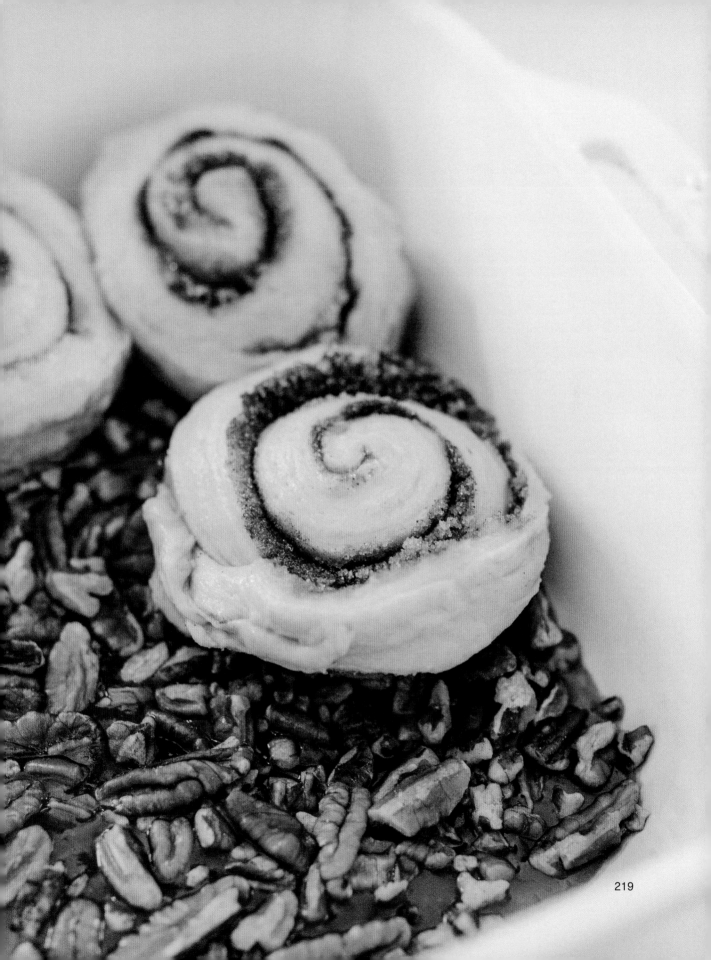

1. **To make the dough:** In the bowl of a stand mixer equipped with a dough hook, combine the starter, water, all-purpose flour, coconut oil, honey, and eggs. Mix on low speed for about 10 minutes, or until the dough is smooth, glossy, and pulls away from the sides of the bowl.

2. Lightly grease a large mixing bowl with coconut oil, then place the dough in the bowl. Cover it tightly and let it rest in a warm spot in your kitchen for at least 8 hours or until doubled.

3. The next morning, preheat the oven to 375°F.

4. Return the dough to the bowl of the stand mixer and add the baking soda, baking powder, and salt. Mix on medium speed for about 5 minutes or knead with your hands until well combined. Cover tightly and set aside while you make the topping and the filling.

5. **To make the filling:** In a small bowl, stir together the butter, brown sugar, and cinnamon until it forms a smooth paste. Set aside.

6. **To make the topping:** In a small saucepan over low heat, stir together the brown sugar, butter, honey, salt, and chopped pecans until the sugar melts. This happens quickly, so do not walk away from your saucepan! Once the sugar is melted, pour the mixture into a cast-iron skillet or a baking dish that you'll use to bake the rolls.

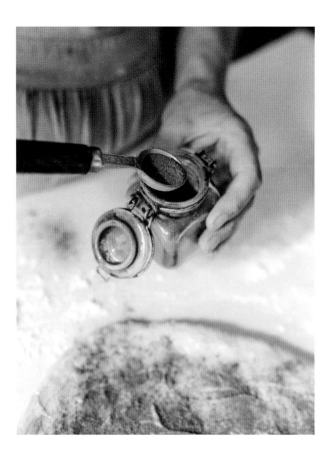

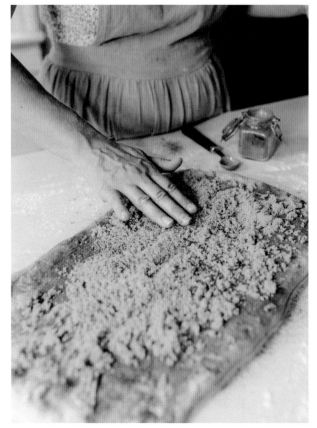

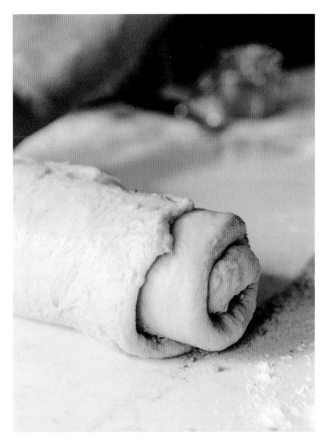

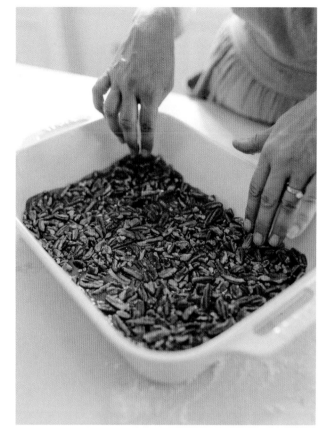

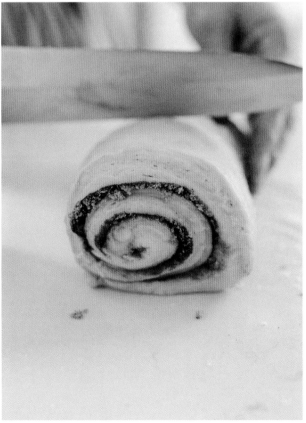

7. Lightly dust your working surface with flour, and then tip the dough out onto it. Roll it into a rectangle about 1/4 inch thick. Spread the filling over the dough.

8. Working from the long edge, roll the dough tightly into a long log and then slice it into twelve equal portions. Place the rolls in the cast-iron skillet or baking dish on top of the pecan mixture.

9. Bake the buns for about 25 minutes, or until lightly brown on top and cooked through. Allow them to cool for about 5 minutes in the pan, then run a knife along the edge of the pan and serve. To store, cover with foil or place inside aan airtight container and keep refrigerated.

PREP TIME:	BAKE TIME:	RISE TIME:	YIELD:
30 MINUTES	**25 MINUTES**	**8 HOURS**	**MAKES 12 ROLLS**

Double Chocolate Sweet Rolls

These sweet rolls celebrate the heady indulgence of chocolate. There's a chocolate dough, sweetened with the lightest swirl of honey. Then comes a sweet, butter-cocoa spread to fill the dough. If that's not enough (is it ever when chocolate is involved?), you top that filling with even more—this time, with coarsely chopped semi-sweet chocolate chunks. A sweet cream glaze tops the rolls, and the result is beyond delicious.

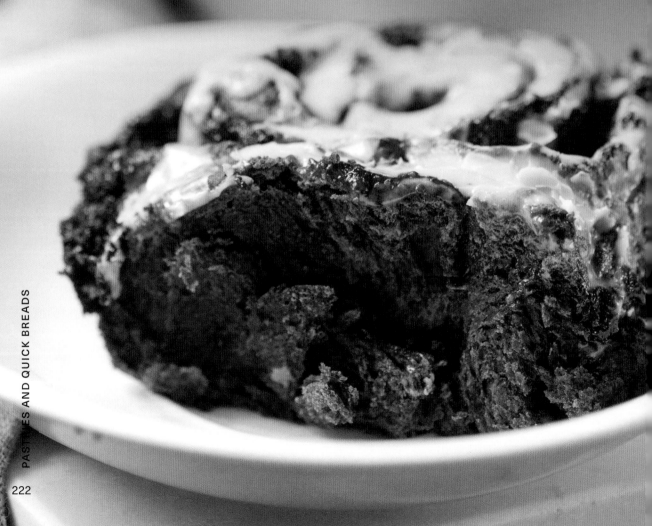

FOR THE DOUGH

1/2 cup (100 grams) active sourdough starter

1/2 cup (118 grams) lukewarm water

1/2 cup (113 grams) coconut oil, melted

1/2 (168 grams) honey

2 eggs

3 1/2 cups (490 grams) all-purpose flour

1/2 cup (45 grams) natural cocoa powder

1 teaspoon (5 grams) baking soda

1 teaspoon (5 grams) baking powder

1/2 teaspoon salt

FOR THE FILLING

1 cup (200 grams) sugar

1/2 cup (113 grams) butter, plus more for the baking dish

1/4 cup (23 grams) natural cocoa powder

1 cup (142 grams) semi-sweet chocolate chunks

FOR THE GLAZE

1/4 cup (60 grams) heavy cream

1 1/2 cups (185 grams) powdered sugar

1 teaspoon (5 grams) vanilla extract

1   **To make the dough:** In the bowl of a stand mixer equipped with a dough hook, combine the starter, water, coconut oil, honey, and eggs. Add the flour and cocoa powder and mix on low speed for about 10 minutes, or until the dough is smooth and elastic and pulls away cleanly from the sides of the bowl.

2   Cover the bowl tightly and let it rise overnight for 8 hours, or until doubled.

3   The next day, return the dough to the stand mixer and sprinkle the baking soda, baking powder, and salt over the dough. Mix for 5 minutes, or until the dough becomes stretchy.

4   Preheat the oven to 375°F and lightly grease a 9-by-13-inch baking dish with butter.

5   **To make the filling:** In a small bowl, stir together the sugar, butter, and cocoa powder until a uniform paste forms. Set aside.

6   Lightly dust your working surface with flour, and roll out the dough into a 12-by-16-inch rectangle. Spread filling evenly over the dough, and then sprinkle it with semi-sweet chocolate chunks.

7   Working from the short end, roll the dough into a tight log. Cut the dough at 1-inch intervals to form twelve rolls (see roll-slicing tutorial on page 215). Place them in the prepared baking dish and transfer to the oven. Bake for about 25 minutes, or until cooked through and beginning to brown at the edges.

8   Allow the rolls to cool in their pan for about 10 minutes.

9   **To make the glaze:** While the rolls cool, in a small bowl, mix the cream, powdered sugar, and vanilla until smooth.

10 Pour the glaze over the rolls and serve. Store any leftovers in an airtight container at room temperature for up to 3 days.

PREP TIME:
30 MINUTES

BAKE TIME:
30 MINUTES

RISE TIME:
**10 HOURS, PLUS 8 TO 13 HOURS
CHILLING TIME IN FRIDGE**

YIELD:
**MAKES 5
CROISSANTS**

Chocolate Croissants

Making croissants is a lesson in patience and perseverance. It takes time and attention. These virtues are worth pursuing in a society where instant gratification is the norm. If it comes with the reward of delicate, flaky layers of pastry filled with chocolate, that's all the better.

Allow plenty of time for this recipe, starting it a day ahead. The real trick is managing the temperature of both the butter and dough as you work. The way the two interact is the key to developing ultra-flaky layers, so keep them cool to the touch but pliable.

FOR THE DOUGH

1/2 cup (100 grams) active
sourdough starter

1 1/4 cup (305 grams) milk

1/4 cup (57 grams) butter,
plus more for the bowl

3 1/2 cups (490 grams) flour

1/4 cup (48 grams) sugar

2 teaspoons (12 grams) salt

FOR THE BUTTER LAYER

1 1/2 cups (339 grams) butter

FOR THE FILLING

1/2 cup (90 grams) semi-sweet
chocolate chips

FOR THE EGG WASH

1 egg yolk

1 tablespoon (15 grams) water

1 **To make the dough:** In the bowl of a stand mixer equipped with a dough hook, combine the starter, milk, and butter. Add the flour, sugar, and salt and mix on low speed for about 10 minutes, or until it pulls away from the sides of the bowl and becomes glossy and stretchy.

2 Lightly grease a large mixing bowl with butter. Transfer the dough to the prepared bowl and cover it tightly. Allow the dough to sit at room temperature for about 8 hours.

3 Transfer the dough to the fridge and let it chill for 1 hour. Then, lightly dust your working surface with flour and roll out the dough to a 10-by-16-inch rectangle. Cover tightly and transfer to the fridge for at least 4 hours and up to overnight (at least 8 hours).

(recipe continued on next page)

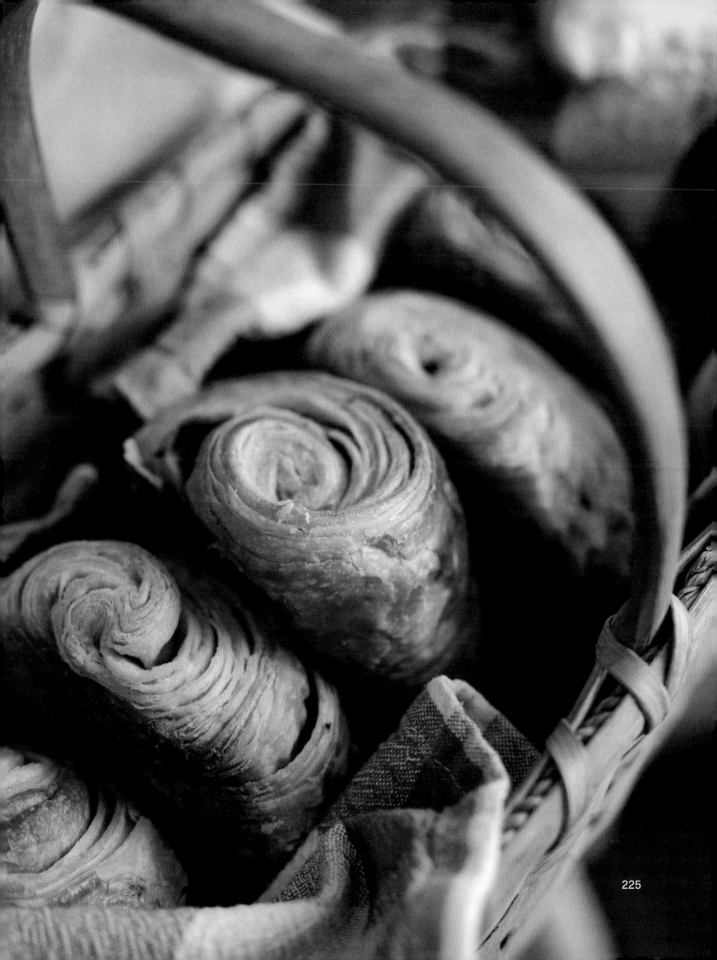

225

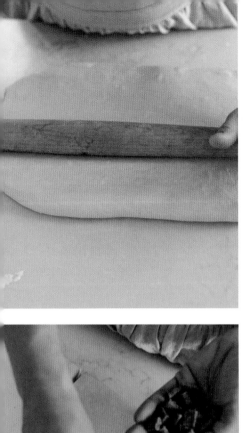
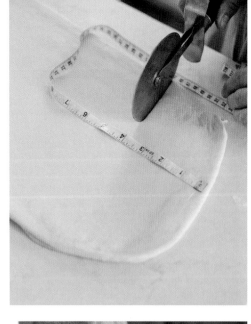
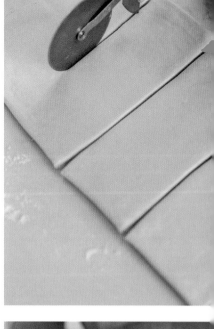
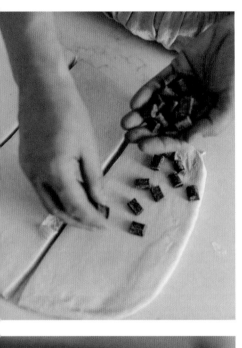
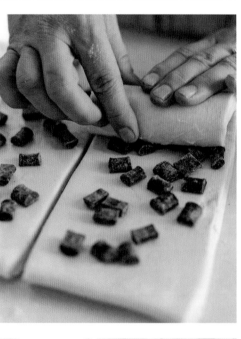
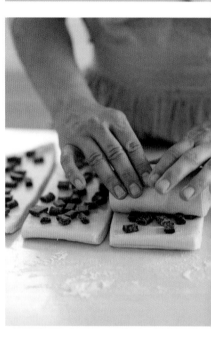
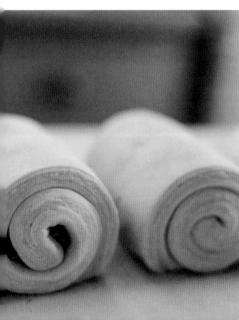
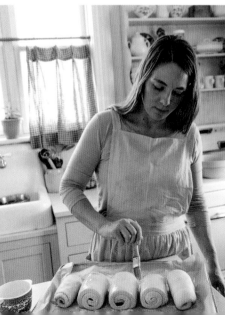
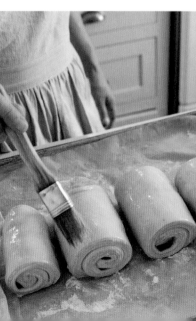

4 **To make the butter layer:** While the dough is in the fridge, cut the butter into slabs about 1/4 inch thick. Lay them out on parchment paper to create an 8-by-10-inch rectangle. Fold the sides of the parchment up around the butter to make a packet that envelops the butter. Using a rolling pin, roll over the packet until the butter forms a uniform slab. Transfer the butter to the fridge and allow it to chill for 15 to 30 minutes, until it's the consistency of the dough.

5 When the dough and the butter have roughly the same consistency, with neither being harder or softer than the other, pull both out of the fridge. Unwrap the dough and the butter, then place the butter in the middle of the dough. Fold the sides over so that the dough envelops the butter. Pinch the edges down so that the dough fully encases the butter.

6 Roll the dough out to a 10-by-16-inch rectangle. If the dough springs back or resists, put it in the fridge to let the gluten relax. Fold the dough into thirds, then tap it with the rolling pin to help soften the butter and make it pliable.

7 Repeat this process twice, ensuring the butter remains pliable but not too warm. Wrap the dough and return it to the fridge for 3 to 4 hours more.

8 **To make the filling:** Roll out the dough into a 10-by-20-inch rectangle. Cut the dough crosswise at 4-inch intervals to form five rectangles of dough. Starting at the short edge, sprinkle chocolate chips at the edge of the dough, and then roll the dough up to create a short, fat log.

9 Place them onto a baking sheet lined with parchment paper. Cover the croissants with a tea towel and allow them to rise for 2 hours at room temperature. Next, transfer them to the fridge for 1 hour.

10 Preheat the oven to 375°F.

11 **To make the egg wash:** In a small bowl, whisk together the egg yolk and water.

12 Remove the baking sheet from the fridge. Brush the croissants with egg wash, then bake them for 30 minutes, or until golden. Allow them to cool, then serve. Store in a ziplock bag or an airtight container with a lid so that they don't dry out.

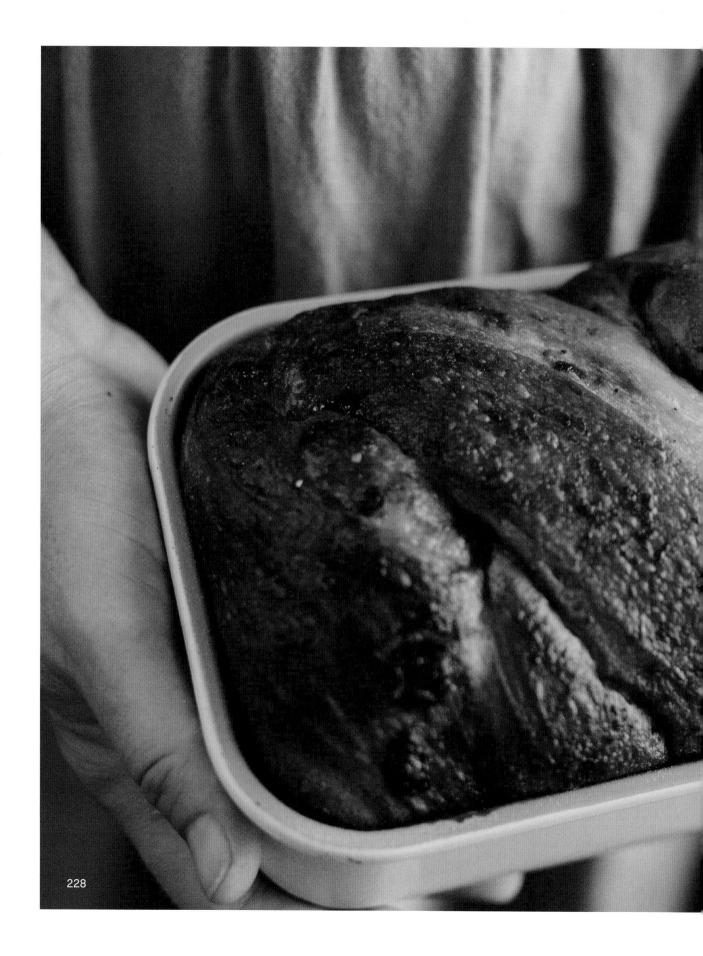

CHAPTER 7

Sweet Treats

THERE'S RARELY A DAY in my home where the kitchen is silent and empty. Our farmhouse seems to constantly buzz with activity. The kitchen is a natural place to congregate. The aroma of baked bread fills the air on most days, and on those that it doesn't, the perfume of freshly baked cookies and sweet treats takes its place.

These treats are also wonderful to share. Crafting something that takes the time and effort brings a better and more complex flavor to many classic sweets. It also shows care for the people you love. Taking the time to bake cookies for a school gathering or a cake for a special birthday instead of stopping by the store is another way to show people that you value them. It shows that they are worth your time, effort, and attention.

For some sweet treats, you'll want to use an active sourdough starter that's bubbly and full of life. Blueberry Babka (page 237) and the Sourdough Chocolate Cake (page 253) benefit from the extra boost that active yeast gives in a proofed starter. For other recipes, such as cookies, sourdough discard is best. These recipes benefit from sourdough's pleasant tart flavor but do not need the boost of lively yeast.

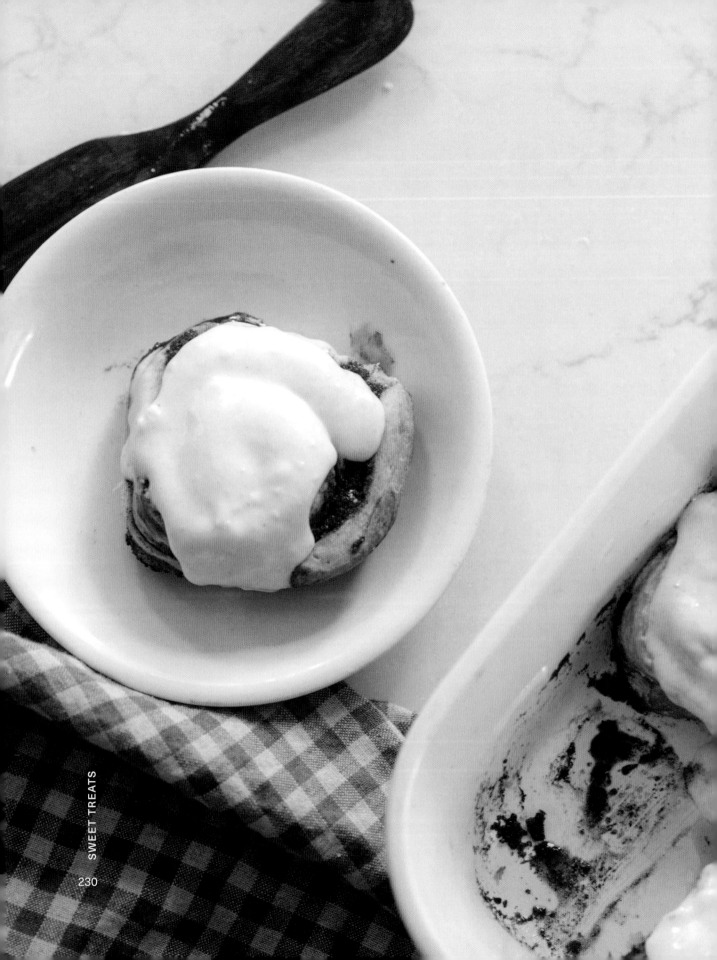

SWEET TREATS

230

PREP TIME:
20 MINUTES

BAKE TIME:
25 MINUTES

RISE TIME:
8 HOURS

YIELD:
MAKES 12 ROLLS

Cinnamon Rolls

These soft rolls with layers of cinnamon sugar baked until golden brown and gooey and topped with cream cheese icing are the ultimate breakfast treat. The fermentation process gives the cinnamon buns a greater depth of flavor for the perfect balance of sweet, sour, and oh, so soft. You have to try this delicious recipe.

Because the dough is quite soft, you'll want to avoid pressing down on it with a knife. I recommend using string or unflavored dental floss to cut the cinnamon rolls (see roll-slicing tutorial on page 215).

FOR THE DOUGH

1/2 cup (100 grams) active sourdough starter

1/2 cup (118 grams) water

1/2 cup (113 grams) melted coconut oil, plus more for the bowl

1/2 cup (168 grams) honey

2 eggs

4 cups (560 grams) all-purpose flour

1 teaspoon baking soda

1 teaspoon baking powder

1/2 teaspoon salt

FOR THE FILLING

1 cup (200 grams) brown sugar

1/2 cup (113 grams) butter, at room temperature

2 tablespoons (16 grams) cinnamon

FOR THE TOPPING

6 ounces (170 grams) cream cheese

1/2 cup (120 grams) heavy cream

1/2 cup maple syrup (160 grams) or honey (168 grams)

2 teaspoons (10 grams) vanilla extract

1   **To make the dough:** In the bowl of a stand mixer equipped with a dough hook, combine the starter, water, coconut oil, honey, and eggs. Add the flour and mix together until smooth, glossy, and the dough passes the windowpane test (see page 13).

2   Grease a large bowl with more coconut oil, add the dough, and cover. Allow to rest in a warm place overnight, at least 8 hours, or until doubled.

3   The next day, preheat the oven to 375°F.

(recipe continued on next page)

4   Return the dough to the bowl of the stand mixer and add the baking soda, baking powder, and salt. Mix on medium speed for about 5 minutes, or knead with your hands, until well combined.

5   **To make the filling:** In a small bowl, stir together the brown sugar, butter, and cinnamon.

6   Lightly dust your working surface with flour and roll out the dough into a 1/4-inch-thick rectangle.

7   Spread the filling evenly over the dough. Roll the dough up as tightly as you can. When you get to the end, pinch the seam closed.

8   Slice to make twelve even rolls, and place them in a well-seasoned 14-inch cast-iron skillet or 9x13 baking dish.

9   Bake for 20 to 25 minutes, or until lightly browned and cooked through. Allow them to cool a bit.

10 **To make the topping:** In a medium saucepan over medium heat, the add cream cheese, heavy cream, maple syrup or honey, and vanilla. Stir until combined. Use an immersion blender to get the frosting extra smooth, if desired.

11 Pour the mixture over the cinnamon rolls and serve. To store, cover with foil or place inside a glass container with an airtight lid and keep refrigerated up to a week.

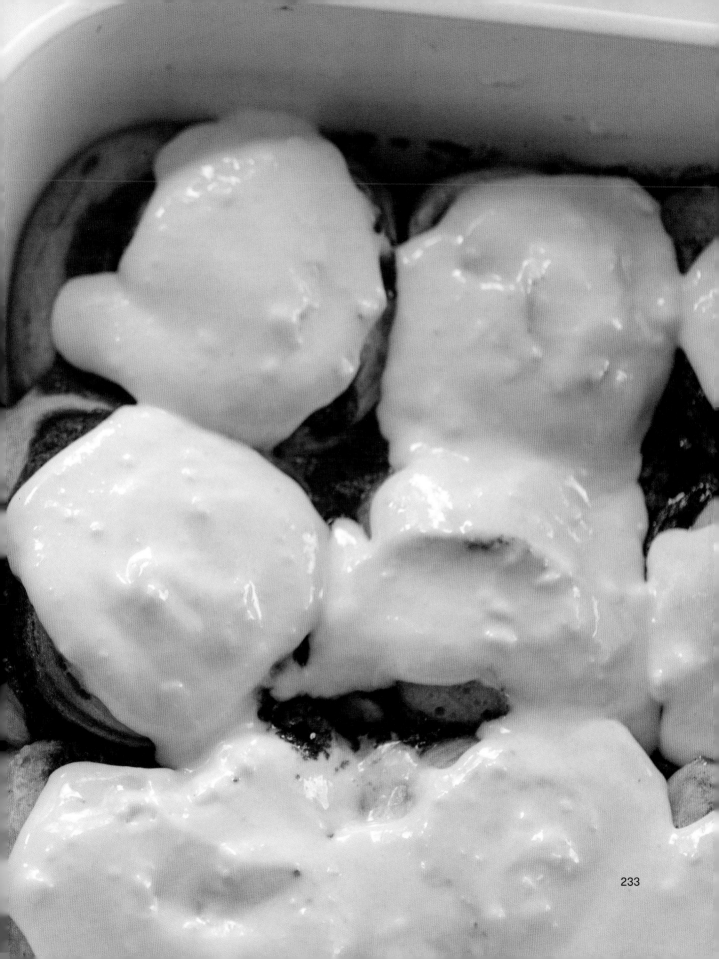

233

Strawberry Shortcakes with Maple Whipped Cream

Early on summer mornings, I head out to milk the cows while it's still dark. The sun begins to rise over the horizon while the veil of morning fog lifts, signaling the beginning of another day. I strain the milk into big mason jars and tuck them into the fridge. Within a few hours, the cream rises to the top—deliciously sweet and fresh. It's perfect when you combine it with ripe summer strawberries still warm from the early morning sun.

Together, they make the most divine strawberry shortcake. Wait for the shortcakes to cool completely before you slice them; otherwise, they might crumble to pieces. Additionally, ensure your butter is very cold, or you might find the shortcakes dense rather than tender.

FOR THE SHORTCAKES

3 cups (420 grams) all-purpose flour

4 1/2 teaspoons (21 grams) baking powder

1 teaspoon (6 grams) salt

3/4 cup (170 grams) cold butter, cut into pieces

1/3 cup (83 grams) sourdough discard

1/2 cup (160 grams) maple syrup

1/3 cup (80 grams) cold heavy cream, plus more for brushing

1 large egg

2 teaspoons (10 grams) vanilla extract

Coarse sugar, for sprinkling

FOR THE STRAWBERRY SAUCE

2 cups (300 grams) strawberries, coarsely chopped

1 tablespoon (20 grams) maple syrup

FOR THE WHIPPED CREAM

2 cups (480 grams) heavy cream

2 tablespoons (40 grams) maple syrup

(recipe continued on next page)

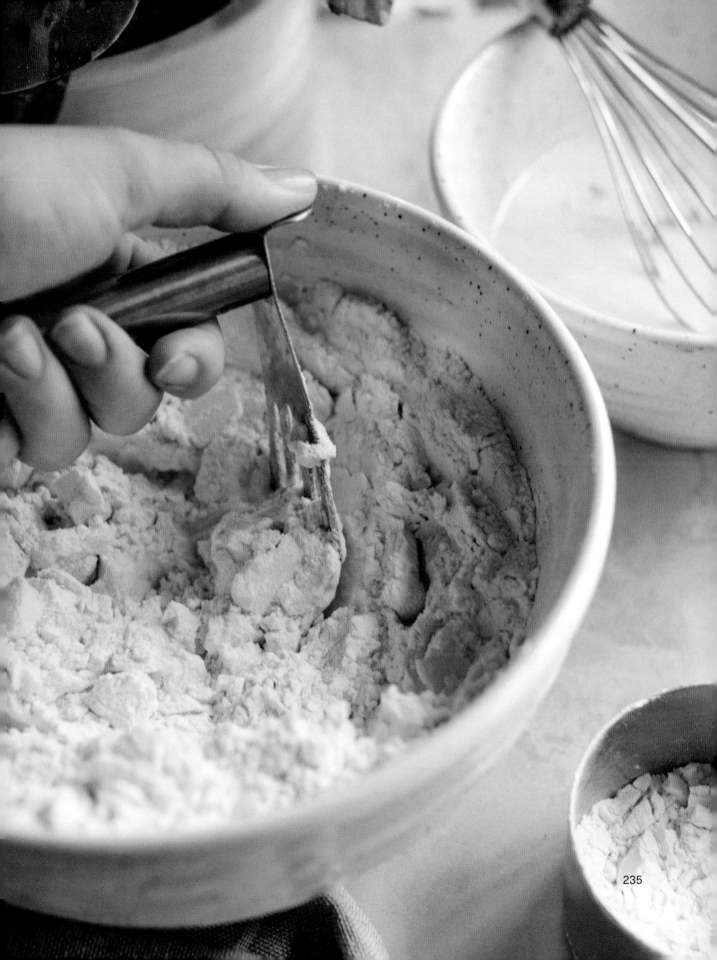

1   Preheat the oven to 375°F and line a rimmed baking sheet with parchment paper.

2   **To make the shortcakes:** In a large mixing bowl, stir together the flour, baking powder, and salt. Cut in the diced butter with a pastry blender or by hand until the texture turns coarse with pea-sized bits of butter.

3   In a separate large bowl, whisk together the sourdough discard, maple syrup, heavy cream, egg, and vanilla until they form a smooth slurry. Pour the cream mixture into the dry ingredients, then stir with a fork to bring it together. Knead by hand to incorporate any dry bits of flour until you form a uniform dough.

4   Scoop up a 1/2 cup of dough, then tap it onto the prepared baking sheet. Repeat with the rest of the dough. Brush a little cream onto the top of the biscuits and sprinkle generously with coarse sugar.

5   Bake for 20 to 25 minutes, or until the shortcakes are lightly golden on the top. Place them on a wire rack to cool while you prepare the strawberry sauce and whipped cream.

6   **To make the sauce:** In a medium saucepan, add the berries and maple syrup and crush the berries lightly with a wooden spoon. Bring to a simmer for a few minutes, stirring frequently until the sauce thickens slightly. Allow to cool before serving.

7   **To make the whipped cream:** In the bowl of a stand mixer fitted with the whisk attachment, whip the heavy cream and maple syrup on medium-high speed until it forms stiff peaks.

8   Slice the shortcakes in half and then top them with strawberry sauce and whipped cream. Serve immediately.

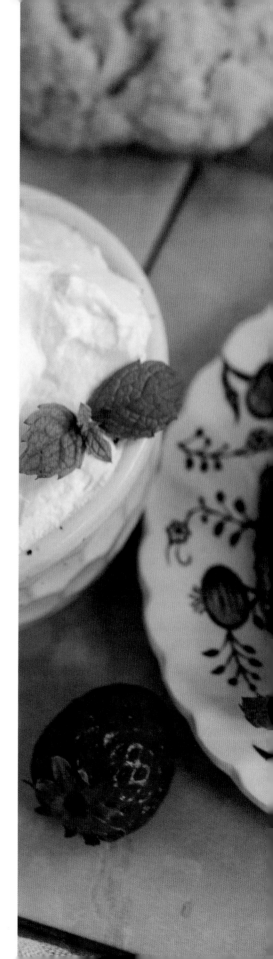

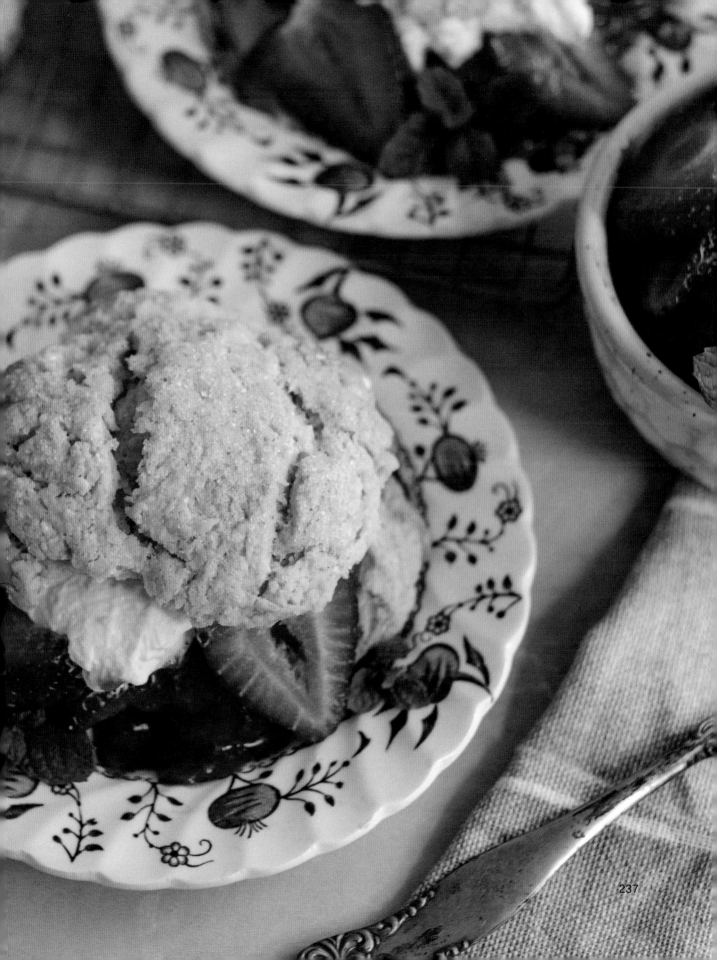

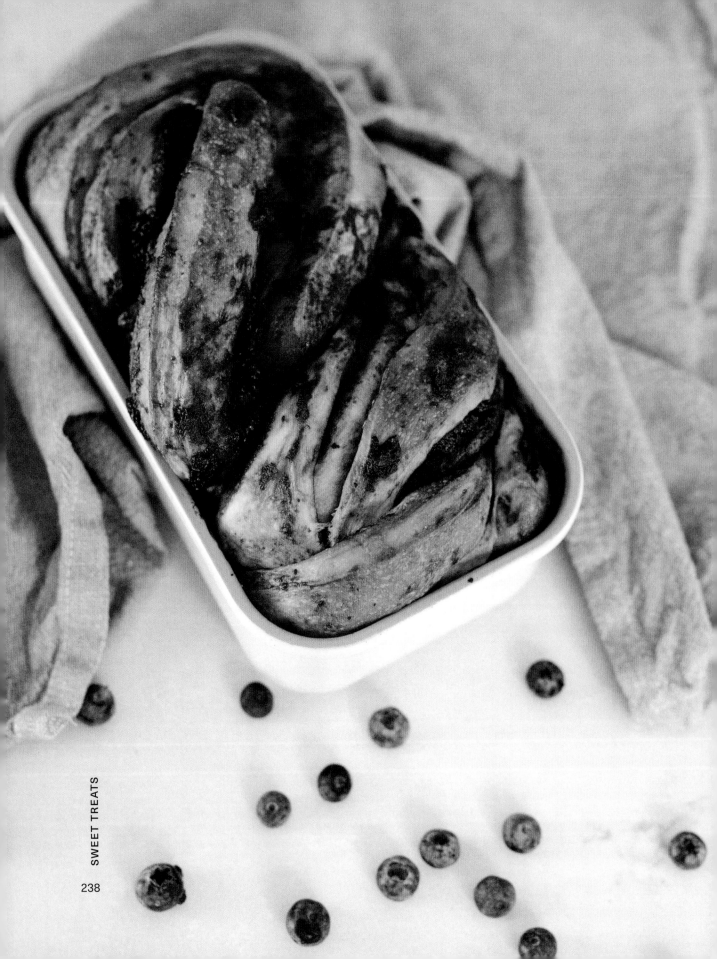

PREP TIME:
45 TO 60 MINUTES

BAKE TIME:
45 MINUTES

RISE TIME:
**12 HOURS, PLUS 8 TO 12
HOURS OF CHILLING TIME**

YIELD:
MAKES 2 LOAVES

Blueberry Babka

Blueberries are at their peak in late summer, during those final hot days before the season fades to fall. Baskets of them fill the kitchen, and we relish the simple pleasure of eating them by the handful. There are too many, of course, and sooner or later, they find their way into baked goods.

This babka starts as a basic sourdough sweet bread—fortified with milk, eggs, and plenty of butter. Then, you simmer the berries with a few spoonfuls of sugar, just long enough so they lose their form to the heat and turn into a luscious filling. Once baked, the blueberry seeps into the crumb of the babka, creating gorgeous purple stripes. It's sensational, especially served with a mug of hot coffee touched with fresh cream.

FOR THE DOUGH

1 cup (200 grams) active
    sourdough starter

1/2 cup (122 grams) milk

10 tablespoons (140 grams)
    butter, plus more for the pan

4 eggs

3 1/2 cups (490 grams) bread flour

1/4 cup (48 grams) sugar

1 1/2 teaspoons (9 grams) salt

FOR THE FILLING

16 ounces (450 grams)
    blueberries

1 cup (200 grams) sugar

FOR THE EGG WASH

1 egg yolk

1 tablespoon (15 grams) water

1 **To make the dough:** In the bowl of a stand mixer equipped with the dough hook, combine the starter, milk, butter, and eggs. Add flour, sugar, and salt and mix on low speed for 10 to 15 minutes, or until the dough turns glossy and pulls away from the sides of the bowl.

2 Cover the bowl tightly and let it sit in a warm spot in your kitchen for 8 hours, or until doubled. Transfer to the fridge overnight, about 8 to 12 hours. The dough should feel stiffer but still be pliable.

3 **To make the filling:** While the dough chills, in a medium saucepan over low heat, combine the blueberries and sugar. Cook, stirring occasionally, for about 30 minutes, or until thickened. Transfer to the fridge and chill until cold.

4 Dust your working surface lightly with flour and grease two loaf pans with butter.

(recipe continued on next page)

5 Tip the dough out onto your working surface, and then divide it into two equal portions. Working with one portion of dough at a time, roll it out to form a 10-by-14-inch rectangle. Spread the filling to the edge, allowing 1 inch of bare dough on the short end. Roll up your dough tightly from the opposite end, and then cut the roll down the middle and twist.

6 Place your babkas in the prepared loaf pans, cover them with a towel, and allow them to rise until doubled, about 4 hours.

7 Preheat the oven to 350°F.

8 **To make the egg wash:** In a small bowl, beat together the egg yolk and water.

9 Brush the babkas lightly with the egg wash and then transfer them to the oven and bake for 40 to 45 minutes, or until beautifully browned. Allow them to cool in the pan for 10 minutes, then transfer them to a wire rack to finish cooling completely before slicing and serving. Store in an airtight container or ziplock bag so the babka doesn't dry out. You can also throw them in the freezer for longer storage.

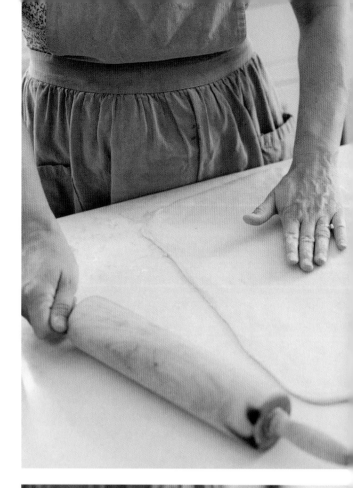

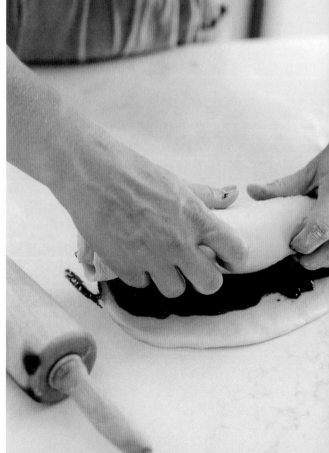

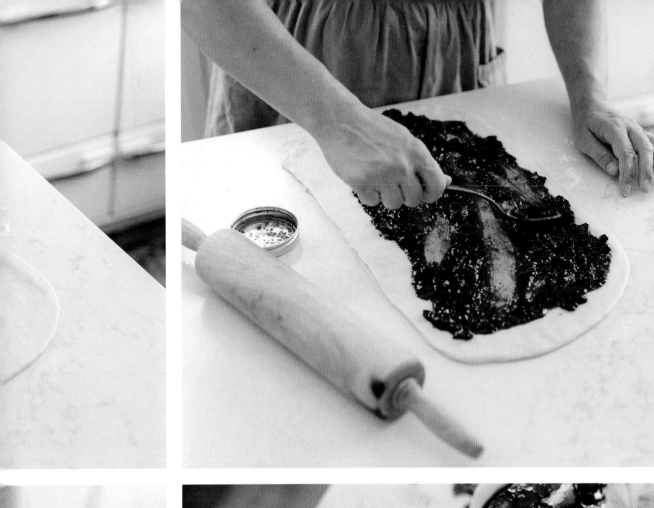

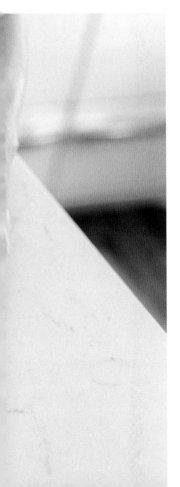

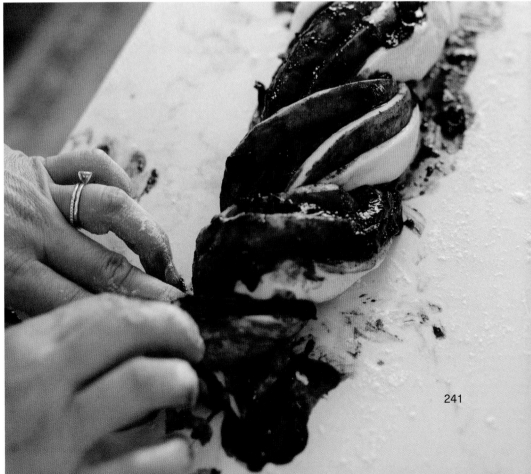

PREP TIME:
15 MIN

BAKE TIME:
45 MIN

RISE TIME:
0 MINUTES

YIELD:
**MAKES 1 CAKE
(ABOUT 16 SERVINGS)**

Einkorn Coffee Cake

I love the leisurely embrace of weekend mornings and the soft and unhurried warmth of the kitchen. When I can, I like to make something memorable that my family will enjoy. This coffee cake is a beautiful example. It's a vanilla-scented cake permeated with cinnamon sugar and topped with a delicate crumb. This recipe is excellent for a crowd—perfect for a weekend brunch or a holiday breakfast. There's certainly plenty to go around.

Einkorn flour gives the cake a lovely depth of flavor. Its nutty notes work well with the cinnamon and brown sugar. Cakes made with this ancient grain develop a soft, tender structure. Sourdough starter adds a subtle touch of acidity, which helps balance the cake's sweetness.

FOR THE CINNAMON FILLING

1 cup (130 grams)
   all-purpose einkorn flour

1/2 cup (100 grams) brown sugar

1 tablespoon (8 grams) cinnamon

FOR THE CRUMB TOPPING

1 1/2 cups (195 grams)
   all-purpose einkorn flour

3/4 cup (150 grams) brown sugar

1/2 cup (113 grams) butter, melted,
   plus more for the baking dish

2 tablespoons (16 grams) cinnamon

FOR THE CAKE

1 cup (225 grams) melted coconut oil

1 cup (192 grams) granulated sugar

1/2 cup (100 grams) brown sugar

1 cup (244 grams) milk

1/2 cup (100 grams) sourdough starter

1/2 cup (118 grams) water

3 eggs

2 teaspoons (10 grams) vanilla extract

3 1/2 cups (455 grams)
   all-purpose einkorn flour

3 teaspoons (17 grams) baking soda

1 teaspoon (6 grams) salt

1   Preheat the oven to 350°F and grease a 9-by-13-inch baking dish with butter.

2   **To make the cinnamon filling:** In a small bowl, stir together the flour, brown sugar, and cinnamon. Set aside.

3   **To make the crumb topping:** In medium bowl, stir together the flour, butter, sugar, and cinnamon. Set aside.

4   **To make the cake:** In the bowl of a stand mixer fitted with a paddle attachment, cream together the coconut oil, granulated sugar, and brown sugar until light and fluffy. Beat in the milk, starter, water, eggs, and vanilla. Then, slowly beat in the flour, salt, and baking soda until it forms a smooth batter.

5   Pour half the cake batter into the prepared baking dish, then spoon the cinnamon filling evenly over it. Pour the remaining cake batter over the filling. Sprinkle the crumb topping over the batter.

6   Bake for 45 minutes, or until a toothpick inserted into the center of the cake comes out clean and the cake turns golden at the edges.

7   Allow it to cool completely before slicing and serving. Store any leftovers in an airtight container at room temperature for up to 3 days.

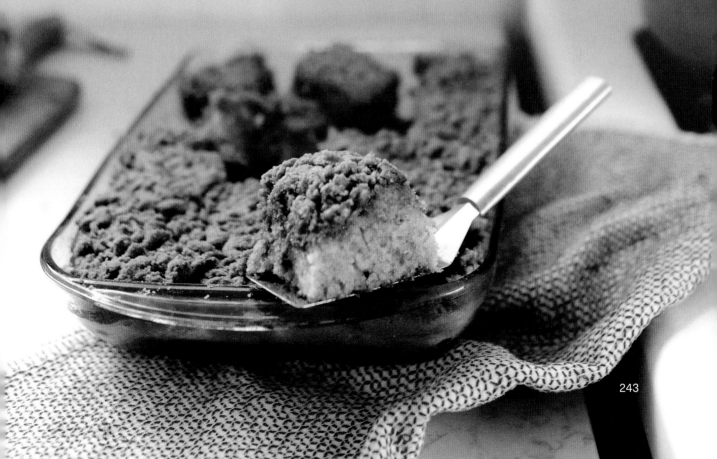

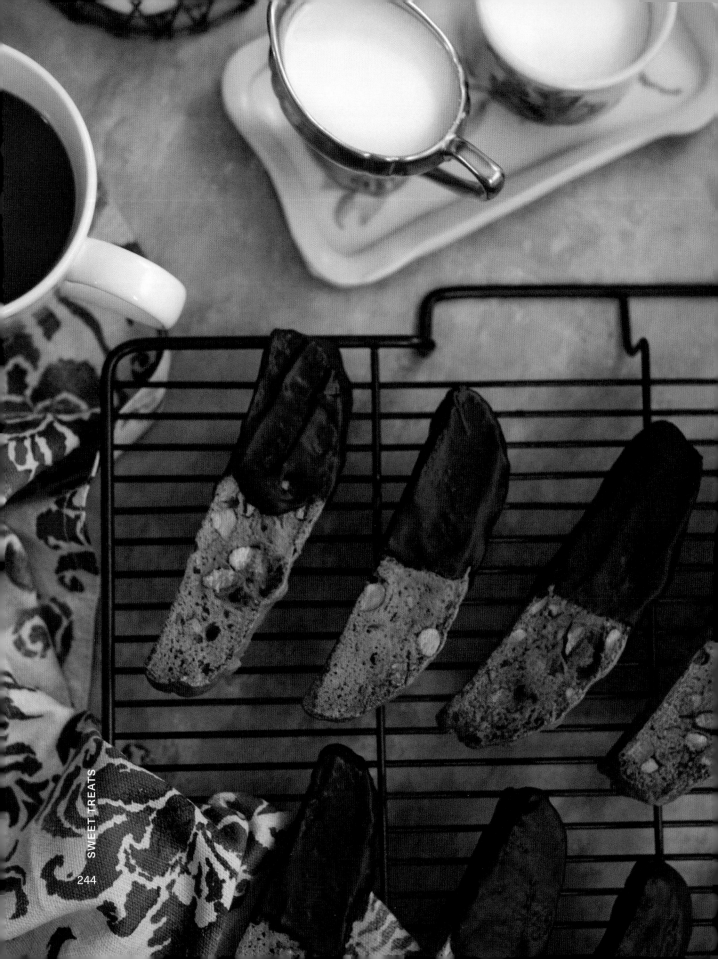

PREP TIME:
10 MINUTES

BAKE TIME:
55 MINUTES

RISE TIME:
30 MINUTES OF CHILLING TIME

YIELD:
MAKES ABOUT 24 BISCOTTI

Toasted Almond Biscotti

If I have a spare moment, I enjoy sitting at the kitchen table on a chilly autumn afternoon with a homemade pumpkin spice latté and a couple of these chocolate-dipped biscotti. The delicate cookie flavor pairs well with coffee. It lacks the overwhelming sweetness found in many other treats.

There are a few things that make this recipe irresistible. Toasting the almonds releases the nuts' oils and gives them a warm, buttery flavor. The sourdough starter lends a complex acidity that balances the biscotti's sweetness. Like traditional biscotti, you'll first bake them as a loaf, then slice them and bake them a second time, which allows them to crisp. It also helps preserve their shelf life.

FOR THE BISCOTTI

1 cup (140 grams)
   raw, whole almonds

1 1/3 cups (267 grams)
   packed brown sugar

1/4 cup (56 grams) olive oil

1/2 cup (125 grams) sourdough
   discard

2 large eggs

1 teaspoon (5 grams) vanilla extract

1 tablespoon (15 grams)
   almond extract

2 1/2 cups (350 grams)
   all-purpose flour

3/4 teaspoon (5 grams) salt

FOR THE CHOCOLATE COATING

2/3 cup (226 grams) semi-sweet
   chocolate chunks

1/4 teaspoon coconut oil

1   Preheat the oven to 325°F and line a rimmed baking sheet with parchment paper.

2   **To make the biscotti:** Spread the almonds evenly onto the prepared baking sheet and bake them for 8 to 12 minutes, or until toasted. Let the almonds cool to room temperature and then chop them coarsely.

3   In the bowl of a stand mixer equipped with the paddle attachment, combine the brown sugar and olive oil. Add the eggs one at a time and mix well, occasionally scraping down the sides of the bowl. Beat in the sourdough discard, vanilla, and almond extract. Working a little at a time, slowly incorporate the flour and salt until just combined. Add the almonds to the bowl and fold them in, taking care not to overmix the dough.

(recipe continued on next page)

4 Lightly dust your working surface with flour, then tip the dough onto it. Divide it into two equal portions, then form them into logs 3 1/2 to 4 inches wide. Cover the logs tightly in plastic wrap, then transfer them to the fridge and allow the dough to chill for 30 minutes.

5 Increase the oven temperature to 350°F. Transfer the chilled dough logs to a parchment-lined baking sheet and bake the biscotti dough for 30 minutes.

6 Let the biscotti loaves cool on the baking sheet for 15 to 20 minutes. Then, use a serrated bread knife to carefully cut the loaves crosswise into 1/2- to 3/4-inch-thick slices. Arrange the slices about 1 inch apart on the baking sheet. Return them to the oven and continue baking for another 10 minutes. Then, flip them and continue baking for 10 to 15 minutes more, or until crisp and baked through. Transfer the biscotti to a wire rack to cool completely.

7 **To make the coating:** While the biscotti cool, ina double boiler, combine the chocolate and coconut oil and stir until melted. (If you don't have a double boiler handy, put a glass bowl over a small saucepan with boiling water. The important thing is to gently melt the chocolate and coconut oil together!)

8 Dip the ends of the biscotti into the coating and then set on a square of parchment paper to cool.

9 Store in an airtight container at room temperature for up to 10 days.

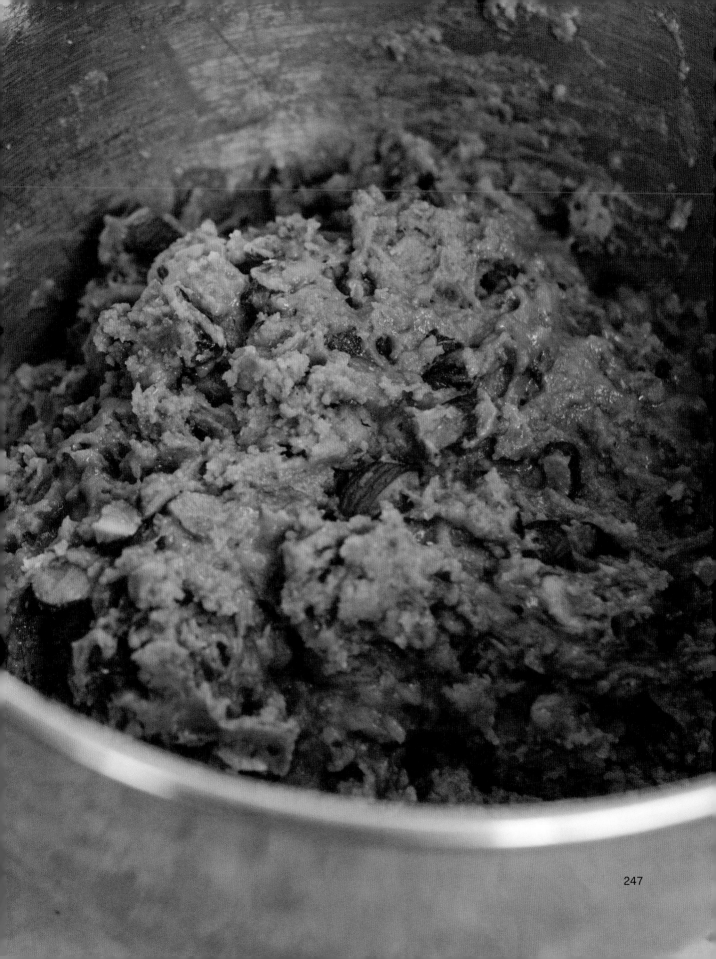

PREP TIME:
30 MINUTES

BAKE TIME:
10 MINUTES

RISE TIME:
**AT LEAST 1 HOUR
OF CHILLING TIME**

YIELD:
**MAKES ABOUT
24 COOKIES**

Sourdough Shortbread

At first glance, this shortbread may seem a little plain. There are no toasted nuts or indulgent pops of dark chocolate, nor any fancy glazes or frostings. It's simple, and that simplicity is precisely what makes this shortbread delightful. Every ingredient can shine. The rich, creamy flavor of butter comes through immediately, followed by a pointed, sharp, tart note from a spoonful of sourdough starter that provides depth. Finally, there's sweetness—just a little, and definitely not too much.

But perhaps the neatest aspect of this recipe is its flexibility. After mixing up the dough, you can shape it into a rectangle and store it in the fridge for up to 3 days before baking. This makes it perfect for planning ahead or for those times when you want freshly baked shortbread at a moment's notice. When you're ready to indulge, simply slice the chilled dough, pop it in the oven, and in no time, you'll be enjoying crisp, buttery shortbread cookies. Sometimes, when I'm feeling particularly indulgent, I might dip them in a little melted chocolate. You could, too.

1 1/2 cups (340 grams) butter, at room temperature

1 cup (192 grams) sugar

1/2 cup (125 grams) sourdough discard

2 teaspoons (10 grams) vanilla extract

3 1/2 cups (490 grams) all-purpose flour

1 teaspoon (6 grams) salt

1 In the bowl of a stand mixer equipped with the paddle attachment, whip the butter and sugar for about 5 minutes, or until light and fluffy. Add the sourdough discard and vanilla and mix until well combined.

2 Scrape down the bowl, then add in the flour and salt. Beat on low speed until the ingredients just come together, about 1 minute.

3 Lightly dust your working surface with flour, and then tip the dough out onto it. Press it into a rectangle about 1 inch thick. Wrap it tightly in plastic wrap and then transfer it to the fridge for at least 1 hour and up to 3 days.

4 When ready to bake, preheat the oven to 350ºF and line a rimmed baking sheet with parchment paper.

SWEET TREATS

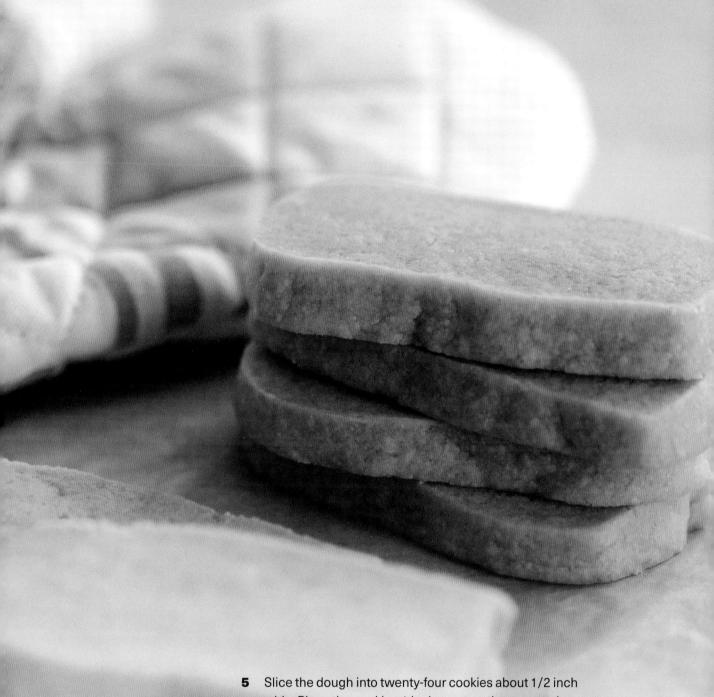

5   Slice the dough into twenty-four cookies about 1/2 inch wide. Place the cookies 1 inch apart on the prepared baking sheet and then transfer to the oven. Bake for 10 minutes, or until cooked through and beginning to turn golden at the edges.

6   Transfer the cookies to a wire rack and let them cool completely before serving. Store any leftovers in an airtight container at room temperature for up to 1 week.

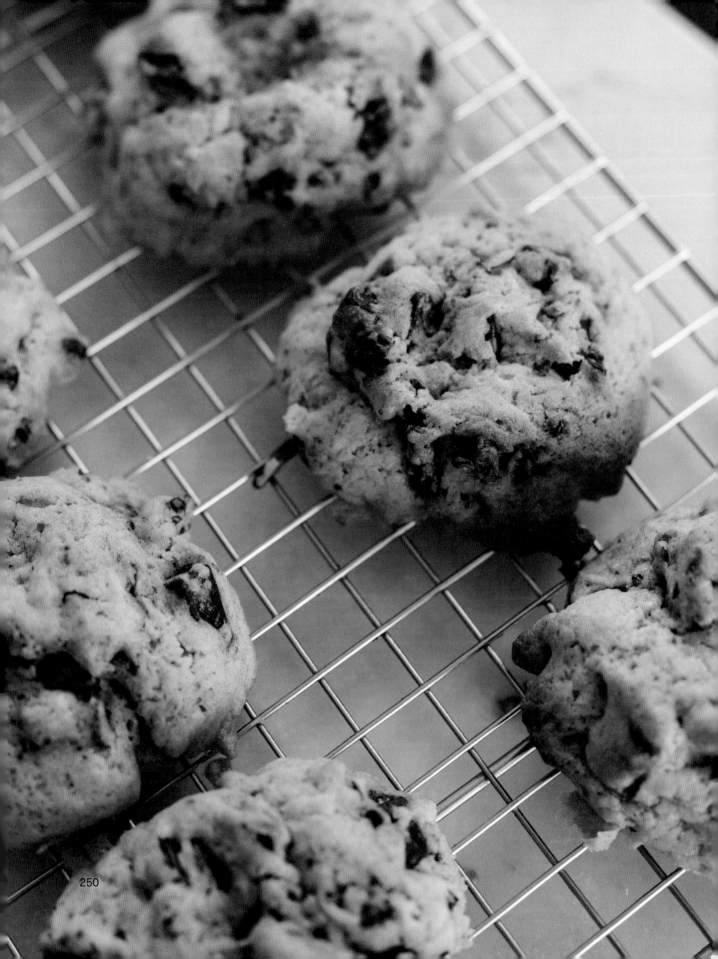

250

PREP TIME:
10 MINUTES

BAKE TIME:
10 MINUTES

RISE TIME:
0 MINUTES

YIELD:
**MAKES ABOUT
24 COOKIES**

Toasted Pecan and Chocolate Chunk Cookies

It's hard to improve upon the iconic chocolate chip cookie. In this version, toasted pecans, dense chunks of dark chocolate, and a little sourdough discard completely transform this classic American treat. It tastes divine. The sourdough discard brings a hint of acidity that balances the chocolate's sweet, bitter notes. The cookies have a delicious, soft, buttery quality that works with a mug of coffee just as well as a glass of fresh milk.

If you're pressed for time, tuck the cookie dough in the fridge for up to 3 days and bake the cookies when you can. It's a lifesaver in a busy household like mine.

1 cup (about 100 grams) pecan halves

1 cup (226 grams) butter

1/2 cup (96 grams) granulated sugar

1/2 cup (100 grams) brown sugar

1 egg

3/4 cup (188 grams) sourdough discard

2 teaspoons (10 grams) vanilla extract

2 cups (280 grams) all-purpose flour

1 teaspoon (6 grams) salt

1/2 teaspoon baking soda

1/4 teaspoon baking powder

2 cups (about 340 grams) semi-sweet chocolate chunks

1. Preheat the oven to 325°F and line a rimmed baking sheet with parchment paper.

2. Spread the pecan halves evenly onto the tray and bake for 8 to 12 minutes, or until toasted. Let the pecans cool to room temperature and then chop them coarsely.

3. Increase the oven's temperature to 350°F and line the rimmed baking sheet with a piece of parchment paper.

4. In the bowl of a stand mixer equipped with the paddle attachment, cream together the butter, granulated sugar, and brown sugar for a few minutes, until light and fluffy. Add the egg and beat until well incorporated. Add the sourdough discard and vanilla and mix until just combined.

5. In a separate medium bowl, whisk together the flour, salt, baking soda, and baking powder.

6. Add the dry ingredients to the wet ingredients about one-third at a time and mix until just incorporated. Then, fold in the chocolate.

7. Scoop the dough into 2-tablespoon balls and drop them on the prepared baking sheet about 2 inches apart. Bake for 10 minutes, or until the edges turn golden.

8. Transfer to a wire rack to cool completely before serving. Store the cookies in an airtight container at room temperature for up to 1 week.

Snickerdoodles

When I'm feeding my starter, I like to save the discard—folding it into cookie batter seems like a perfect solution. There's no waste, and, instead, you have a lovely treat to share. These crisp-edged, cinnamon-coated cookies are ready just in time for an afternoon snack.

Snickerdoodles taste sharp and tangy thanks to the inclusion of cream of tartar. Still, a little sourdough starter goes a long way to amplify that flavor. This version is a favorite in our house.

FOR THE COOKIES

2 3/4 cups (385 grams) all-purpose flour

2 teaspoons (10 grams) cream of tartar

1 1/2 teaspoons cinnamon

1 teaspoon (5 grams) baking soda

1 teaspoon (6 grams) salt

1 1/2 cups (288 grams) sugar

1 cup (226 grams) butter

2 eggs

1/2 cup (125 grams) sourdough discard

2 teaspoons (10 grams) vanilla extract

FOR THE CINNAMON-SUGAR COATING

1/4 cup (50 grams) sugar

1 tablespoon (8 grams) cinnamon

1   Preheat the oven to 400°F and line a baking sheet with parchment paper.

2   **To make the cookies:** In a medium bowl, whisk together the flour, cream of tartar, cinnamon, baking soda, and salt. Set aside.

3   In the bowl of a stand mixer equipped with the paddle attachment, cream together the sugar and butter for 3 to 5 minutes on high, or until light and fluffy. Add the eggs and beat until well incorporated. Add the sourdough discard and vanilla and beat until just combined.

4   Slowly add the dry ingredients to the wet ingredients, mixing well and scraping down the sides of the bowl as needed.

SWEET TREATS

5 **To make the coating:** In a small bowl, stir together the sugar and cinnamon and set aside.

6 Scoop the dough into 2-tablespoon balls and then roll it in the cinnamon-sugar mixture. Repeat for the rest of the dough, placing the coated dough balls about 2 inches apart on the prepared baking sheet.

7 Bake the cookies for 10 to 12 minutes, or until they begin to turn golden at the edges.

8 Remove from the oven and immediately transfer to wire racks to cool. Store at room temperature in an airtight container for up to 1 week.

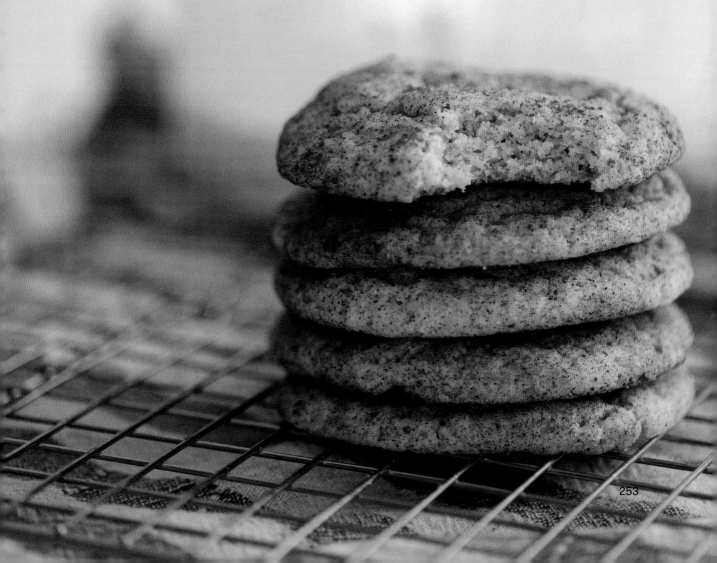

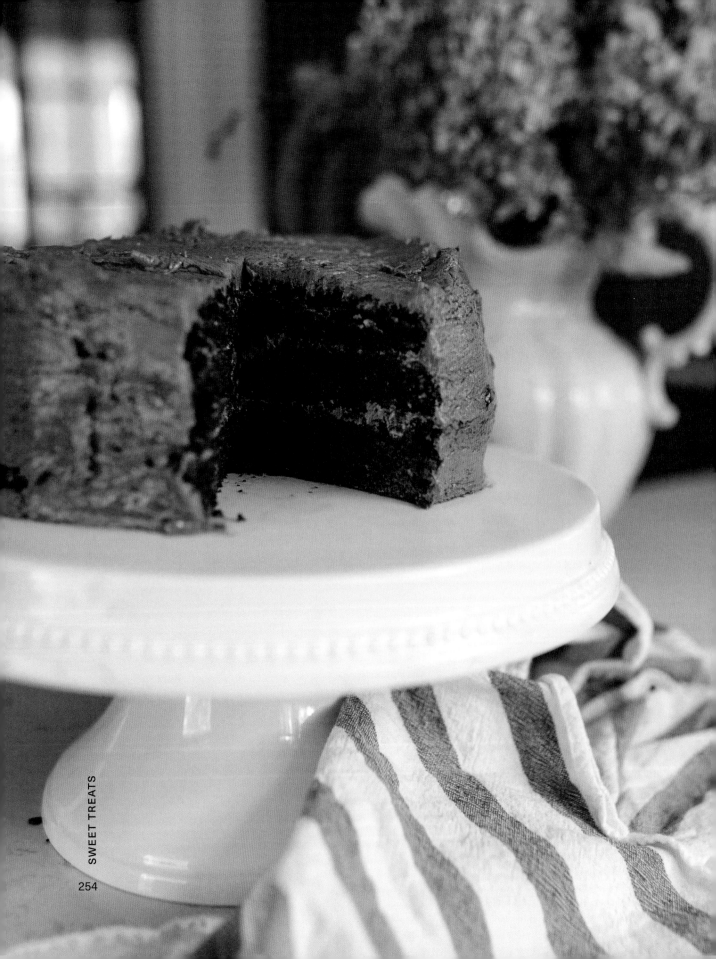

PREP TIME:
20 MINUTES

BAKE TIME:
35 MINUTES

RISE TIME:
12 HOURS

YIELD:
**MAKES 2 (9-INCH)
CAKE LAYERS**

Sourdough Chocolate Cake

While it may seem like an odd combination, chocolate and sourdough are truly made for each other. Sourdough's tart, acidic flavor adds a complex depth to chocolate's deep, bitter notes while also balancing its innate sweetness. As a result, you'll find that this chocolate cake somehow tastes richer and more complex than most. It's perfect for birthdays and potlucks.

Starting the cake batter the night before might seem like extra work, but it helps the batter develop flavor, tenderness, and structure. It also makes the cake easier to digest. When you slather it with a butter-rich cocoa frosting, you'll realize that the extra effort comes with its rewards. I like to use rapadura sugar in this cake, a minimally processed cane sugar with a lovely amber color and mineral-like flavor that lends complexity to the cake. You can certainly substitute granulated sugar in a pinch.

FOR THE CAKE

2 cups (280 grams) all-purpose flour

1 cup (236 grams) water

1/2 cup (113 grams) coconut oil,
   plus more for the pans

1/2 cup (100 grams) sourdough starter

2 cups (384 grams) rapadura sugar

1 teaspoon (6 grams) salt

1 teaspoon (5 grams) finely ground coffee

1 cup (244 grams) whole milk

3/4 cup (75 grams) cocoa powder

2 eggs

2 teaspoons (10 grams) vanilla extract

2 teaspoons (10 grams) baking soda

FOR THE FROSTING

1 cup (226 grams) salted butter, at room
   temperature

3 cups (360 grams) powdered sugar

1/2 cup (48 grams) cocoa powder

3 tablespoons (45 grams) heavy cream,
   plus more as needed

2 teaspoons (10 grams) vanilla extract

(recipe continued on next page)

1   **To make the cake:** In a medium mixing bowl, stir together the flour, water, coconut oil, and sourdough starter. Cover the bowl tightly and allow it to sit for 12 hours.

2   Preheat the oven to 350°F and grease two 9-inch cake pans.

3   In a separate large bowl, stir together the rapadura sugar, salt, and coffee. Beat in the milk, cocoa powder, eggs, and vanilla. Next, whisk in the sourdough mixture and baking soda into the cocoa mixture until it forms a smooth batter.

4   Pour the cake batter evenly into the two cake pans. Bake for 30 to 35 minutes, or until a toothpick inserted into the center of the cake comes out clean. Allow the cakes to cool in their pans for 10 minutes, then turn them onto a wire rack to cool completely.

5   **To make the frosting:** While the cake cools, inthe bowl of a stand mixer equipped with a whisk attachment, beat the butter on high speed for a few minutes until it becomes light and fluffy. Turn the mixer speed to low and slowly beat in the powdered sugar, cocoa powder, heavy cream, and vanilla until uniformly incorporated. Increase the speed to medium and whip the frosting until light and fluffy, adding more heavy cream if the frosting seems stiff.

6   Frost the cake and serve. Save the leftover cake by storing in an airtight plastic or glass container to prevent it from drying out and store for 1 to 2 days at room temperature.

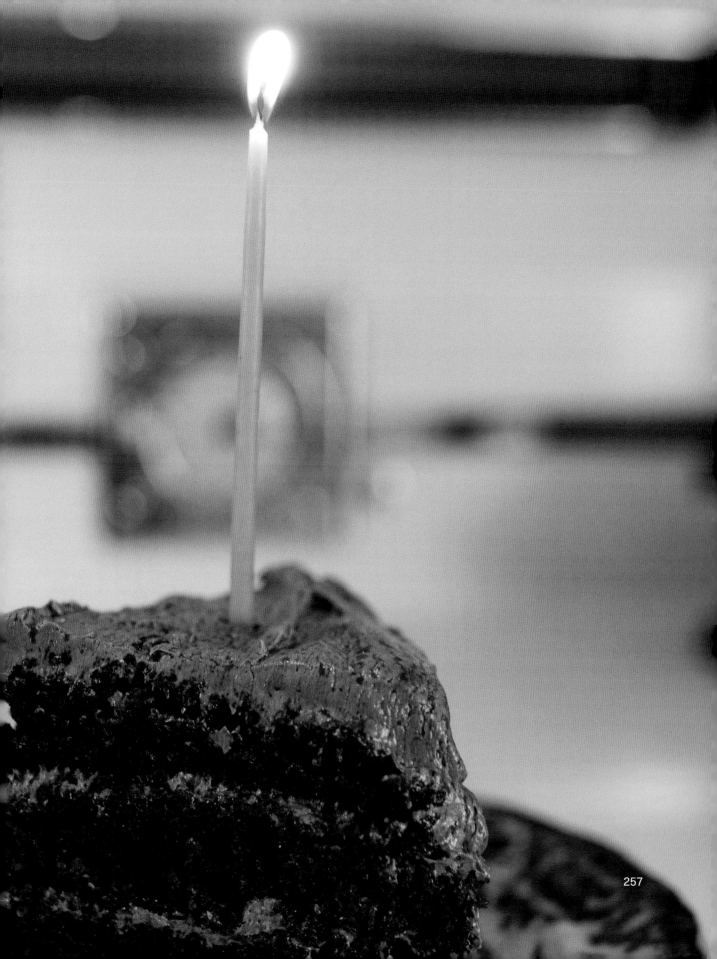

PREP TIME:
20 MINUTES

BAKE TIME:
40 MINUTES

RISE TIME:
0 MINUTES

YIELD:
MAKES 12 BROWNIES

Fudge Walnut Brownies

This sourdough brownie recipe has been a favorite for years. Using both chocolate and cocoa powder deepens the brownies' flavor. The secret is the sourdough discard, which cuts the sweetness with a pleasant punch of acid. As a result, these brownies taste slightly tangy. That beautiful complex flavor makes you want to go back to the plate again and again.

This recipe is easy to adjust. All-purpose flour works well, but you can also use whole-wheat pastry flour or spelt flour. Both will add a pleasant wheat flavor to the brownies but won't impact their soft texture. Toasting the walnuts gives them a deliciously buttery flavor with notes of caramel. You'll find that the little bit of extra effort is worthwhile.

1/2 cup walnuts, coarsely chopped

1/2 cup (113 grams) butter

1 cup (170 grams) semi-sweet chocolate chips

1 tablespoon (15 grams) vanilla extract

1 1/4 cups (240 grams) sugar

3/4 cup (105 grams) all-purpose flour

1/2 cup (40 grams) cocoa powder

1/2 teaspoon salt

1/2 cup (125 grams) sourdough discard

2 eggs, at room temperature

1 Preheat the oven to 325ºF and line a rimmed baking sheet with parchment paper.

2 Spread the chopped walnuts evenly onto the prepared baking sheet and bake them for 8 to 12 minutes, or until toasted. Let the nuts cool to room temperature and set them aside.

3 Increase the oven's temperature to 350ºF. Grease a 9x9 pan with butter.

4 In a medium saucepan over medium-low heat, melt the butter. Add the chocolate chips and vanilla, then stir together until melted.

5 In a medium mixing bowl, whisk together the sugar, flour, cocoa powder, and salt. Pour the chocolate-butter mixture into the dry ingredients. Add the sourdough discard and eggs and beat together until it forms a smooth batter with no clumps.

6 Pour the batter into the prepared pan. Bake for 40 minutes, or until a toothpick inserted into the center of the brownies comes out clean.

7 Allow the brownies to cool completely before slicing and serving. Store any leftovers in an airtight container at room temperature for up to 5 days.

SWEET TREATS

258

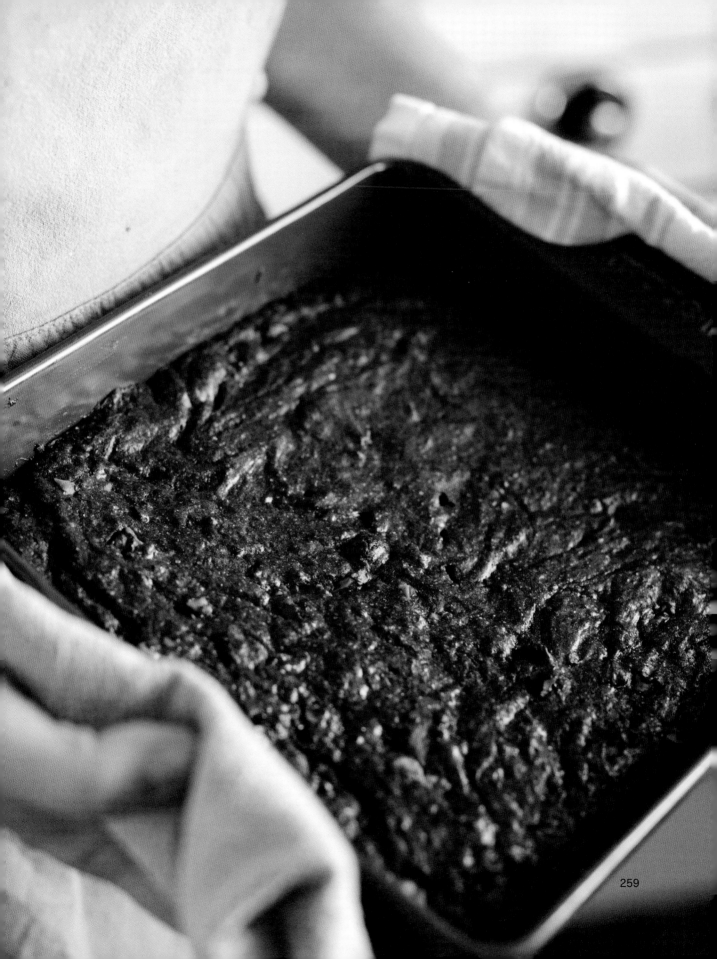

PREP TIME:
30 MINUTES

BAKE TIME:
20 MINUTES

RISE TIME:
8 TO 12 HOURS

YIELD:
MAKES ABOUT 8 SERVINGS

Cherry Cobbler

On late-summer afternoons, my kids and I head out to the cherry trees with buckets in hand. We spread out, each looking for the juiciest and ripest cherries. It's like a scavenger hunt, and we fill our buckets with the best picks. When we get home, we pit the cherries by hand. It's a tedious task, to be sure, but there's a delightful rhythm to it. We chat, we giggle, and, most importantly, we share this moment, engulfed in the beautiful, simple monotony of old-fashioned tasks. We're together, undistracted.

It's one of many lessons I want to impart to my kids: giving importance to the little things and doing even the smallest tasks well. Another is patience—the idea that some things are worth waiting for. From picking cherries to mixing the cobbler batter the night before, it takes time and is worth every moment.

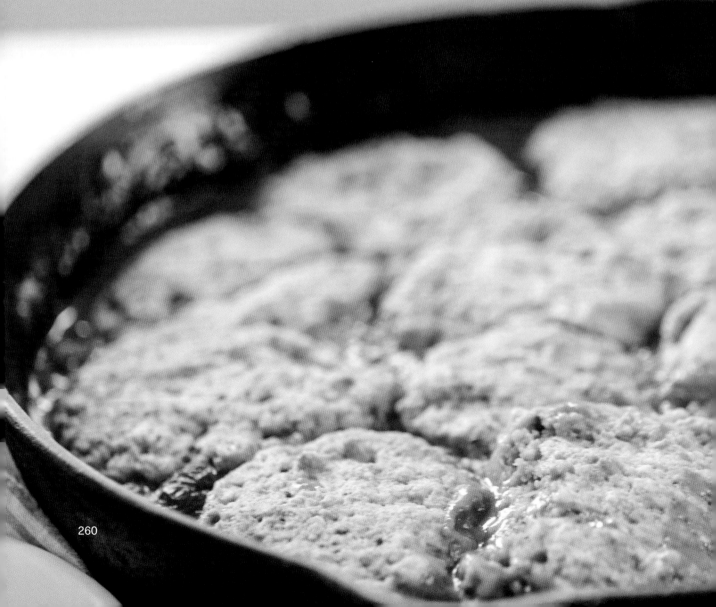

FOR THE BISCUIT TOPPING

2 cups (280 grams) all-purpose flour

1/2 cup (100 grams)
  active sourdough starter

1/3 cup (75 grams) butter, melted

1/4 cup (84 grams) honey

1/2 cup (120 grams) heavy cream

1/4 cup (50 grams) brown sugar

1 teaspoon (5 grams) baking soda

1 teaspoon (5 grams) baking powder

1/2 teaspoon salt

FOR THE FILLING

4 cups (about 600 grams)
  pitted sour cherries

1/4 cup (33 grams)
  all-purpose einkorn flour

1/3 cup (113 grams) honey

3 tablespoons (42 grams) butter

1   **To make the topping:** In a large mixing bowl, combine the all-purpose flour and starter. Beat in the butter and honey. Cover the bowl tightly with plastic wrap, a beeswax wrap, or a damp tea towel and let it sit in a warm spot in your kitchen for 8 to 12 hours.

2   The next day, preheat the oven to 350°F.

3   **To make the filling:** In a cast-iron skillet over medium-low heat, add the cherries and top with the all-purpose einkorn flour, honey, and butter. Stir continuously until the butter melts and the ingredients are well combined with no clumps of flour remaining. Turn off the heat and set aside while you finish the cobbler topping.

4   Uncover the bowl and mix in the cream, brown sugar, baking soda, baking powder, and salt by hand until the ingredients are evenly distributed.

5   Lightly flour a clean working surface and then tip out the dough onto it. Pat it out until it is about 1/2 inch thick. Cut out 3- to 4-inch-diameter biscuits and place them on top of the cherry filling.

6   Transfer the skillet to the oven and bake for about 20 minutes, or until the biscuits turn golden brown and the filling is bubbly.

7   Serve warm. Store any leftovers in an airtight container in the fridge for up to 3 days.

PREP TIME:
20 MINUTES

BAKE TIME:
15 MINUTES

RISE TIME:
8 TO 12 HOURS

YIELD:
**MAKES ABOUT 10
SERVINGS**

Pumpkin Roll

When the winter weather comes, I find myself baking even more. It helps warm up the kitchen on cold mornings. I particularly love the cinnamon-and-spice aroma of this pumpkin roll as it bakes. Like many recipes, this one is best started the night before. Good things take time, and this pumpkin roll is no exception.

Mix the batter the night before and let it ferment. This develops a beautiful, complex acidity that partners well with the soft, earthy undertones of pumpkin. Fermenting the batter also helps break down some complex starches in the flour. As a result, many people find long-fermented baked goods a little easier to digest.

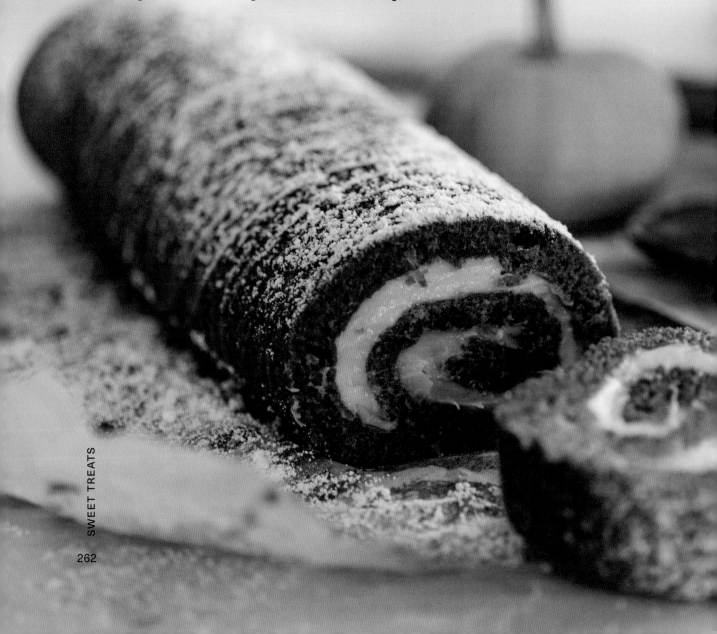

FOR THE CAKE

1 cup (140 grams) all-purpose flour

1/2 cup (122 grams) pumpkin purée

1/2 cup (100 grams)
   active sourdough starter

1/2 cup (168 grams) maple syrup

1/2 cup (96 grams) rapadura sugar

3 eggs

3 teaspoons (15 grams) pumpkin pie spice

2 teaspoons (10 grams) vanilla extract

1/4 teaspoon salt

1 teaspoon (5 grams) baking soda

FOR THE FROSTING

8 ounces (226 grams)
   cream cheese, softened

1/2 cup (168 grams) maple syrup

1/4 cup (57 grams) butter

2 teaspoons (10 grams) vanilla extract

1 **To make the cake:** In a medium mixing bowl, stir together the flour, pumpkin purée, starter, and maple syrup until a smooth batter forms. Cover it tightly and let it rest in a warm spot in your kitchen for at least 8 and up to 12 hours.

2 Preheat the oven to 375°F and line a 10-by-15-inch rimmed baking sheet with parchment paper.

3 Uncover the sourdough mixture and add the rapadura sugar, eggs, pumpkin pie spice, vanilla, and salt, stirring until well incorporated. Sprinkle baking soda evenly across the batter and then stir it in.

4 Spoon the batter onto your prepared baking sheet, then spread it evenly with a rubber spatula. Tap the baking sheet gently on the counter to distribute the batter and remove any large air bubbles.

5 Transfer to the oven and bake for 15 minutes, or until the cake is baked through and a toothpick inserted into the center of the cake comes out clean.

6 Starting from the short side, roll the cake in the parchment paper as soon as it comes out of the oven, taking care not to burn yourself. Allow the cake to cool while rolled.

7 **To make the frosting:** While the cake is cooling, in a medium mixing bowl, beat together the cream cheese, maple syrup, butter, and vanilla until smooth and fluffy.

8 Carefully unroll the cooled cake. Then, evenly spread the cream cheese frosting across the cake and roll it back up. Slice and serve or cover tightly and refrigerate for up to 3 days.

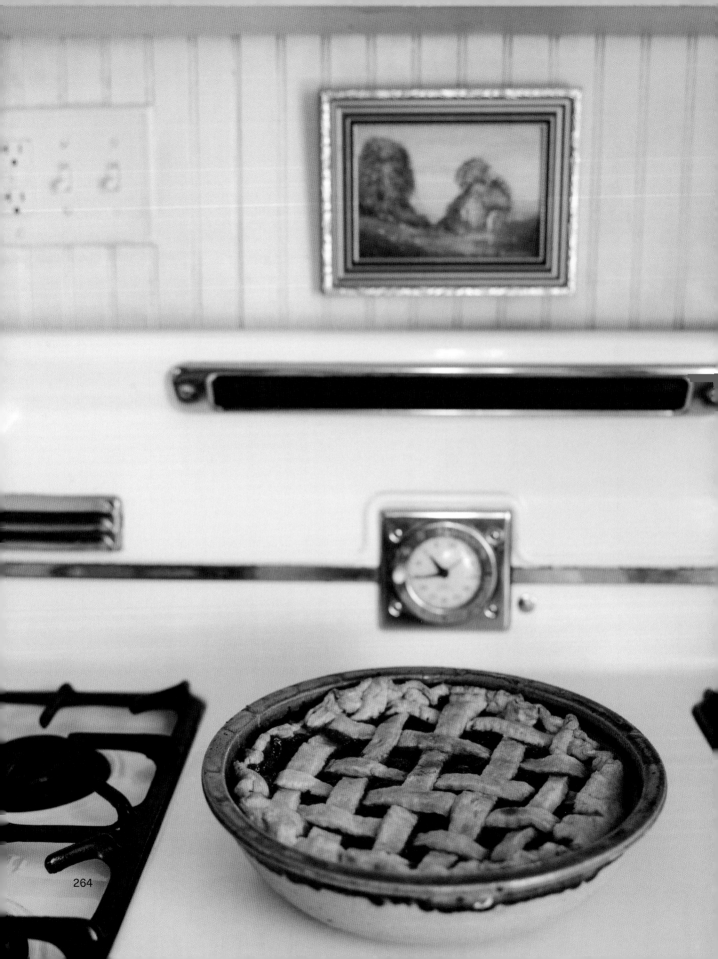

PREP TIME:
15 MINUTES

BAKE TIME:
**15 MINUTES + 45 MINUTES
OR UNTIL THE FILLING IS
BUBBLY AND COOKED**

RISE TIME:
**2 HOURS OF
CHILLING TIME
FOR THE CRUSTS**

YIELD:
**MAKES 1
(9-INCH) PIE**

Blackberry-Vanilla Pie

Berry season is so reliable you can almost set your clock by it. It starts with strawberries, fresh from the garden. When they're exhausted, our friend's farm is bustling with the blueberry crop, and we head there to pick what we can. Later come the raspberries. Finally, the blackberries arrive. They are a sort of last hurrah of summer. Their boisterous flavor is somehow bright, sweet, and bracingly sour all at once. We eat so many they stain our fingertips.

They're delicious in pie. A little lemon brings out the berries' bright, acidic notes. Vanilla's soft, floral flavor perfectly complements blackberries' inky sweetness.

FOR THE CRUST

2 cups (280 grams) all-purpose flour

2 teaspoons (8 grams) sugar

1 teaspoon (6 grams) salt

1 cup (226 grams) cold butter, cubed

1 cup (250 grams) sourdough discard

FOR THE PIE FILLING

1 lemon

6 cups (750 grams)
    fresh or frozen blackberries

3/4 cup (145 grams) rapadura sugar

1/3 cup (46 grams) all-purpose flour

1 teaspoon (5 grams) vanilla extract

2 tablespoons (28 grams)
    cold butter, cubed

FOR THE EGG WASH

1 egg yolk

1 tablespoon (15 grams) water

1   **To make the crust:** In a large mixing bowl, combine the flour, sugar, and salt. Work in the butter, being careful not to overmix. Add in the sourdough discard and stir until combined.

2   Dust your working surface lightly with flour, and then tip the dough out onto it. Divide it into two equal portions and pat them into thick discs. Wrap them tightly with plastic wrap and transfer them to the fridge for at least 2 hours and up to 3 days.

3   Heat the oven to 425°F.

4   **To make the filling:** In a small bowl, grate the zest of 1 lemon, avoiding the bitter white pith. Then, cut the lemon in half and juice it. In a large bowl, stir together the lemon zest, lemon juice, blackberries, rapadura sugar, flour, and vanilla. Use a wooden spoon to gently mash the mixture and break up the berries a little.

(recipe continued on next page)

5   Roll out the discs into 11-inch circles about 1/8 inch thick. Arrange one disc in a deep 9-inch pie plate, allowing any excess dough to fall over the edges. Spoon the filling into the dough-lined pie plate, then dot it with the cubed butter.

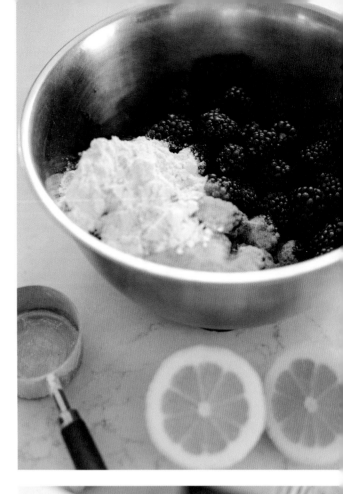

6   Then, use a pizza cutter to slice the second dough circle into 1-inch strips. Arrange four of the dough strips parallel to each other across the pie, about 1 inch apart. Fold back every other strip, and layer on one of the remaining dough strips across the pie, perpendicular to the first strips. Unfold the strips that were folded back, and then fold back the alternate strips. Layer on another strip perpendicular to the original strips. Continue to alternate the original strips, as a new perpendicular strip is placed in, creating a beautiful weave pattern. Crimp the pie firmly at the edge, trimming any excess.

7   **To make the egg wash:** In a small bowl, whisk the egg yolk with water and brush it over the pie crust.

8   Transfer the pie to the oven and bake for 15 minutes, or until the crust begins to brown. Turn the heat down to 350°F and continue baking for 45 minutes, or until the filling is bubbly and cooked.

9   Serve warm or keep covered and store in the fridge for up to 3 days.

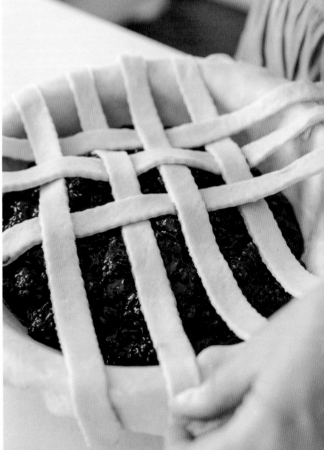

SWEET TREATS

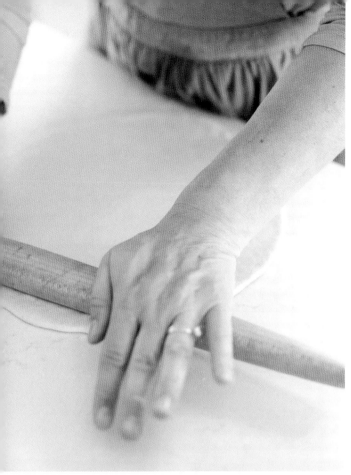
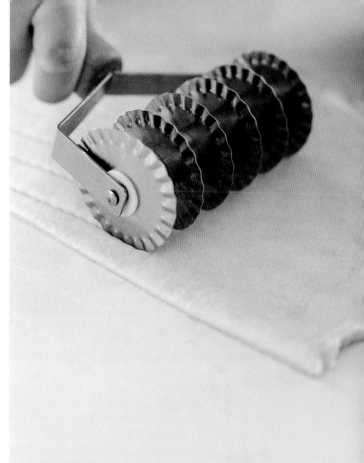
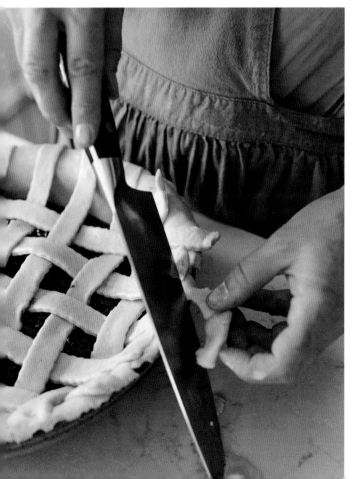
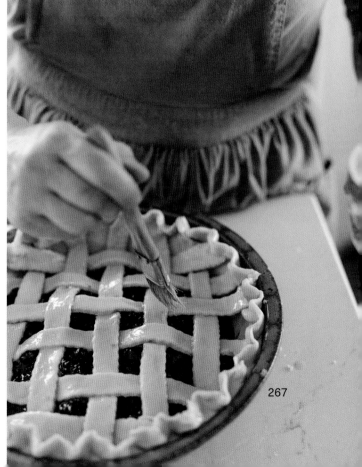

267

PREP TIME:
15 MINUTES

BAKE TIME:
30 MINUTES

RISE TIME:
**2 HOURS OF
CHILLING TIME**

YIELD:
**MAKES ABOUT
18 HAND PIES**

Sourdough Hand Pies

Many of us hold a nostalgic place in our hearts for Pop-Tarts—the stiff pastry, the too-sweet filling, the icing, and sprinkles. Here's a secret: You can make something even better at home with a little jam and some pie crust. These hand pies fit the bill: a buttery crust, real fruit, and none of the junk.

They're fun to make with children. My little ones love filling the pastries with their favorite jams, jellies, and fruit butter before crimping the edges tight. Plus, the hand pies pack up easily for picnics, potlucks, and snacks on the go.

FOR THE CRUST

2 cups (280 grams)
    all-purpose flour

2 teaspoons (8 grams)
    sugar

1 teaspoon (6 grams) salt

1 cup (226 grams) cold
    butter, cubed

1 cup (250 grams)
    sourdough discard

FOR FINISHING THE PIES

3/4 cup (about 255 grams)
    jam, jelly, pie filling, or fruit
    butter

1 egg yolk

1 tablespoon (15 grams)
    water

1 tablespoon (about 16
    grams) coarse sugar,
    such as demerara or
    pearl sugar

1   **To make the crust:** In a large mixing bowl, combine the flour, sugar, and salt. Work in the butter with a fork, pastry cutter, or your fingers (my preference!), being careful not to overmix. Add in the sourdough discard and stir until combined.

2   Dust your working surface lightly with flour, and then tip the dough out onto it. Divide it into two equal portions and pat them into thick discs. Wrap them tightly with plastic wrap and transfer them to the fridge for at least 2 hours and up to 3 days.

3   Roll out the discs into 10-by-13-inch rectangles. Then, using a ruler and a pizza cutter or sharp knife, trim the rectangles to 9 by 12 inches, discarding the excess and ensuring the edges are square. Slice the rectangles into nine smaller rectangles, approximately 3 by 4 inches.

4   Preheat the oven to 350°F and line a baking sheet with parchment paper.

5   **To finish the pies:** Working one at a time, spoon 1 tablespoon of filling onto the center of a small rectangle of pie dough. Cover it with a second piece of dough and crimp the edges tightly. Continue working until you've made all the hand pies. Cut three vertical slits to allow for ventilation.

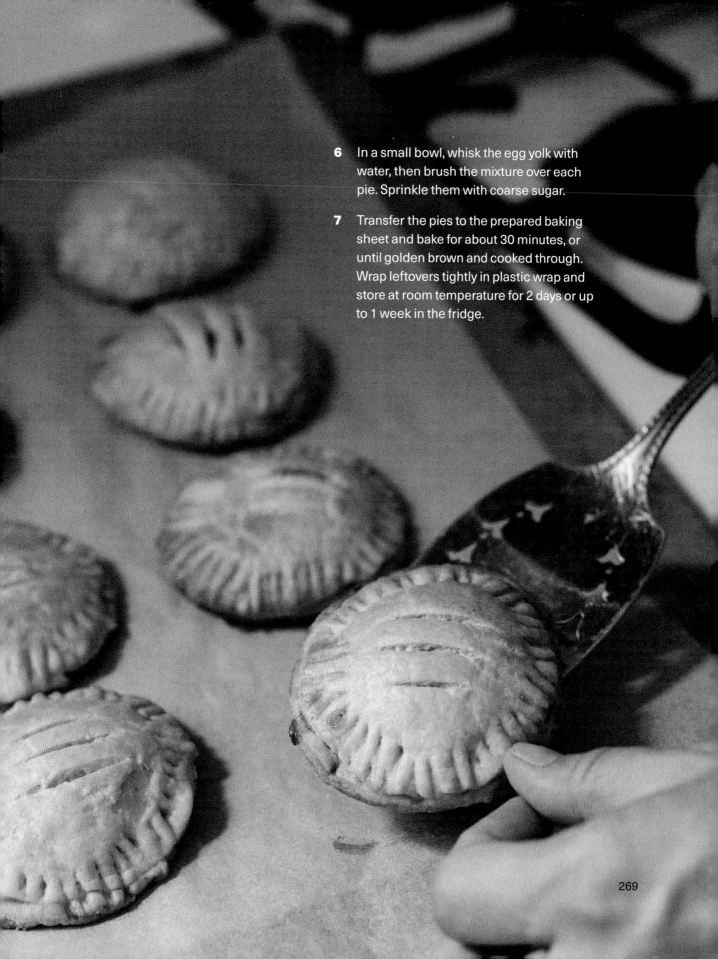

6 In a small bowl, whisk the egg yolk with water, then brush the mixture over each pie. Sprinkle them with coarse sugar.

7 Transfer the pies to the prepared baking sheet and bake for about 30 minutes, or until golden brown and cooked through. Wrap leftovers tightly in plastic wrap and store at room temperature for 2 days or up to 1 week in the fridge.

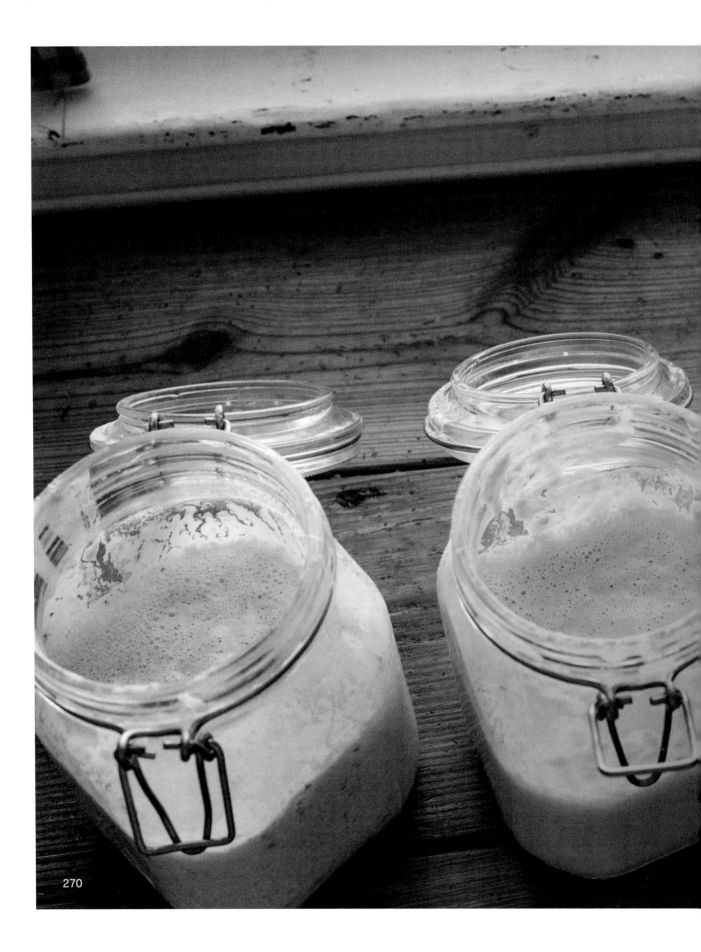

CHAPTER 8

Keep the Discard

THERE ARE A GREAT many life lessons sourdough will teach you. Patience. Planning. Care. Diligence. Perhaps one of the most valuable is economy—making use of every little bit of what you have. At the farmhouse, nothing goes to waste. Sourdough discard always finds a home in meals and treats.

When you bake sourdough bread long enough, you'll find you end up with more starter than you can use. Every time you feed your starter to prepare it for baking, you're left with a little discard. It's certainly sour, but not quite bubbly. Sure, you can spoon it into the compost bin and move on to your loaves of bread. Better than that, try these ingenious ways to use every bit. In skilled hands, sourdough discard evolves from an afterthought to an essential kitchen ingredient. It lends a pleasant complexity to crêpes and pancakes, offers a bright punch of acidity to homemade crackers, and can even be the foundation for easy one-pan dinners on busy nights.

Sourdough Crêpes with Whipped Cream Cheese

Crêpes are an excellent use for sourdough discard. You don't need to add extra flour; instead, you just beat in some eggs and a little milk and butter. This means it's deliciously tangy and super easy to digest since the flour has been fermented for so long. We like to serve them with billowy spoonfuls of maple-infused whipped cream cheese and fresh fruit. Vibrant summer berries are a favorite in the summer. Cinnamon-dusted sautéed apples are perfect for fall.

If you make crêpes often, it's worth investing in a crêpe pan. These wide, short-sided pans are perfect for swirling the batter and flipping the crêpes. A well-seasoned cast-iron skillet works, too. On busy mornings, I sometimes have four batter-filled pans on my stove. This speeds up the process and satisfies hungry bellies more quickly.

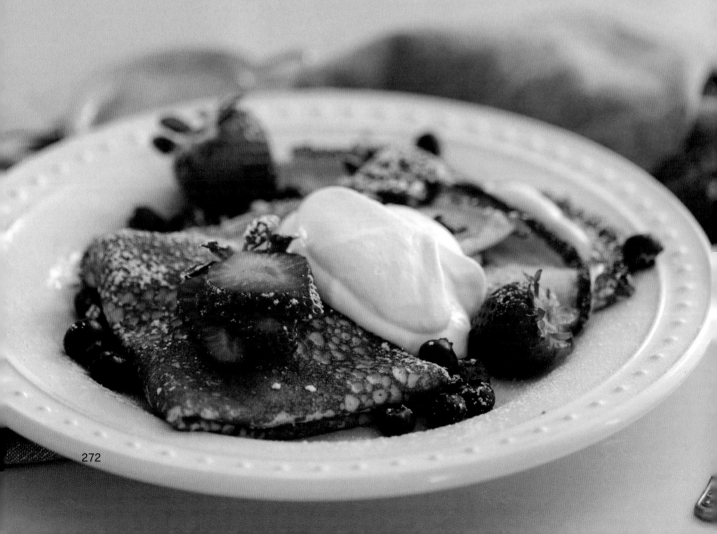

FOR THE CRÊPES

1 cup (200 grams)
  sourdough discard

8 eggs

3/4 cup (183 grams) milk

3 tablespoons (42 grams)
  melted unsalted butter,
  plus more for the pan

1/4 teaspoon salt

FOR THE FILLING

4 ounces (113 grams) cream
  cheese, at room temperature

1/4 cup (84 grams) maple syrup

1/2 teaspoon vanilla extract

1/2 pint (240 grams) heavy cream

FOR THE TOPPING (OPTIONAL)

Strawberries

Blueberries

1 **To make the crêpes:** In a medium mixing bowl, beat together the starter, eggs, milk, butter, and salt until they form a smooth batter.

2 **To make the filling:** In a medium mixing bowl, beat together the cream cheese, maple syrup, and vanilla until smooth.

3 In a separate large bowl, whip the cream until it forms stiff peaks, then fold it into the cream cheese mixture. Set it aside while you prepare the crêpes.

4 Warm a 10-inch crêpe pan, well-seasoned cast-iron skillet, or a nonstick pan over medium heat. Hold your hand a few inches above the pan. When you can feel warmth radiating from the pan, it's ready.

5 Brush your pan with a little melted butter, then pour about 1/2 cup batter into the pan. Lift the pan and swirl the batter to fill the pan's surface up to the edges. Allow it to cook undisturbed for a few minutes or until it's nearly cooked through and golden. Then, gently dislodge it from the pan using a rubber spatula, flip, and continue cooking for about 1 minute more.

6 Set the finished crêpes on a plate until you've worked through all the batter. Dab a little of the cream cheese mixture in the center of each crêpe, fold them into quarters, and serve. Top with strawberries or blueberries, if desired. You can store leftovers, with filling and crêpe separate, in an airtight container in the fridge for up to 3 days.

PREP TIME:
5 MINUTES

BAKE TIME:
15 MINUTES

RISE TIME:
0 MINUTES

YIELD:
**MAKES ABOUT
6 SERVINGS**

Dutch Baby Pancakes

Dutch baby pancakes like to make an entrance. The thin, eggy batter puffs up magnificently in a hot oven, forming an airy custard-like pillow. While they look complicated and fussy, with all their drama, they're actually a breeze to make. When you're feeding a crew of hungry kids, it can make all the difference between a morning of chaos and one of order.

Serve it with fresh seasonal fruit. In the winter, consider squeezing some fresh lemon juice over the pancake and drizzling it with honey. In the summer, berries and cream or homemade yogurt are the perfect companions.

Timing is the trick to getting the recipe right, so pay attention while it's in the oven. As soon as it puffs up, it's ready. You should serve it immediately because it deflates like a popped balloon once it comes out of the oven.

2 cups (500 grams) sourdough discard

6 eggs

1/3 cup (81 grams) milk

2 tablespoons (42 grams) honey

1 teaspoon (5 grams) vanilla extract

1/2 teaspoon salt

6 tablespoons (84 grams) butter

1 Preheat the oven to 425°F.

2 To the pitcher of a blender, add the sourdough discard, eggs, milk, honey, vanilla, and salt and blend until smooth.

3 Drop the butter in a 12-inch cast-iron skillet and place it in the oven to melt. When the butter has melted, carefully swirl it around the pan, then pour in the batter. Bake for 15 to 20 minutes, or until puffed up and golden.

4 Serve right away with with your choice of toppings. My favorites are butter, fruit, maple syrup, or honey.

KEEP THE DISCARD

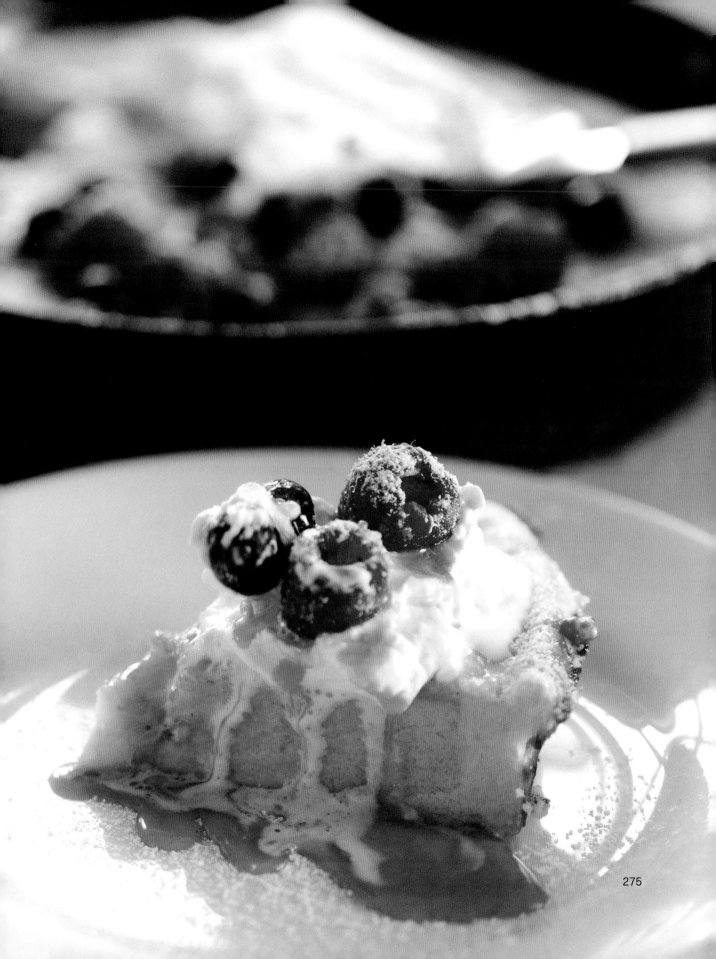

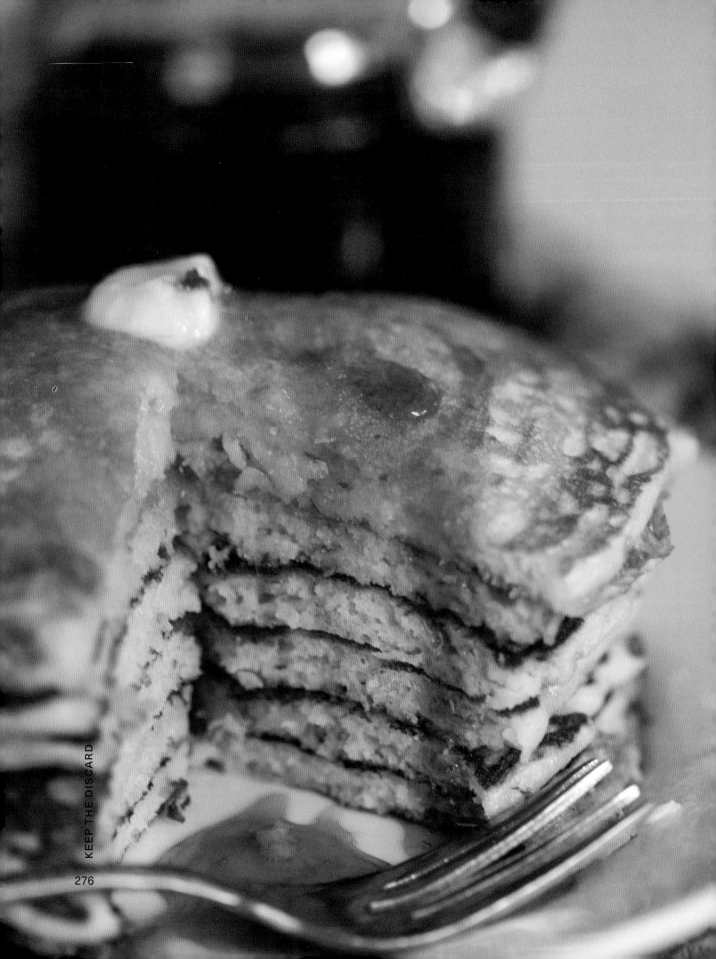

PREP TIME:
5 MINUTES

COOK TIME:
60 MINUTES

RISE TIME:
0 MINUTES

YIELD:
MAKES 12 PANCAKES

Sourdough Pancakes

Everyone loves pancakes. They're the perfect vehicle for butter and maple syrup, and sourdough gives them a beautifully complex flavor that is rich and tart. They're also fun to make. I love watching the batter bubble up as I mix in the baking soda. It's a natural chemical reaction as the acidic starter meets the alkaline baking soda. You feel like a cross between an alchemist and a magician, swirling the bubbly batter together. In many pancake recipes, you'd need to add buttermilk to get this reaction. Fortunately, sourdough starter is acidic enough on its own. It's not only fun to watch the reaction, but all those air bubbles also produce a lighter, fluffier pancake, too.

I like pancakes with crispy edges, so I fry them in plenty of coconut oil. You could also use butter, too. Use less fat in the skillet if you're not a fan of crisp-edged pancakes.

2 cups (400 grams)
   active sourdough starter

2 eggs

1/4 cup (56 grams)
   melted coconut oil, plus
   more for the pan

2 tablespoons (42 grams)
   honey

1 teaspoon (5 grams)
   baking soda

1/2 teaspoon salt

1 In a medium mixing bowl, whisk together the active starter, eggs, coconut oil, honey, baking soda, and salt until they form a smooth batter.

2 Warm a skillet over medium heat and drop in a spoonful of coconut oil. When it melts, pour in about 1/2 cup batter and turn the heat to medium-low. Allow the pancake to cook for a few minutes until you see bubbles appearing in the center of the batter. Then, flip it and continue cooking for another minute or two until it's cooked through. Transfer the pancake to a platter and continue working until you've exhausted the batter.

3 Serve warm, and store any leftovers in the fridge for up to 5 days.

Sweet Potato and Sage Galette

Galettes are free-form pies, so there's no need for a pie plate. Part of their charm is their rustic, imperfect nature. Embrace it. Rest assured, there's no pressure for perfection here. Rather, it's the tiny flaws that make the galette so worthwhile. This is a version I make in the autumn, when we've nearly forgotten all the crisp summer salads and our bodies crave simple, nourishing comfort food. Fresh sage is a natural match for sweet potatoes, although you can use thyme or fresh rosemary if that's what you have. A rimmed baking sheet is a must for this recipe, as it will catch any drips or spills if the galette's filling happens to run over.

FOR THE CRUST

2 cups (280 grams) all-purpose flour

1 teaspoon (6 grams) salt

1 cup (226 grams) cold butter, cubed

1 cup (250 grams) sourdough discard

FOR THE FILLING

1 1/2 tablespoon (21 grams) olive oil, plus more for drizzling

1 large (about 250 grams) leek, thinly sliced white and light green parts only

1/2 teaspoon salt

4 ounces (114 grams) soft goat cheese, at room temperature

6 tablespoons (90 grams) heavy whipping cream, plus more for brushing the dough

1 tablespoon lemon zest

1 small (about 115 grams) sweet potato, peeled and thinly sliced

2 teaspoons chopped fresh sage

1 **To make the crust:** In a large mixing bowl, combine the flour and salt. Use a pastry cutter or your fingers to work in the butter, being careful not to overmix. Add in the sourdough discard and stir until combined.

2 Dust your working surface lightly with flour, and then tip the dough out onto it. Divide it into two equal portions and pat them into thick discs. Wrap them tightly with plastic wrap and transfer them to the fridge for at least 2 hours and up to 3 days.

3 Heat the oven to 400°F and line a rimmed baking sheet with parchment paper.

4 **To make the filling:** In a skillet over medium heat, warm the olive oil. Add the leek and sprinkle them with salt. Sauté until the leek softens and releases its aroma, about 8 minutes. Transfer to a small bowl and set aside while you prepare the remaining ingredients.

KEEP THE DISCARD

5 Pull the galette crusts out of the fridge and roll them into 12-inch circles about 1/8 inch thick.

6 In a small bowl, mix together the goat cheese, cream, and lemon zest. Spread a thin, even layer on each crust, leaving a 1-inch border. Top with the softened leeks, sweet potatoes, and sage. Drizzle with additional olive oil, if desired.

7 Fold the edges of the dough over the filling and then lightly brush the dough with a little extra cream. If you'd like to freeze your galette for a later meal, wrap your galette in plastic wrap and put it in the freezer.

8 Transfer to the oven and bake for 35 to 45 minutes, or until the crusts turn a pale golden brown. Cover leftovers with foil place in a glass container with a silicone lid and store in the fridge. It will keep for up to 1 week. To reheat, cover the galette in foil and bake in the oven at 350° for 6 to 8 minutes or until warmed.

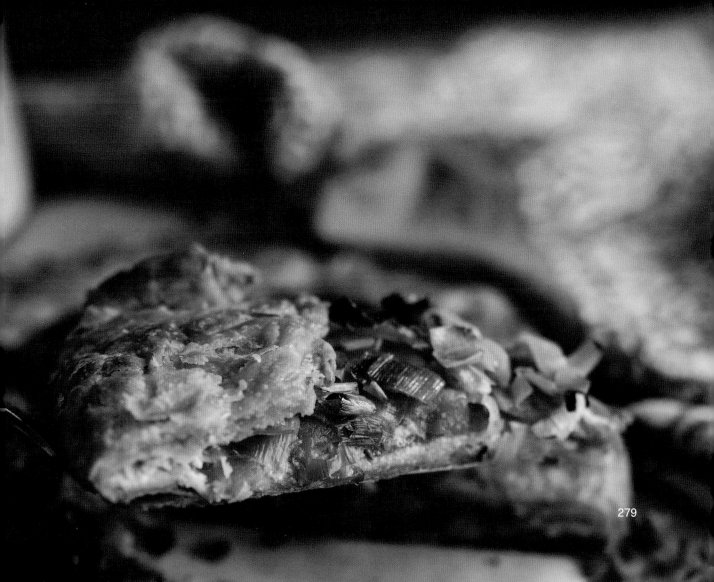

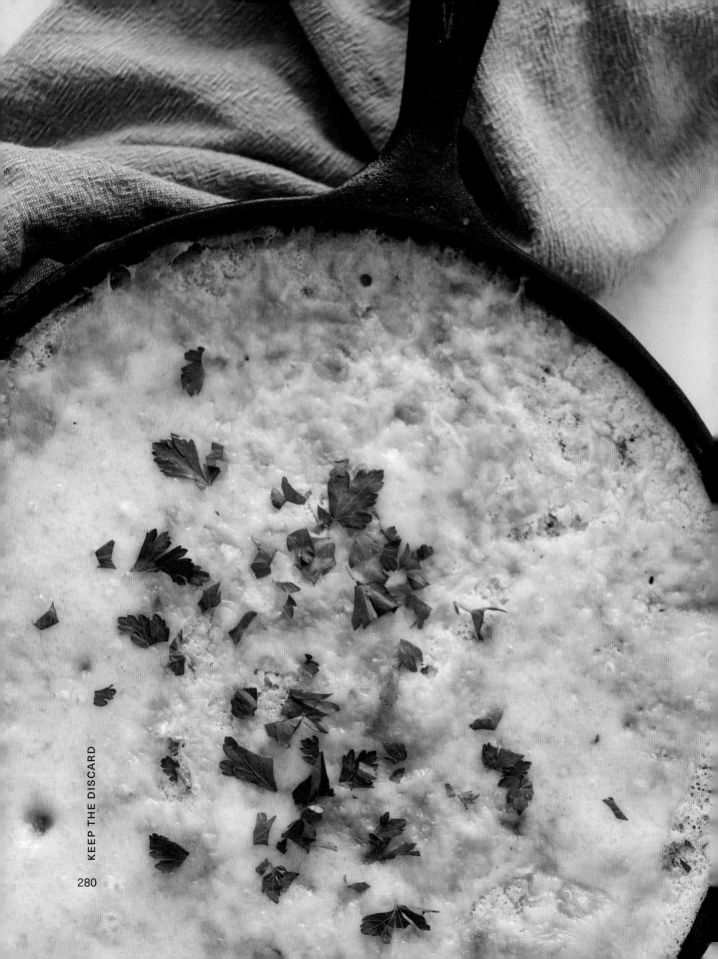

KEEP THE DISCARD

280

PREP TIME:
10 MINUTES

COOK TIME:
40 MINUTES

RISE TIME:
0 MINUTES

YIELD:
MAKES 8 SERVINGS

Farmers' Market Sourdough Skillet

We've all been there: pressed for time, exhausted after a long day. You wonder how you'll feed your family when you just can't muster any extra energy. Everyone needs an easy weeknight dinner recipe. You can count on it when you're stressed or short on time and just need to get dinner on the table. Sourdough skillets are a standby in our kitchen for times just like these. It's a reliable recipe that you can make in a single pan. Better yet? It never disappoints.

I make them when there's a jumble of ingredients in the kitchen. I scrounge through the fridge, hoping to find a few vegetables, some ground meat, and maybe a little cheese or some fresh herbs. You have meat, vegetables, and healthy fats together in a single pan, and cleanup is a cinch.

Fresh summer produce is perfect for this recipe. It's especially good for using up those last few peppers or zucchini that linger in the crisper drawer of your fridge. Remember, this recipe is forgiving. In the wintertime, you can also use butternut squash instead of zucchini. In the spring, use fresh asparagus if you have it. These skillet dinners taste delicious and are easy to make.

FOR THE FILLING

2 tablespoons (30 grams) olive oil

1 small onion (about 100 grams), diced

1 pound (454 grams) loose Italian sausage

1 small zucchini (about 100 grams), sliced

1 medium tomato (about 150 grams), chopped

1 large bell pepper (about 200 grams), diced

1/2 teaspoon salt

FOR THE TOPPING

1 1/2 cups (375 grams) sourdough discard

3 eggs

3 tablespoons (42 grams) melted butter

2 tablespoons (6 grams) chopped fresh parsley

2 teaspoons (10 grams) baking powder

1 teaspoon (6 grams) salt

1/2 teaspoon garlic powder

1/2 cup (85 grams) shredded cheddar cheese

(recipe continued on next page)

1   Preheat the oven to 400°F.

2   **To make the filling:** In a 12-inch cast-iron skillet over medium heat, warm the olive oil. Add the onion and sauté for about 7 minutes, or until fragrant and translucent. Add the sausage, breaking it up with your spatula, and cook it for about 10 minutes, or until well browned. Stir in the zucchini, tomato, and pepper and sprinkle them with salt. Sauté for about 6 minutes more, or until tender. Turn off the heat while you prepare the topping.

3   **To make the topping:** In a medium mixing bowl, mix the sourdough discard, eggs, butter, parsley, baking powder, salt, and garlic powder until it forms a uniform batter. Pour the sourdough mixture into the skillet over the meat and vegetables. Then, top it with the cheese.

4   Transfer the skillet to the oven and bake for 25 minutes, or until cooked through and golden on top.

5   Serve warm, and store any leftovers in an airtight container in the fridge for up to 5 days.

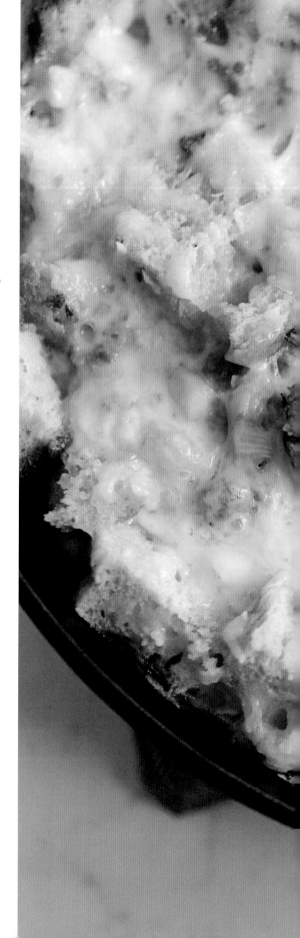

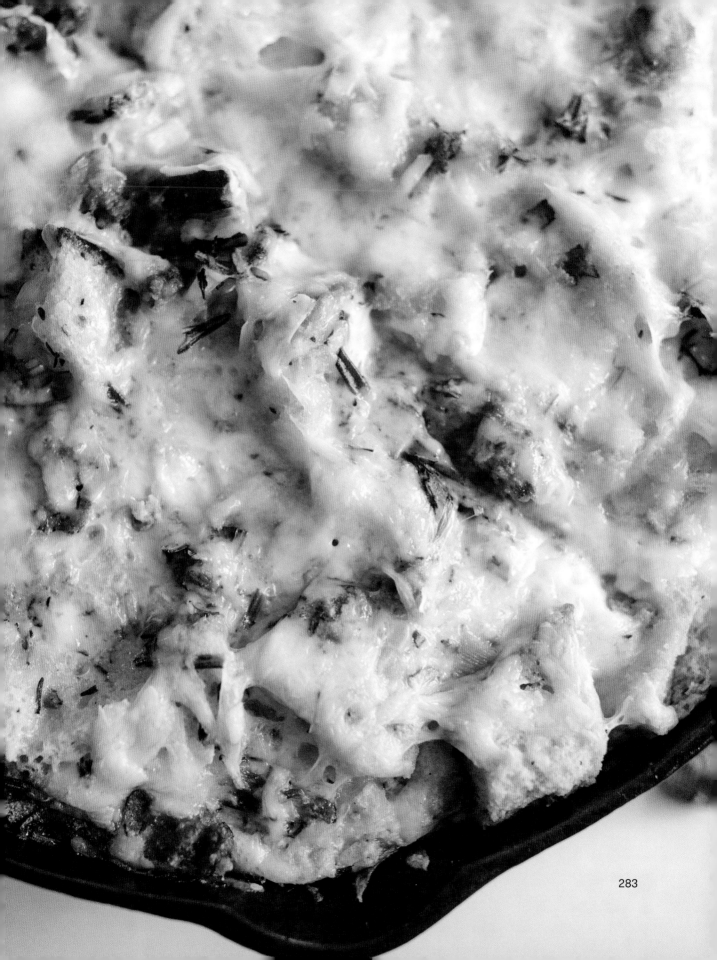

PREP TIME:
25 MINUTES

BAKE TIME:
25 MINUTES

RISE TIME:
10 TO 12 HOURS

YIELD:
MAKES ABOUT 8 SERVINGS

Biscuit-Topped Chicken Potpie

One of my absolute favorite comfort foods to make on the homestead is homemade chicken potpie. It starts with a flavorful chicken stew packed with juicy bits of chicken, sweet peas, carrots, onions, and potatoes. Plenty of good broth and just the right amount of cream pull the filling together. It smells heavenly as it simmers away on the stove.

But what makes this potpie truly special is the topping—sourdough biscuits sweetened with a spoonful of honey. These biscuits have a unique tart quality with just a little sweetness for balance. The secret to their perfect texture and flavor is letting the biscuit dough rise overnight. As the potpie bakes, the biscuits turn golden brown, creating a delicious contrast to the rich stew bubbling away beneath.

FOR THE BISCUIT TOPPING

2 cups (280 grams) all-purpose flour

1/2 cup (113 grams) cold butter, cubed

1 cup (250 grams) sourdough discard

1/2 cup (122 grams) whole milk

1 tablespoon (21 grams) honey

2 teaspoons (10 grams) baking powder

1 teaspoon (5 grams) baking soda

3/4 teaspoon salt

FOR THE FILLING

1/4 cup (57 grams) butter

3 medium red potatoes (about 450 grams), chopped

4 medium carrots (about 250 grams), chopped

1 medium yellow onion (about 100 grams), chopped

4 medium (about 15 grams) garlic cloves, minced

3 cups (720 grams) chicken broth

1/4 cup (35 grams) all-purpose flour

1 tablespoon (15 grams) dried parsley

1 teaspoon (5 grams) garlic powder

1 teaspoon (5 grams) onion powder

1 tablespoon (18 grams) salt

4 cups (450 grams) diced cooked chicken

1 cup (150 grams) fresh or frozen peas

1/2 cup (120 grams) heavy cream

1 **To make the biscuit topping:** To a large mixing bowl, add the flour and work the butter into it with a fork or pastry blender until it comes together. Add the sourdough discard, milk, and honey and stir until well combined.

2 Cover the bowl and let it rest at room temperature for 10 to 12 hours.

3 The next day, preheat the oven to 400°F.

4 **To make the filling:** In a cast-iron skillet over medium-low heat, warm the butter until it froths. Toss the potatoes, carrots, onions, and garlic into the butter and sauté for 10 minutes, or until the vegetables begin to soften. Sprinkle the flour over the vegetables and let them continue cooking for 1 to 2 minutes more.

5 Pour the broth into the skillet and then stir in the dried parsley, garlic powder, and onion powder. Cover with a lid and continue cooking for 10 minutes, or until thickened. Lift the lid and stir in the chicken, peas, and cream. Turn the heat down to low, stirring occasionally, and continue cooking for no more than 10 minutes while you finish the biscuits.

6 To complete the biscuit topping, sprinkle the baking powder, baking soda, and salt over the dough. Mix everything together well to form a rough but pliable dough.

7 Lightly flour your working surface, then turn the dough onto your working surface and pat it into a rectangle about 3/4 inch thick. Dip a biscuit cutter in flour and then cut out the biscuits.

8 Place the biscuits on top of the chicken mixture, and then transfer it to the oven. Bake for 10 to 15 minutes, or until the biscuits are golden brown and the stew is bubbly.

9 Serve hot, and store any leftovers in an airtight container in the fridge for up to 5 days.

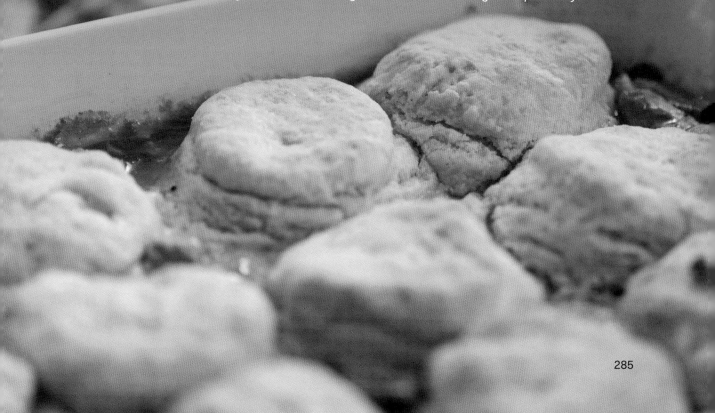

285

PREP TIME:
40 MINUTES

COOK TIME:
5 MINUTES

RISE TIME:
30 MINUTES

YIELD:
MAKES ABOUT 8 SERVINGS

Sourdough Pasta

Making pasta at home is easier than you think—you don't even need a pasta maker. Plenty of fresh eggs lend a beautiful golden color to the pasta, while sourdough starter gives it a rich, complex flavor. It's equally delicious served with a robust, tomato-rich ragù as it is with a little butter and olive oil.

3 cups (420 grams) all-purpose flour

1 cup (250 grams) sourdough discard

4 eggs

Salt, for cooking the pasta

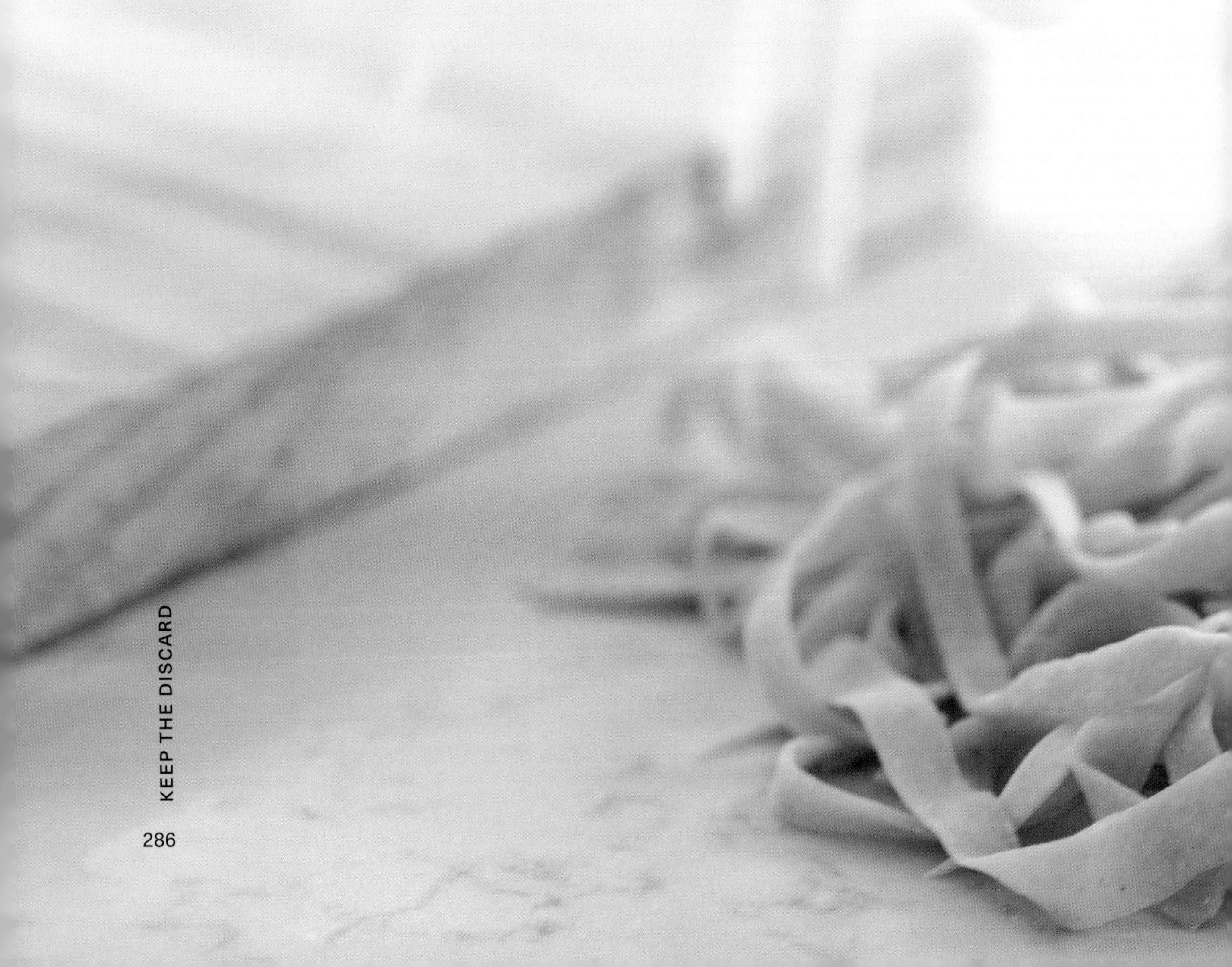

1 In the bowl of a stand mixer equipped with a dough hook, combine the flour, sourdough discard, and eggs. Mix on low speed until the dough is smooth and pliable, about 10 minutes. Cover the bowl tightly and allow the dough to rest for 30 minutes.

2 To shape the dough without a pasta maker, lightly dust your working surface with flour, then turn the dough out onto it. Roll it as thin as possible with a rolling pin, then cut into 1/4- to 1/2-inch-thick strands with a sharp knife or pizza cutter.

3 To shape the dough with a pasta maker, lightly dust your working surface with flour, then turn the dough out onto it. Shape it by hand into a 4-by-4-inch square.

4 Pass the pasta dough through the pasta maker on its thickest setting, catching it as it goes through. Fold the dough into thirds, lengthwise, then run through the widest setting again. Continue running the dough through the pasta maker, changing the setting lower and lower each time. Allow the pasta to dry on a drying rack for at least 30 minutes.

5 Once the dough has passed through the thinnest setting, change out the attachment to the pasta cutter. Run the dough through the cutter, guiding it and catching the pasta strands as they come out. Allow the pasta to dry on a drying rack for at least 30 minutes.

6 To cook the pasta, fill a large pot with water and season it well with salt. Add the fresh pasta to the pot and boil for 4 to 5 minutes, stirring constantly, until the noodles are al dente—just cooked but still with plenty of texture.

7 Store the fresh, uncooked noodles in the fridge for up to 24 hours. Store the cooked noodles in the fridge for up to 3 days.

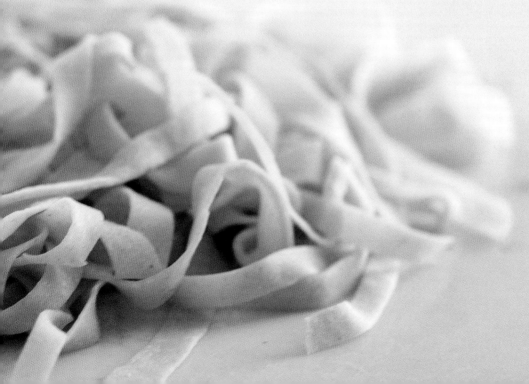

PREP TIME:
15 MINUTES

COOK TIME:
15 MINUTES

RISE TIME:
0 MINUTES

YIELD:
MAKES ABOUT 8 SERVINGS

Chicken Dumpling Soup

In my mind, there's nothing in the world quite as nourishing as a bowl of brothy chicken soup. This one is made all the better by plump sourdough dumplings that float in a golden-yellow broth dotted with carrots, celery, and fresh herbs. It's the perfect soup for using up not only sourdough discard but also leftover chicken.

Serve this soothing soup on a cold winter day when you need a little warmth. Or make it when you need a gentle and loving dish to feed a sniffly loved one. While there may be no cure for the common cold, this nourishing soup comes pretty close.

FOR THE DUMPLINGS

1 1/4 cups (175 grams) all-purpose flour

3 teaspoons (15 grams) baking powder

2 teaspoons (12 grams) salt

1/4 cup (56 grams) cold butter,
  cut into chunks

1 cup (250 grams) sourdough discard

1 egg, beaten

1 tablespoon (5 grams) minced parsley

FOR THE SOUP

2 tablespoons (28 grams)
  extra-virgin olive oil

5 medium (about 250 grams) carrots,
  peeled and chopped

5 medium (about 200 grams)
  celery ribs, chopped

1 medium (about 150 grams)
  yellow onion, chopped

2 teaspoons (12 grams) salt

1 teaspoon (5 grams) dried thyme

6 cups (1,420 grams) chicken broth

2 cups (about 150 grams) shredded
  cooked chicken

1/2 cup (about 15 grams)
  chopped flat-leaf parsley, loosely packed

(recipe continued on next page)

KEEP THE DISCARD

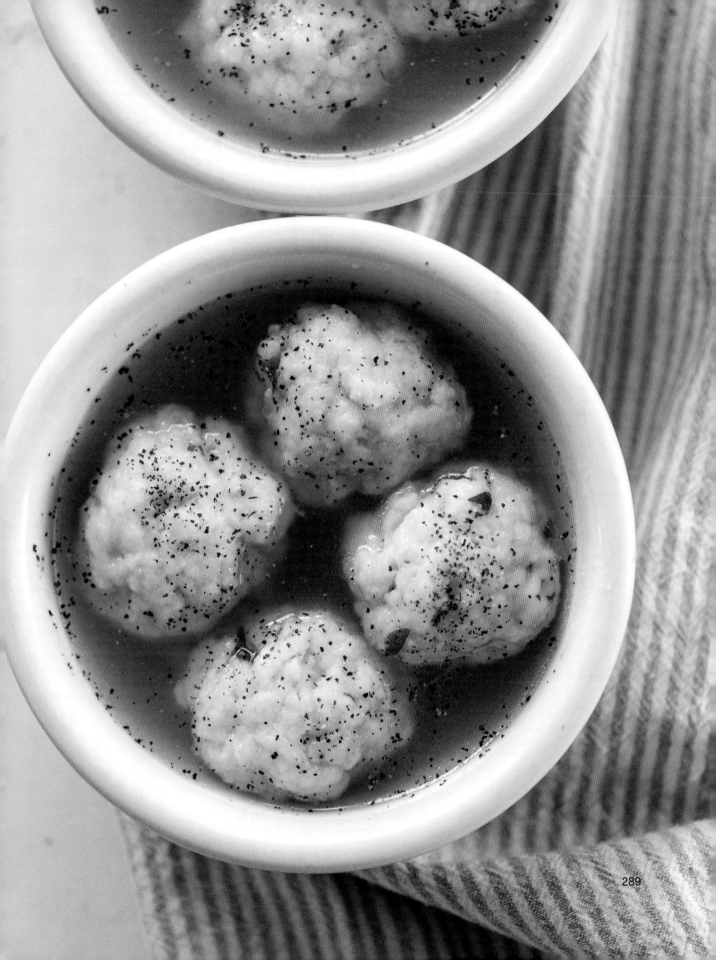

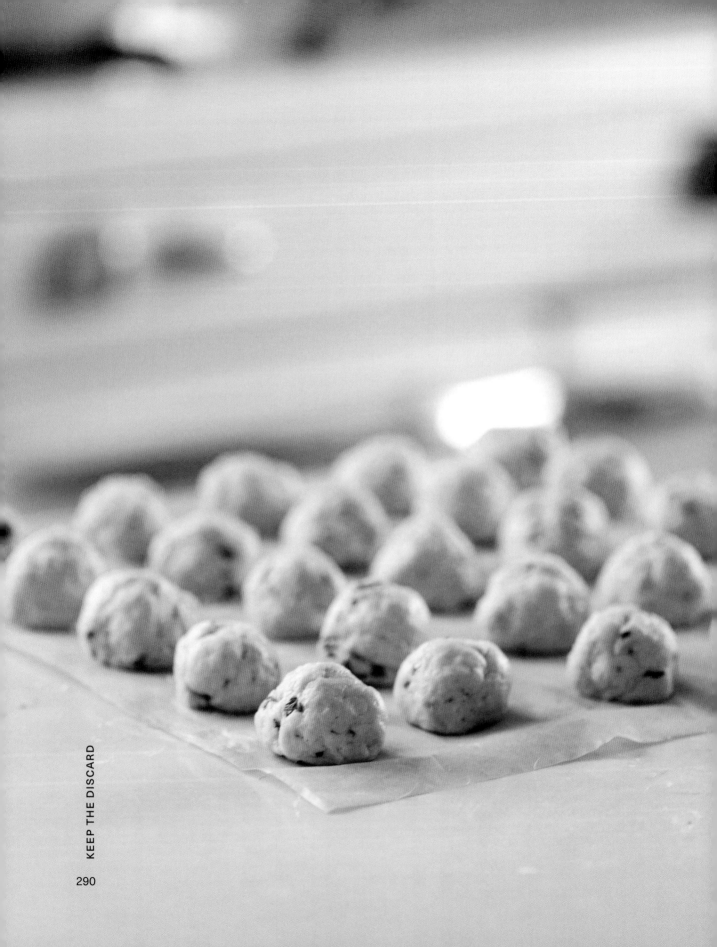

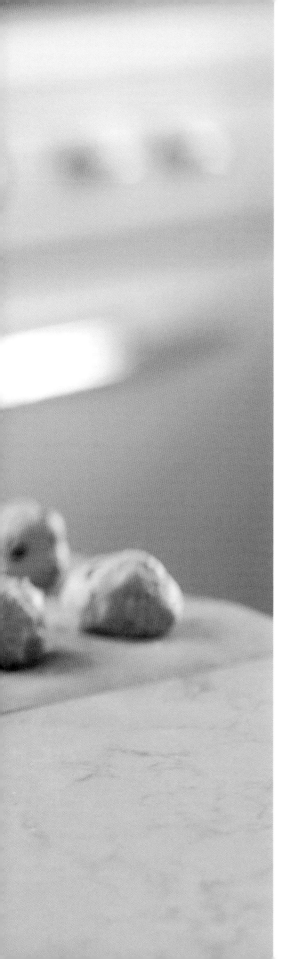

1. **To make the dumplings:** In a large mixing bowl, stir together the flour, baking powder, and salt. Cut in the butter with a fork or pastry knife until the mixture resembles cornmeal. Stir in the sourdough discard, egg, and parsley until it forms a smooth, uniform dough.

2. Line a rimmed baking sheet with parchment paper. Scoop about 1 tablespoon of dough and form it into a ball. Set it on the prepared baking sheet and continue working through the batter until you've used it all. Set the dough balls on the counter while you prepare the soup

3. **To make the soup:** In a Dutch oven over medium heat, warm the olive oil. Stir in the carrots, celery, and onions and sauté for about 5 minutes, or until fragrant. Stir in the salt and thyme, continue cooking for 1 or 2 minutes more, and then pour in the broth. Turn up the heat to medium-high, bring the contents of the pot to a boil, then turn down the heat to medium and simmer for 10 minutes, or until the vegetables lose their bite.

4. Stir in the chicken and then drop the dumplings into the pot one at a time. Stir gently to prevent them from sticking together. Cover the pot and continue simmering for about 15 minutes, or until the dumplings are cooked through and float on the surface of the soup.

5. Serve immediately and store any leftovers in an airtight container in the fridge for up to 3 days.

PREP TIME:
10 MINUTES

BAKE TIME:
20 MINUTES

RISE TIME:
8 TO 12 HOURS

YIELD:
**MAKES ABOUT
9 SERVINGS**

Fresh Corn Cornbread

On hot summer weekends, we like to host barbecues. It's perfect for showcasing all the favorites of the season. Salads have robust heirloom tomatoes dressed in herbs and olive oil. We also serve baked beans touched with molasses, fresh watermelon dripping with juice, and grilled chicken or ribs. Cornbread, naturally, makes it onto the menu, too—especially when fresh corn is in season.

Folding corn kernels into the batter gives the cornbread a delicate freshness and a delightful texture. It also imparts a distinct summery essence, as though each bite celebrates all the good the season has to offer.

Like many sourdough recipes, this cornbread needs a little extra time. You'll mix the batter the night before and let it ferment. The lengthy fermentation time gives the cornbread a richer flavor. It also helps increase its nutritional value.

1 cup (150 grams) yellow cornmeal

1/2 cup (70 grams)
   all-purpose flour

1/2 cup (96 grams) sugar

1/2 cup (125 grams)
   sourdough discard

1/2 cup (122 grams) milk

1/4 cup (56 grams) melted butter,
   plus more for the baking dish

2 teaspoons (10 grams)
   baking powder

1 teaspoon (5 grams) baking soda

1 teaspoon (6 grams) salt

1 large egg, beaten

1 cup (174 grams) fresh or frozen
   corn kernels

1   In the bowl of a stand mixer equipped with a paddle attachment, combine the cornmeal, flour, and sugar. Add the sourdough discard, milk, and butter and mix until well combined. Cover tightly, and allow it to ferment for 8 to 12 hours.

2   Preheat the oven to 400°F and lightly grease an 8-by-8-inch baking dish with butter.

3   Return the dough to the stand mixer equipped with a paddle attachment. Sprinkle the baking powder, baking soda, and salt over the dough. Add an egg and beat on low until it forms a smooth and uniform batter. Pour the batter into the prepared pan and then bake for 20 minutes, or until a toothpick comes out clean and the edges of the cornbread begin to brown.

4   Allow the cornbread to cool completely before slicing and serving. Store the leftovers in an airtight container at room temperature for up to 3 days.

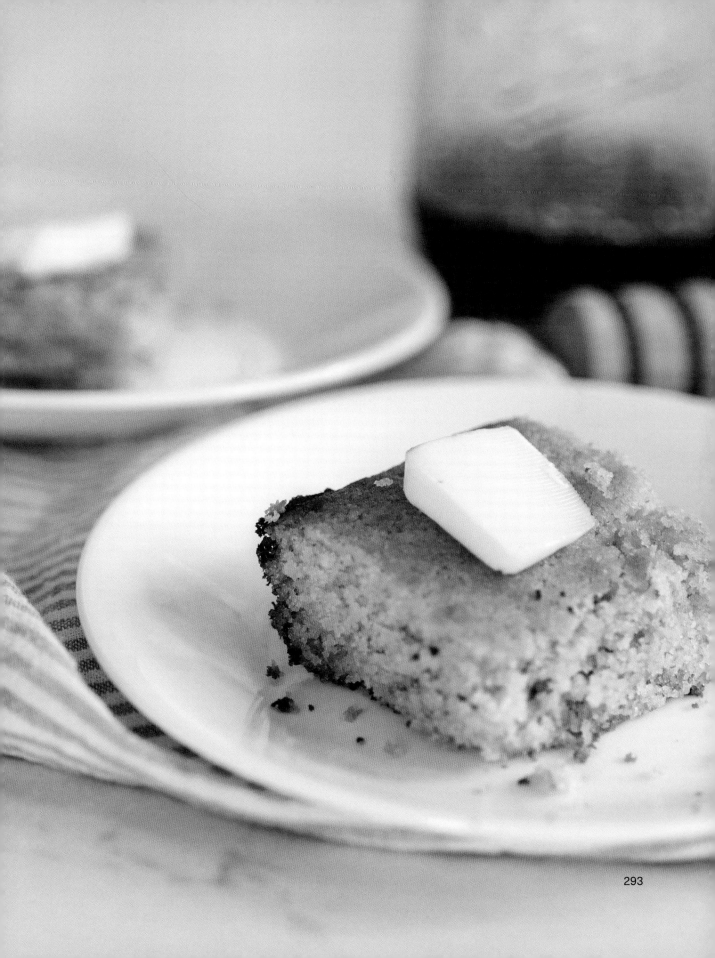

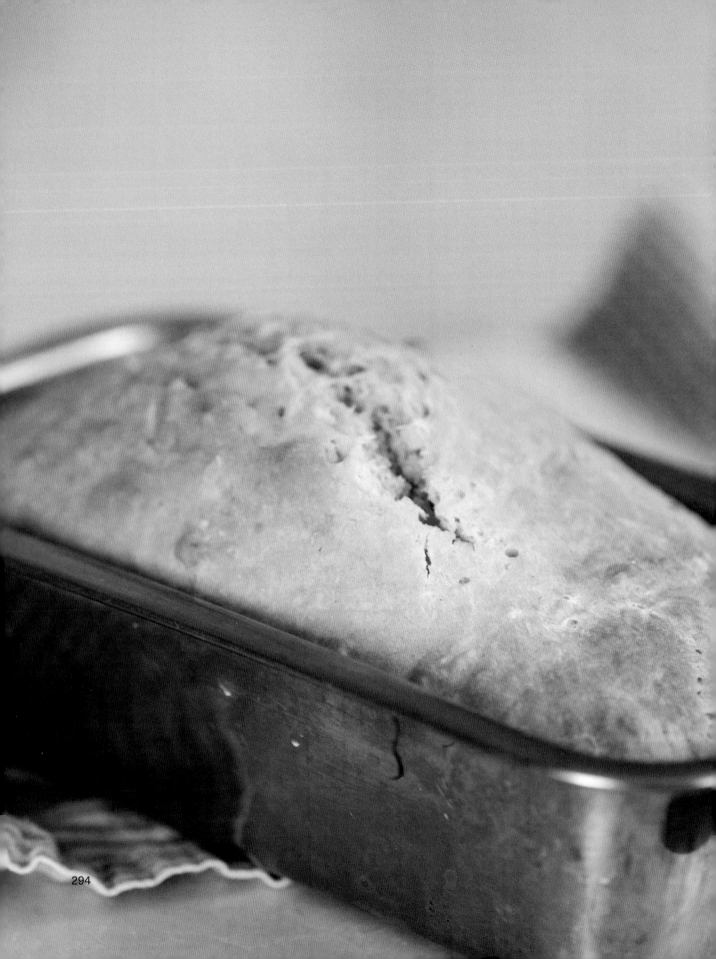

PREP TIME:
15 MINUTES

BAKE TIME:
45 MINUTES

RISE TIME:
0 MINUTES

YIELD:
MAKES 1 LOAF

Beer Bread

I love long, slow-rise artisan-style bread but don't always have time to plan ahead. When pressure is mounting, you often need something that comes together a little quicker. This beer bread ticks the mark. It has a luscious, rich, malty flavor, and it comes together in under an hour from start to finish. This makes it the perfect last-minute addition to lunch or dinner.

I love to serve it at the table with plenty of butter and sharp, raw-milk cheddar. The salty cheese is the perfect match for the yeasty, wheaten loaf. It's also delicious served alongside a big bowl of tomato soup.

3 cups (450 grams) all-purpose flour

1/4 cup (48 grams) sugar

2 teaspoons (10 grams) baking powder

1 teaspoon (6 grams) salt

12 ounces beer

1/2 cup (125 grams) sourdough discard

4 tablespoons (57 grams) melted unsalted butter, divided, plus more for the pan

1. Preheat the oven to 375°F, then lightly grease a 9-by-5-inch loaf pan with butter.

2. In a large mixing bowl, gently stir together the flour, sugar, baking powder, and salt. Add the beer, sourdough discard, and 3 tablespoons (45 grams) of the butter and stir until a uniform batter forms. Pour the batter into the prepared pan and drizzle the top with the remaining 1 tablespoon (12 grams) of butter.

3. Bake for 45 to 50 minutes, or until a toothpick inserted into the center of the bread comes out clean.

4. Allow to cool completely, and then slice and serve. Store leftovers in an airtight container at room temperature for up to 3 days.

PREP TIME:	BAKE TIME:	RISE TIME:	YIELD:
5 MINUTES	**30 MINUTES**	**0 MINUTES**	**MAKES ABOUT 6 POPOVERS**

Popovers

Popovers are magic. You start with a thin, eggy batter, and in no time, they puff up and make the most ethereal, delicate roll. I love to break them open when they're still warm and serve them with herb butter and a little homemade jam.

Temperature is the key to making good popovers great. If you're not careful, you'll find that your popovers will never puff up. Make sure that all your ingredients are at room temperature and take the time to preheat your tin in the oven. You can use a standard muffin tin if you do not have a popover tin.

Butter, for greasing the pan

1 cup (244 grams) milk, at room temperature

3 eggs, at room temperature

1/2 cup (125 grams) sourdough discard

1 teaspoon (6 grams) salt

1 cup (140 grams) all-purpose flour

1 Lightly brush a little butter on your popover or standard muffin tin and tuck it in the oven. Preheat the oven to 450°F.

2 In a large mixing bowl, beat together the milk, eggs, sourdough discard, and salt, and then whisk in the flour until it forms a smooth batter. Pour the batter into the prepared tin, filling the cups about two-thirds full.

3 Bake for 20 minutes, then turn the heat down to 350°F and continue baking for 10 minutes more, or until the popovers puff up and are golden brown. Store leftover popovers in an airtight container or ziplock bag at room temperature for up to 3 days.

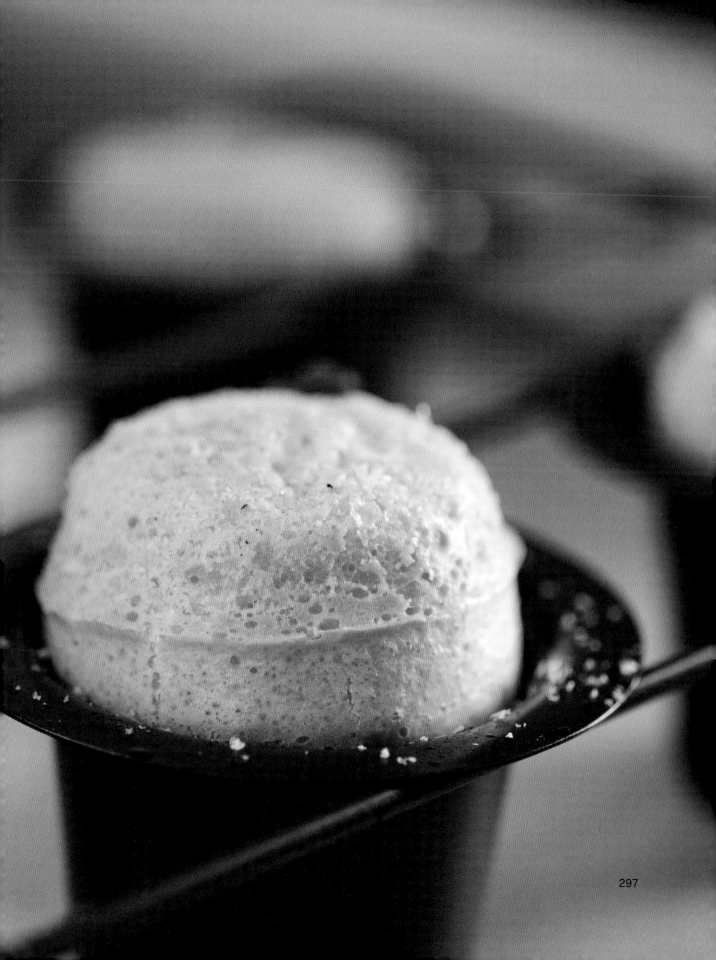

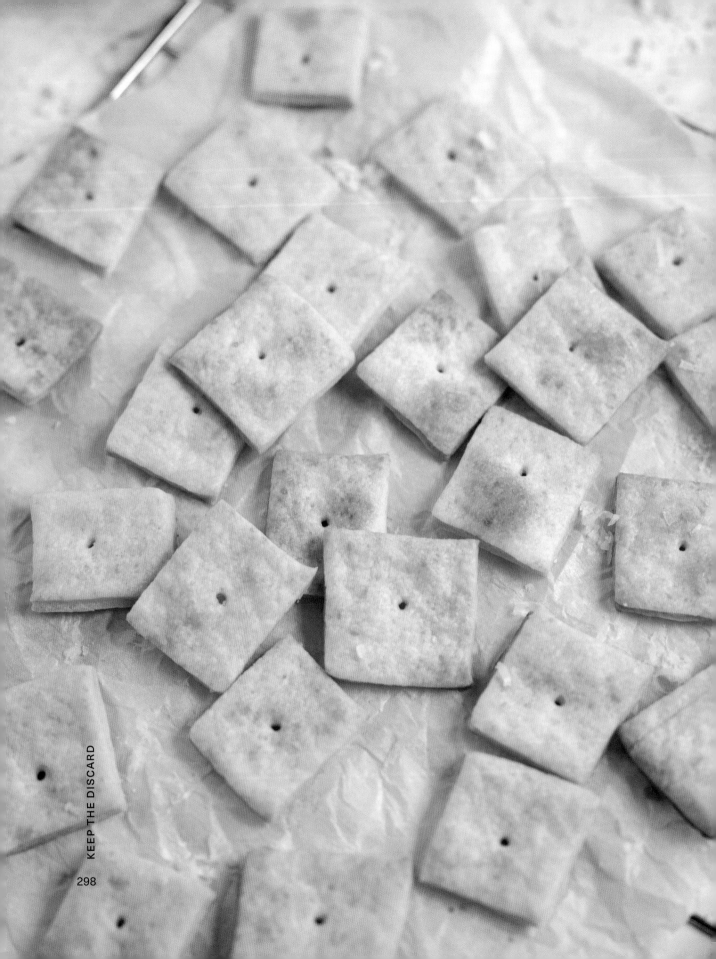

PREP TIME:
5 MINUTES

BAKE TIME:
10 MINUTES

RISE TIME:
0 MINUTES

YIELD:
**MAKES ABOUT
6 SERVINGS**

Parmesan Crackers

These rustic, wafer-thin crackers are delicious served with soup or on a charcuterie board. They have an intense, savory, salty flavor thanks to the inclusion of parmesan cheese, while sourdough starter lends its characteristic sharpness. Instead of rolling the crackers out and cutting them into neat little squares, I enjoy baking the whole sheet of dough and breaking it apart by hand. The crackers take on beautiful rustic shapes.

1 cup (250 grams)
  sourdough discard

3/4 cup (105 grams)
  all-purpose flour

1/2 cup (45 grams) freshly
  grated parmesan cheese

1/4 cup (56 grams) butter,
  at room temperature, plus
  melted butter for brushing
  the crackers, optional

1 teaspoon (6 grams) salt

1 Preheat the oven to 450°F and line a rimmed baking sheet with parchment paper.

2 In a medium mixing bowl, combine the sourdough discard, flour, cheese, butter, and salt until it comes together.

3 Place the dough between two pieces of parchment paper and roll it out as thinly as possible, about 1/16 inch. Transfer dough on the parchment to a baking sheet.

4 Remove the top piece of parchment paper and brush with melted butter, if desired. Transfer the baking sheet to the oven and bake for 10 minutes, or until crispy.

5 Cool to room temperature. Break them apart and store them in an airtight container for about 1 week.

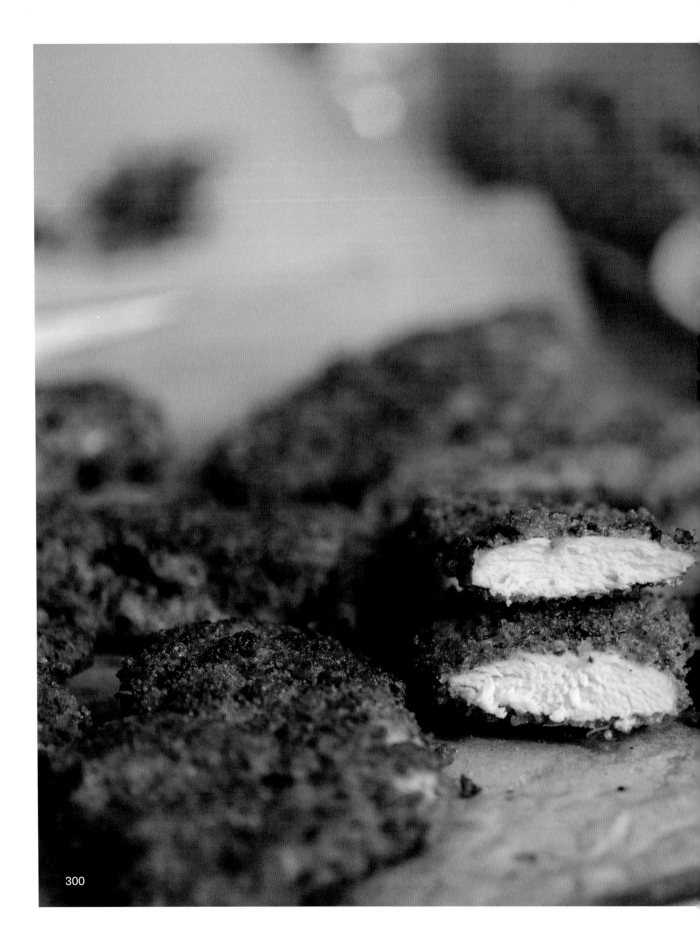

CHAPTER 9

Don't Throw It Away!

AS A BAKER, you're bound to have a few stale loaves lurking in your kitchen. And as a beginning baker, you're also likely to have a few loaves that don't turn out quite right. But don't toss them! Even bread that is stiff, dry, or didn't turn out well can find new life with a little know-how and a few ingenious hacks. In a well-tended kitchen, nothing goes to waste. Old bread is an ingredient in its own right like olive oil or butter or garlic.

It's a rebirth of sorts. What was once a waste is now a luxury. Stale bread is what lays the foundation for luscious, custardy French toast. Tossed with a little olive oil and garlic and toasted in the oven, stale bread becomes the croutons that give texture to dull lettuce salads or creamy soups. Crumbled into bread crumbs, it gives bulk to meatloaf and lends a crisp coating to fried chicken. Nestled into a baking dish with plenty of vegetables and some beaten eggs, it becomes a breakfast strata that can feed a crowd.

It's a lesson in resourcefulness, and a lesson I want to impart to my children. We should all waste less. But more importantly, we should find pleasure in resourcefulness, too.

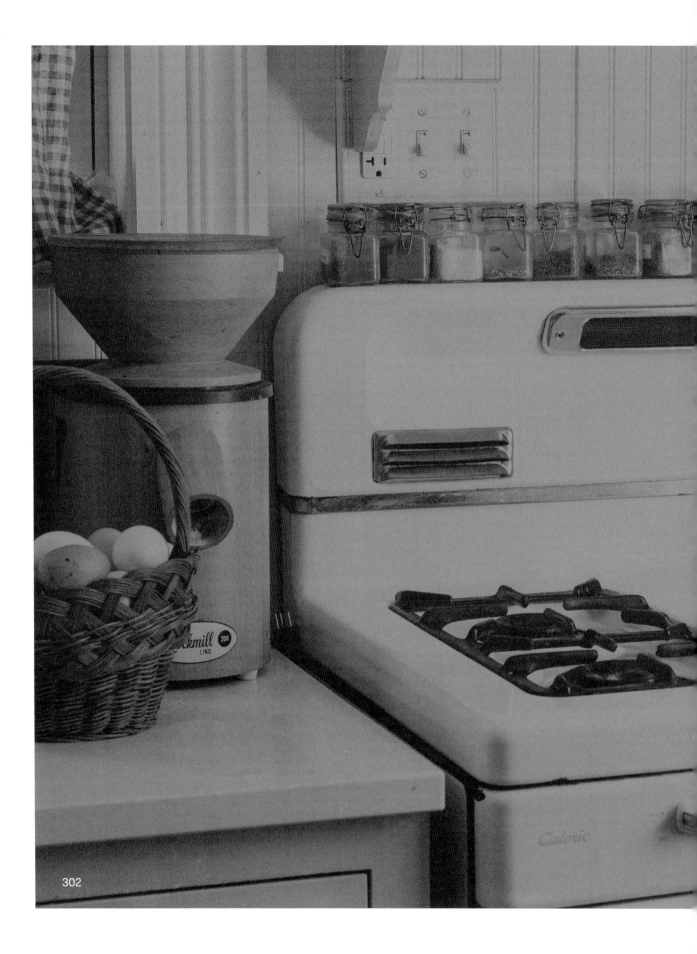

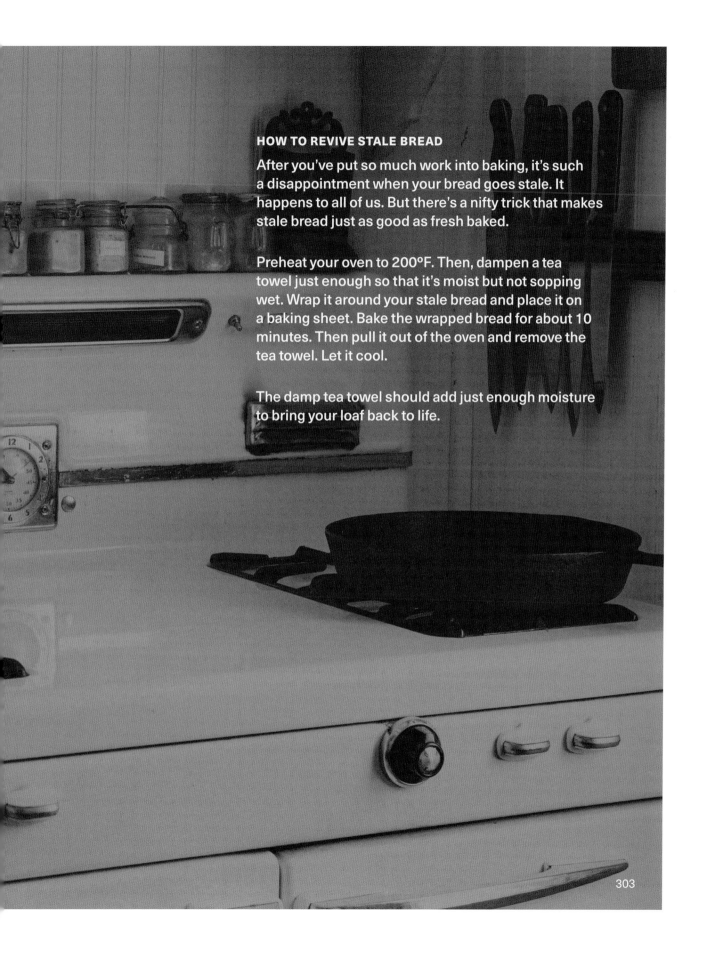

HOW TO REVIVE STALE BREAD

After you've put so much work into baking, it's such a disappointment when your bread goes stale. It happens to all of us. But there's a nifty trick that makes stale bread just as good as fresh baked.

Preheat your oven to 200°F. Then, dampen a tea towel just enough so that it's moist but not sopping wet. Wrap it around your stale bread and place it on a baking sheet. Bake the wrapped bread for about 10 minutes. Then pull it out of the oven and remove the tea towel. Let it cool.

The damp tea towel should add just enough moisture to bring your loaf back to life.

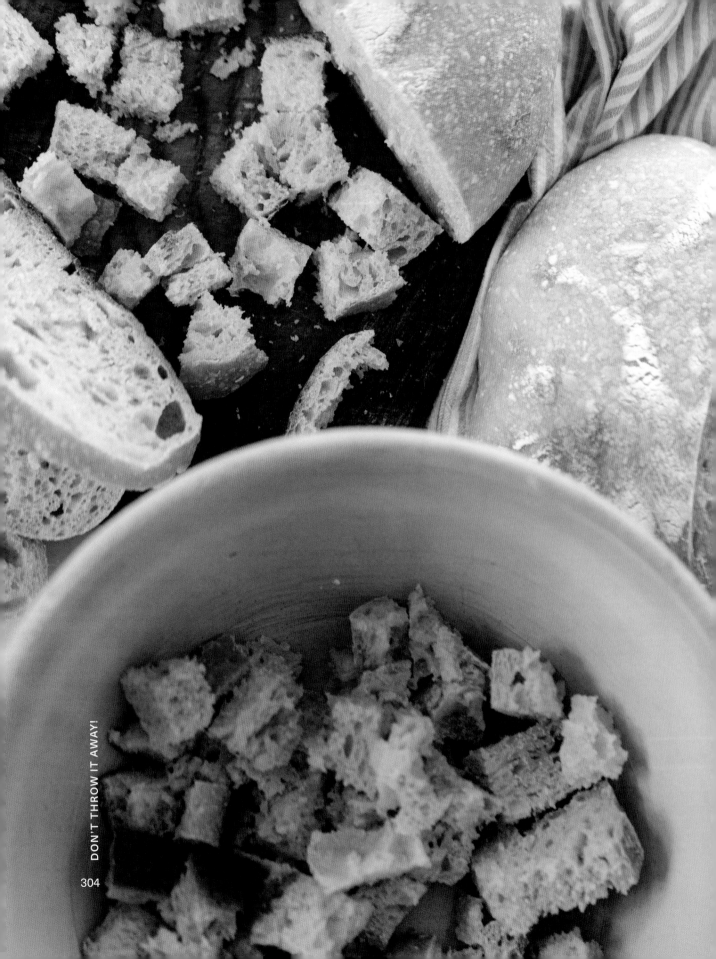

PREP TIME:
10 MINUTES

BAKE TIME:
15 MINUTES

RISE TIME:
0 MINUTES

YIELD:
**MAKES ABOUT
10 SERVINGS**

Croutons

Once you find yourself baking regularly, you're bound to end up with a few extra loaves here or there. The best way to use them is to make croutons. They're the perfect way to rescue a stale loaf and give it new life. Add them to fresh vegetable salads in the summertime or to wholesome, nourishing soups in the winter.

They're so easy to make. You just toss cubed bread in a bowl with some oil, salt, and herbs and then bake them until crisp. That's it. If you prefer a more rustic approach to cooking, you can tear the bread by hand instead of cubing it with a knife. They become super crunchy, with lots of nooks and crannies for the oil to seep into.

1 loaf day-old sourdough bread, cut into 3/4-inch cubes

1/4 cup (60 grams) extra-virgin olive oil

3 teaspoons (15 grams) herbes de Provence or Italian seasoning

1/2 teaspoon salt

1 Preheat the oven to 350ºF and line a rimmed baking sheet with parchment paper.

2 In a large mixing bowl, add the bread. Drizzle with olive oil and sprinkle the herbs and salt over top. Toss well or until the olive oil and seasonings evenly coat all the cubes of bread.

3 Arrange the bread in a single layer on the prepared baking sheet. Bake for 15 to 20 minutes, or until the edges turn golden. Allow to cool completely and enjoy. Store any leftovers in an airtight container for up to 5 days.

PREP TIME:
5 MINUTES

BAKE TIME:
30 MINUTES

RISE TIME:
0 MINUTES

YIELD:
**MAKES ABOUT
4 CUPS**

Herbed Bread Crumbs

It's always convenient to keep bread crumbs on hand. You can mix them into meatballs or meatloaf to add moisture or use them to bread Sourdough Fried Chicken (page 309). They're even delicious sautéed in olive oil and sprinkled over salads instead of croutons.

Using stale bread—a day or two old—for this recipe is vital. Fresh bread has too much moisture and may take a long time to dry out or dry unevenly.

1 loaf day-old sourdough bread, cut into 1-inch cubes

1 teaspoon garlic powder

1/2 teaspoon dried oregano

1/2 teaspoon dried thyme

1/2 teaspoon salt

1/4 teaspoon ground black pepper

1 Preheat the oven to 325°F and line a rimmed baking sheet with parchment paper.

2 Arrange the bread in a single layer on the prepared baking sheet. Bake for 20 to 30 minutes, or until completely dry, stirring about halfway through the cooking time to promote even cooking.

3 Transfer the bread cubes to a food processor. Add the garlic powder, oregano, thyme, salt, and pepper. Pulse until they form coarse crumbs.

4 Store in an airtight container at room temperature for up to 3 months.

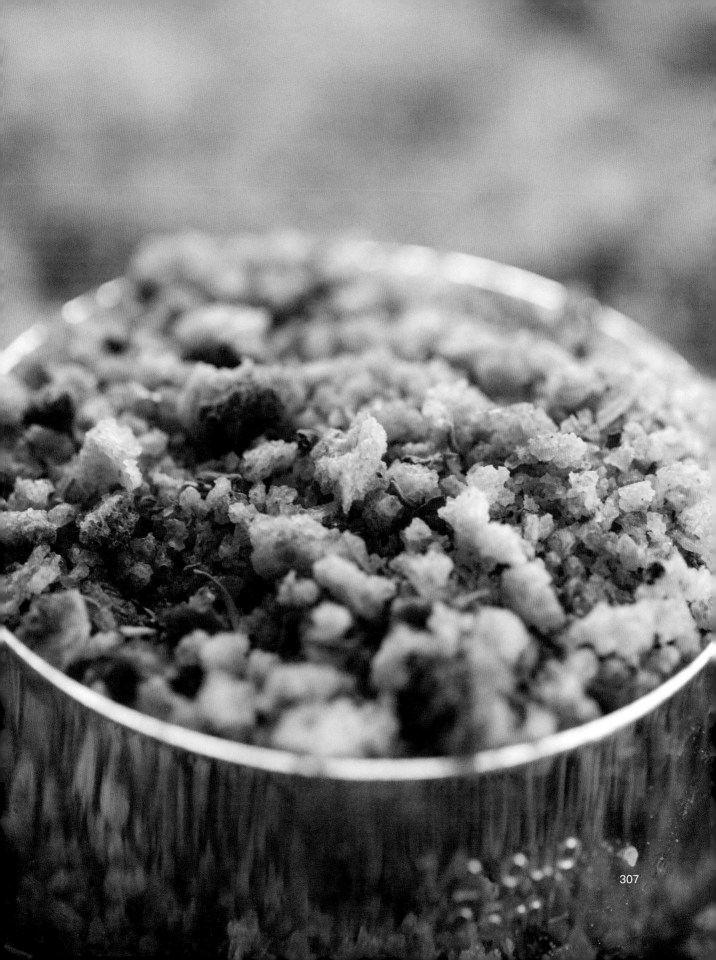

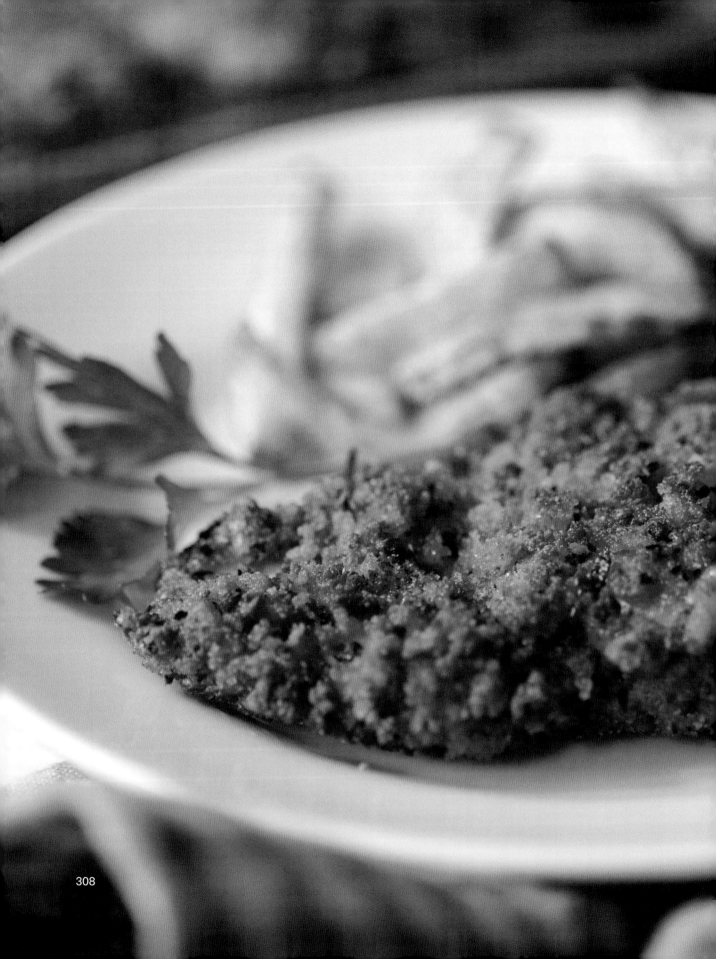

PREP TIME:
15 MINUTES

COOK TIME:
10 MINUTES

RISE TIME:
0 MINUTES

YIELD:
**MAKES ABOUT
6 SERVINGS**

Sourdough Fried Chicken

Fried chicken is one of my favorite foods, although we don't eat it too often. Instead, it's a special treat in our house, and I love to serve it with Fresh Corn Cornbread (page 292), crispy potatoes, and fresh vegetables straight from the garden.

I like to fry chicken in lard, an old-fashioned cooking fat that's perfect for fried chicken. But you can substitute an alternative such as beef tallow, refined coconut oil, or avocado oil.

Lard, for frying

2 cups (180 grams) Herbed Bread Crumbs (page 306)

2 teaspoons (12 grams) salt

2 teaspoons (10 grams) Italian seasoning

2 eggs

4 large (about 800 grams) boneless, skinless chicken breasts, halved horizontally.

1. Add enough lard to a cast-iron skillet to reach a depth of 3/4 inches. Heat over medium heat until it reaches a temperature of about 350ºF. Line a rimmed baking sheet with paper towels.

2. In a shallow bowl, whisk together the bread crumbs, salt, and herbs together.

3. In a separate small bowl, beat the eggs.

4. Pat the chicken dry with a clean kitchen towel or paper towel. Working one at a time, dip pieces of chicken into the beaten eggs, taking care to coat both sides evenly. Next, dip them in the bread crumbs.

5. Working in small batches, gently place the chicken into the hot fat and fry for about 5 minutes. Turn to the other side and cook for another 5 minutes, or until the crust is golden brown and the internal temperature is 165ºF.

6. Transfer to the prepared baking sheet to allow the oil to drain and continue frying the remaining chicken pieces.

7. Serve warm, and store any leftovers in an airtight container for up to 5 days.

PREP TIME:
10 MINUTES

BAKE TIME:
55 TO 60 MINUTES

RISE TIME:
0 MINUTES

YIELD:
**MAKES ABOUT
6 SERVINGS**

Old-Fashioned Glazed Meatloaf

When I'm after old-fashioned comfort food, I make meatloaf. There are no fancy ingredients, no complex techniques. It's just simple, wholesome food at its best. You can mix it up in about 5 minutes flat and then set it in the oven while you prepare any side dishes you might want. It's a crowd-pleaser, especially with its sweet glaze that begins to caramelize just a bit toward the end of baking.

FOR THE MEATLOAF

2 pounds (907 grams)
   ground beef

1 medium (about 100 grams)
   yellow onion,
   finely chopped

3/4 cup (60 grams) Herbed
   Bread Crumbs (page 306)

1/3 cup (80 grams) ketchup

2 eggs, beaten

1 1/2 teaspoons (9 grams)
   salt

FOR THE GLAZE

3/4 cup (180 grams) ketchup

3 tablespoons (45 grams)
   brown sugar

1 Preheat the oven to 375°F.

2 **To make the meatloaf:** In a large mixing bowl, combine the beef, onion, bread crumbs, ketchup, eggs, and salt and mix until the ingredients just come together. Form the meat mixture into a loaf and place it into a 9-by-5-inch loaf pan.

3 Transfer the meatloaf to the oven and bake for 40 minutes. Make the glaze while the meatloaf is baking.

4 **To make the glaze:** In a small bowl, combine the ketchup and brown sugar and set it aside.

5 Remove the meatloaf from the oven, brush it with the ketchup mixture, and return it to the oven for 15 to 20 minutes more, or until it reaches an internal temperature of 160°F.

6 Serve warm, and store any leftovers in an airtight container in the fridge for up to 5 days.

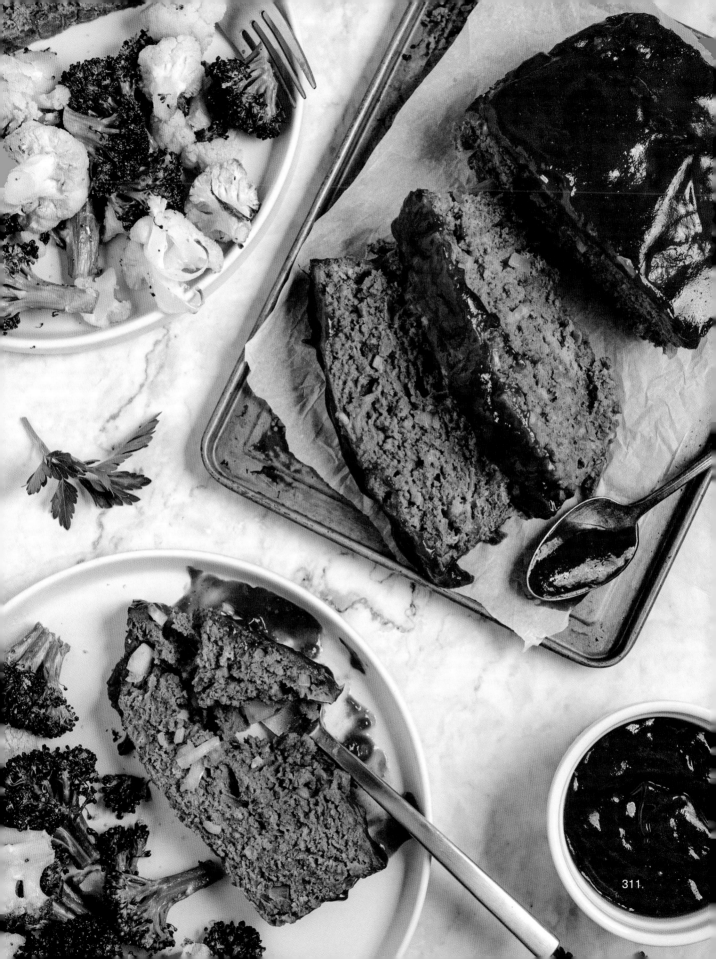

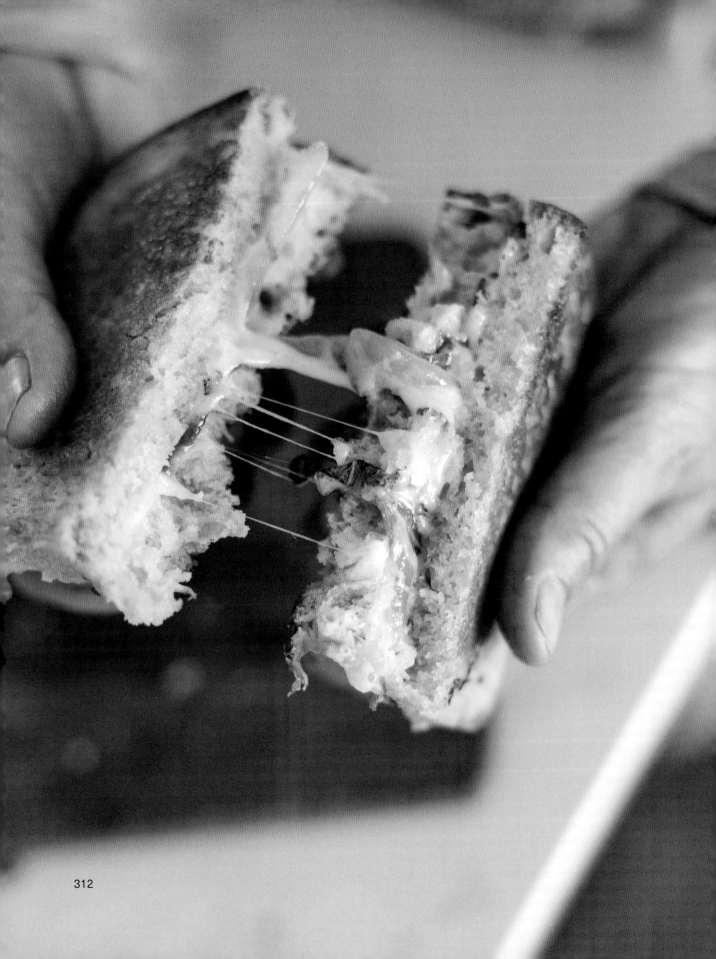

PREP TIME:
45 MINUTES

COOK TIME:
6-8 MINUTES

RISE TIME:
0 MINUTES

YIELD:
**MAKES
4 SANDWICHES**

Caramelized Onion and Herb Grilled Cheese

One of the best things about cooking at home is transforming the classics into something new. Sweet caramelized onions and vibrant fresh herbs transform a basic grilled cheese into something exquisite. Two kinds of cheese (Gruyère and cheddar) add to the deliciousness. The result is magnificent: French onion soup flavors masquerading as grilled cheese.

Best of all, once you've made the caramelized onions, the rest of the recipe is a snap. Make them in advance and then tuck them into the fridge, where they'll keep for about a week. Then, they're ready for whenever you have a hankering for this sandwich. It's so easy. You just butter the bread, fill the sandwiches, and let them cook until the cheese melts to a beautiful consistency and the bread crisps in the butter.

FOR THE CARAMELIZED ONIONS

2 tablespoons (28 grams) extra-virgin olive oil

4 medium (about 400 grams) yellow onions, thinly sliced

1 teaspoon (6 grams) salt

1 teaspoon (5 grams) sugar

FOR THE SANDWICHES

8 slices Basic Sandwich Bread (page 144)

2 tablespoons (28 grams) butter

12 ounces (340 grams) grated Gruyère cheese

8 ounces (226 grams) grated white cheddar cheese

2 teaspoons chopped fresh sage

2 teaspoons fresh thyme leaves

2 teaspoons chopped fresh rosemary

(recipe continued on next page)

1 **To make the caramelized onions**: Heat a cast-iron skillet over medium-low heat. Drizzle in the olive oil, add the onions, and sprinkle them with salt and sugar. Cook, stirring occasionally to prevent scorching or uneven cooking, for about 40 minutes, or until sweet and meltingly tender. Set the onions aside, or transfer them to an airtight container and store in the fridge for up to 1 week.

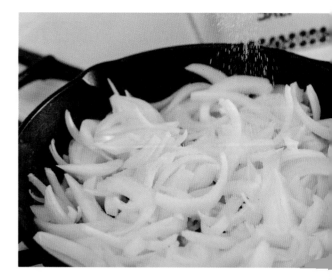

2 **To make the sandwiches:** Wipe your skillet clean, and then heat it over medium heat.

3 Slather each slice of bread with butter on one side only. Then, top 4 slices of the bread with Gruyère, cheddar cheese, caramelized onions, sage, thyme, and rosemary. Top each with a second slice of bread, buttered side out.

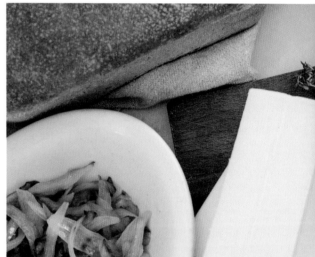

4 Place the sandwiches in the skillet and cover. Allow the sandwiches to cook for 3 to 4 minutes, or until the bread starts to turn golden on one side and the cheese starts to melt. Flip and cook for 3 to 4 minutes more, or until the bread begins to turn golden. Remove from the skillet and slice. Serve warm.

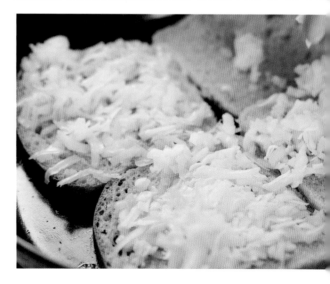

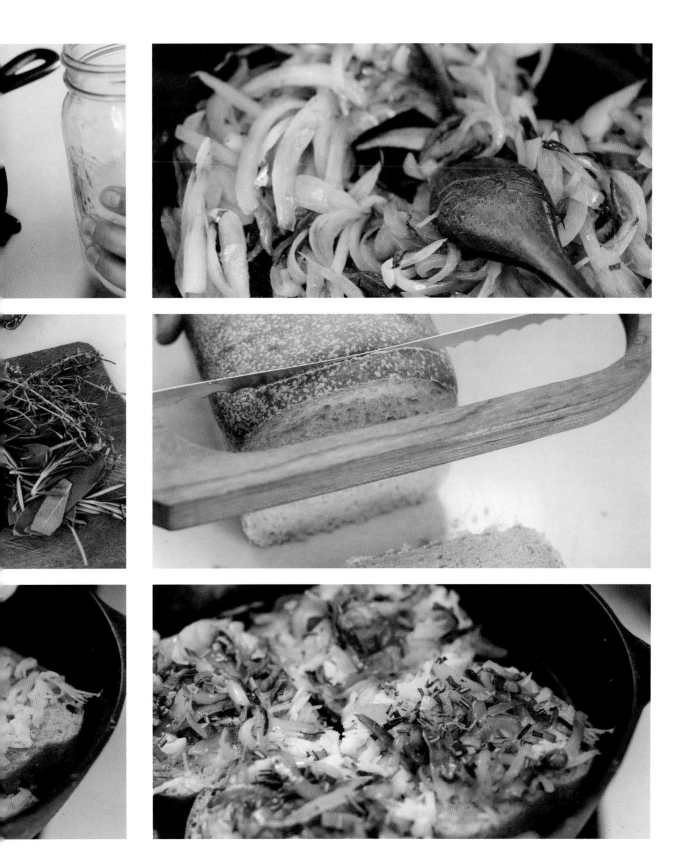

PREP TIME:
5 MINUTES

COOK TIME:
10 MINUTES

RISE TIME:
0 MINUTES

YIELD:
MAKES 4 SANDWICHES

Breakfast Sandwiches

Hearty and filling, breakfast sandwiches are a great way to start the day. We love when we have extra English muffins in our pantry. They're perfect for using up extra eggs, especially in the springtime when the chickens lay frequently. We can hardly seem to keep up with them.

You can easily customize the sandwiches. Skip the bacon in favor of ham, or use Swiss cheese or Havarti instead of cheddar. I often like adding sliced tomato and avocado to the sandwiches.

4 English Muffins (page 187)

4 teaspoons (19 grams) butter, divided, plus more for the pan

4 eggs

8 slices (about 96 ounces) crisp bacon, divided

4 slices (about 120 grams) cheddar cheese, divided

1 Warm a large skillet over medium heat.

2 Cut the English muffins in half horizontally, then toast in the skillet for a few minutes, or until golden. Spread each muffin wth 1 teaspoon of butter and set them aside.

3 Add a little butter to the skillet and then cook the eggs to your liking.

4 Divide the eggs evenly on 4 of the English muffins, then top each muffin with 2 slices of bacon and 1 slice of cheese. Top with the remaining halves of the English muffins and serve warm.

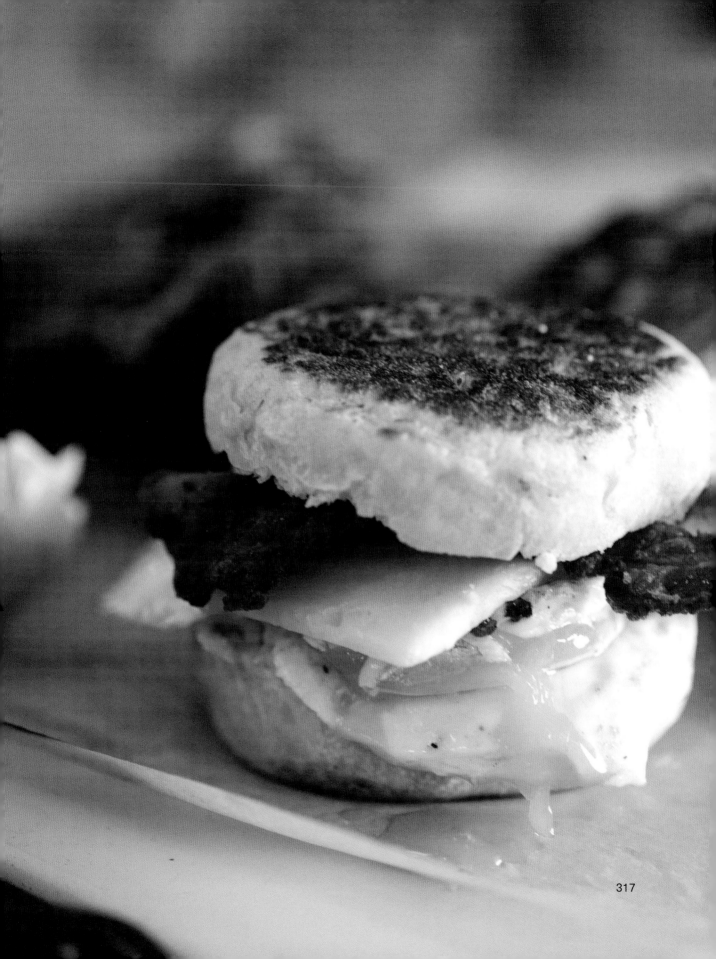

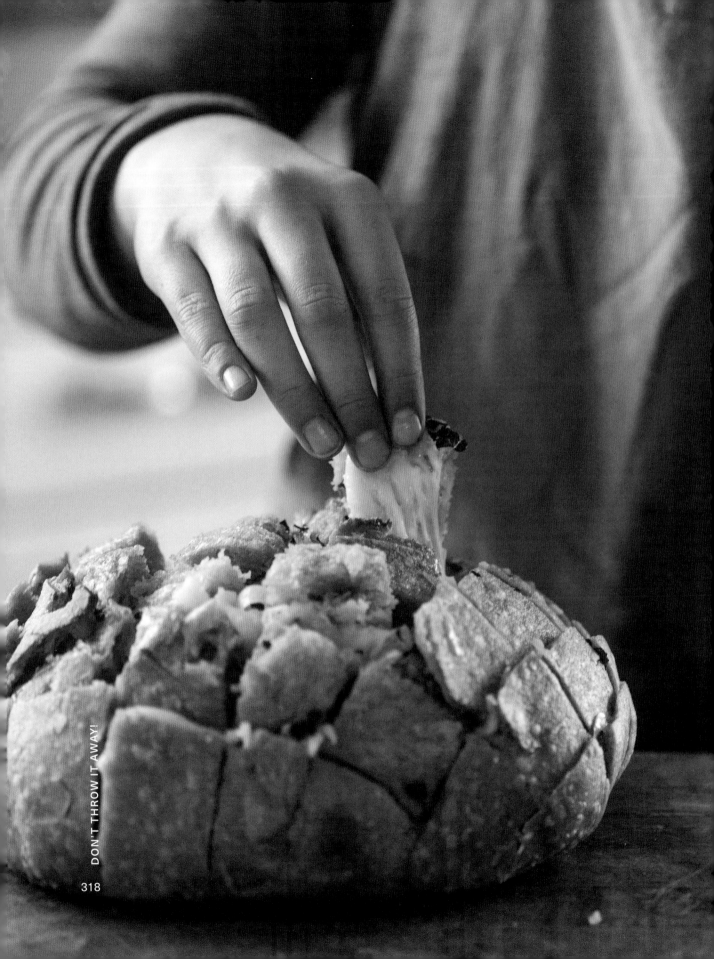

PREP TIME:
10 MINUTES

BAKE TIME:
35 MINUTES

RISE TIME:
0 MINUTES

YIELD:
MAKES 1 LOAF

Cheesy Pull-Apart Bread

All it takes is some melted butter, fresh herbs, garlic, and lots of mozzarella cheese to turn ordinary bread into something indulgent. As the bread warms in the oven, garlic-herb butter seeps into all the nooks and crannies, drenching every crumb with flavor. The mozzarella melts, covering each little piece of bread in cheese. The best part? You can use day-old bread for this recipe, so there's no need to bake a special loaf.

If you prefer, you can substitute another cheese for mozzarella. Any cheese that melts well works, including cheddar, fontina, Havarti, and Gruyère.

1 loaf No-Knead Sourdough Bread (page 120)

8 tablespoons (114 grams) melted butter

1/4 cup (about 8 grams) coarsely chopped fresh parsley

3 medium (about 15 grams) garlic cloves, minced

1/2 teaspoon salt

8 ounces (226 grams) shredded low-moisture mozzarella cheese

1 Preheat the oven to 350°F.

2 Slice the bread diagonally at 1-inch intervals, taking care to slice to the bottom of the bread without slicing completely through it. Rotate the bread a quarter turn, and make another series of diagonal cuts to create a crisscross pattern.

3 In a small bowl, stir the butter, parsley, garlic, and salt together. Brush the garlic-herb butter inside the cuts throughout the bread so that it deeply penetrates. Then, pack shredded cheese into the cuts.

4 Wrap the bread in foil and set it on a rimmed baking sheet. Bake for 35 minutes, or until the herbs are fragrant and the cheese has melted completely. Serve warm. Store in an airtight container or a ziplock bag in the fridge for up to 1 week.

PREP TIME:
5 MINUTES

BAKE TIME:
10 MINUTES

RISE TIME:
0 MINUTES

YIELD:
MAKES 8 SERVINGS

Sourdough Garlic Bread

You know when you just need that perfect "back pocket" recipe that will always, and I mean *always*, complement dinner? The same recipe that will always impress a crowd, no matter where you take it? Well, this sourdough garlic bread is the ticket.

We're talking sourdough bread that has been long fermented to develop all that amazing tangy goodness, then slathered with a garlic-herb butter and topped with cheese. It's toasted to perfection—where all the little edges and the parmesan cheese start to turn golden and crisp. It's delicious partnered with robust soup for lunch, a bright summer salad, or a big plate of pasta and tomato sauce.

1 loaf Sourdough French Bread (page 143)

1/2 cup (113 grams) butter, at room temperature

4 medium (about 15 grams) cloves garlic, minced

3 tablespoons (about 8 grams) chopped fresh parsley

2 tablespoons (28 grams) extra-virgin olive oil

1/4 teaspoon salt

1/4 cup (25 grams) grated parmesan cheese

1 Preheat the oven to 400°F and line a rimmed baking sheet with parchment paper.

2 Slice the bread lengthwise through the middle, so that you have two even, long halves. Set it on the prepared baking sheet.

3 In a small bowl, beat together the butter, garlic, parsley, olive oil, and salt until they form a uniform paste. Generously spread both halves of the bread with the garlic-herb butter and then sprinkle with parmesan cheese.

4 Transfer to the oven and bake for 10 minutes or until the cheese melts and the bread is lightly toasted at the edges. Allow it to cool for about 5 minutes until it's comfortable to handle, then slice and serve. Store in an airtight container or a ziplock bag in the fridge for up to 1 week.

DON'T THROW IT AWAY!

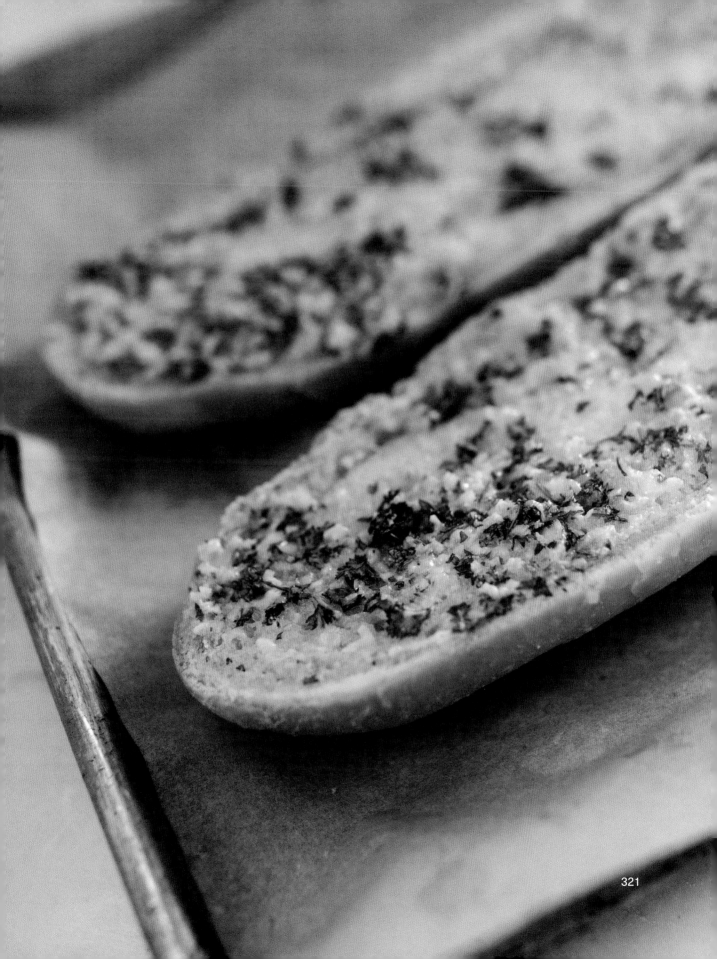

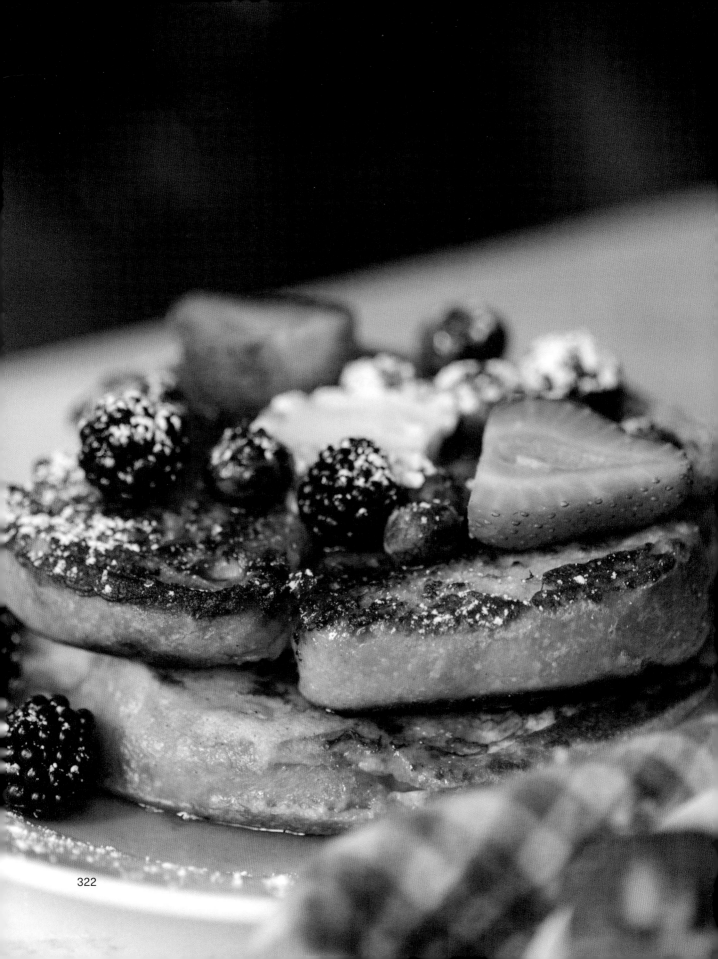

PREP TIME:
15 MINUTES

COOK TIME:
20 MINUTES

RISE TIME:
0 MINUTES

YIELD:
MAKES 8 SERVINGS

French Toast

Day-old brioche bread makes perfect French toast. The soft, pillowy bread turns delightfully custardy in a hot skillet. In the cold months, I'll often serve it with maple syrup and plenty of butter. In the summer, fresh berries and plenty of whipped cream seem like the right fit.

8 eggs

1/2 cup (120 grams) milk

1/4 cup (50 grams) sugar

2 teaspoons (6 grams) cinnamon

1 teaspoon (5 grams) vanilla extract

1 loaf Sourdough Brioche (page 150), cut into 8 slices

Butter, for frying

Maple syrup, jam, berries, and whipped cream, for serving

1   Heat a cast-iron skillet over medium heat.

2   In a shallow dish, whisk the eggs, milk, sugar, cinnamon, and vanilla until smooth. Dip the bread slices into the egg mixture and soak for a few minutes on both sides. The bread should be soaked through, having absorbed much of the egg mixture.

3   Melt the butter in the hot pan, then turn down the heat to medium-low.

4   Working one at a time, carefully place the egg-soaked brioche into the skillet and fry for a few minutes on each side or until browned and cooked through.

5   Serve warm with maple syrup, jam, or berries and freshly whipped cream. Store any leftovers in the fridge for up to 3 days.

PREP TIME:
10 MINUTES

BAKE TIME:
30 MINUTES

RISE TIME:
0 MINUTES, PLUS 8-24 HOURS CHILLING TIME

YIELD:
MAKES ABOUT 4 SERVINGS

French Toast Casserole with Apples and Raisins

French toast casserole is the perfect make-ahead breakfast. It has all the flavor and richness of French toast without the fuss of hovering over a hot skillet. You prepare the casserole the night before and let it set in the fridge overnight. The following day, put it in the oven to bake. It will be ready in about half an hour.

I love the combination of apples and raisins, but you can also swap in fresh or frozen berries or other fruit, depending on the season.

2 cups (240 grams) whole milk

1/2 cup (160 grams) maple syrup

10 eggs

1 teaspoon (5 grams) vanilla extract

1/2 teaspoon cinnamon

1 loaf day-old No-Knead Sourdough Bread (page 120), cubed

4 medium (about 300 grams) apples, peeled, cored, and chopped

1/2 cup (85 gram) raisins

1/2 cup (113 grams) melted butter

1   Preheat the oven to 350°F.

2   In a medium mixing bowl, whisk the milk, maple syrup, eggs, vanilla, and cinnamon until they form a uniform mixture.

3   Arrange the cubed bread, chopped apples, and raisins in a 9-by-13-inch baking dish. Pour the egg mixture over the bread, cover it tightly with foil or plastic wrap, and transfer it to the fridge for at least 8 and up to 24 hours or until the bread is fully saturated.

4   The next day, preheat the oven to 350°F.

5   Drizzle the butter over the top of the bread mixture, transfer it to the oven, and bake for 30 minutes, or until cooked through and golden brown on top.

6   Serve warm, and store any leftovers in an airtight container in the fridge for up to 3 days.

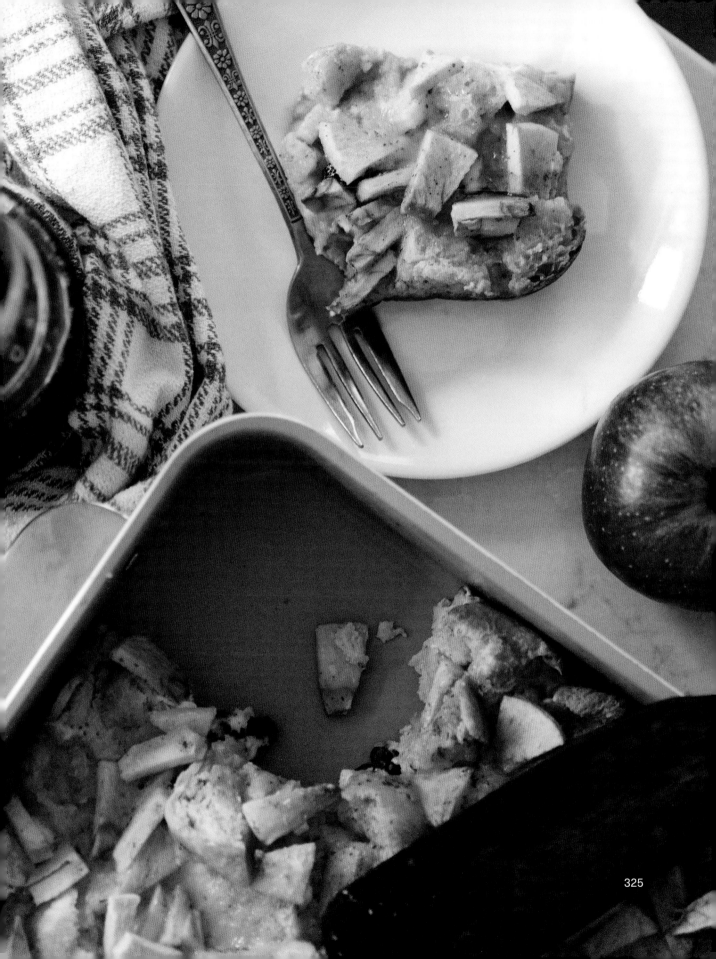

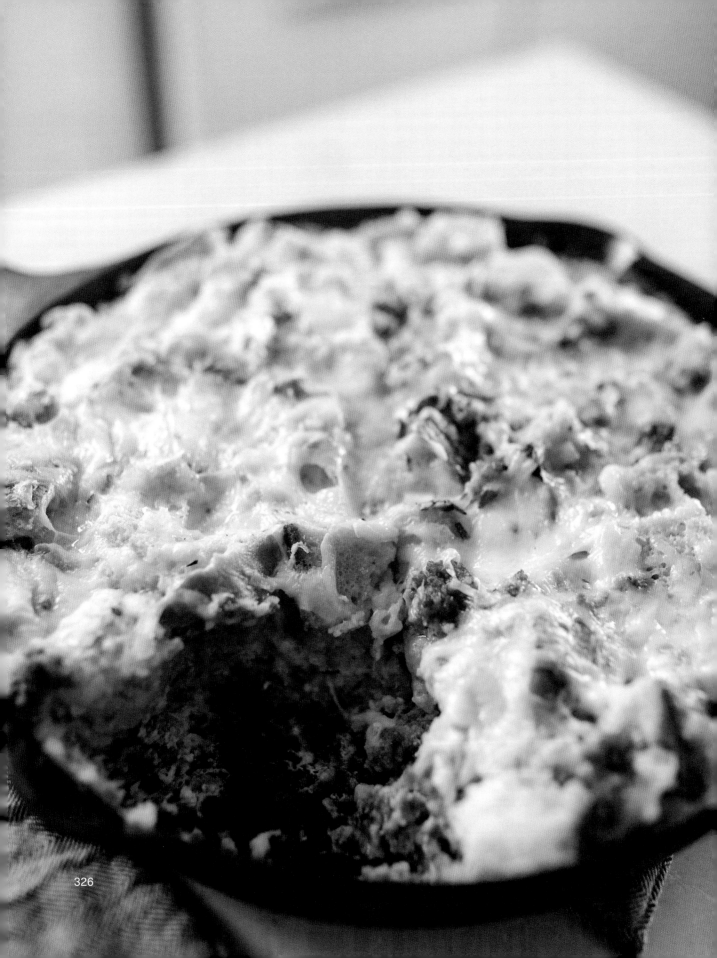

PREP TIME:
20 MINUTES

COOK TIME:
1 HOUR

RISE TIME:
**0 MINUTES + 8 TO 12
HOURS CHILLING TIME**

YIELD:
MAKES ABOUT 8 SERVINGS

Sausage and Herb Breakfast Strata

Every morning, no matter the weather, farm chores await. Goats need milking. Animals need feeding. The chickens need moving, and the cows must be turned out to fresh pasture. It's hard and gratifying work that drives a deep hunger. We need something hardy to fill bellies made hungrier by the work and something warm to take the chill away.

We are always grateful to come inside for a warm, filling meal on winter mornings. This strata feels heaven-sent at times like those. It's fuel for hard work, but it tastes delicious, too. Fresh herbs lend a little brightness to the rich, robust flavor of sausage and cheese. It's also a great way to use sourdough bread leftover from the previous day.

1 loaf day-old Same-Day Sourdough Bread (page 118), about 6 cups, cubed

1 tablespoon (14 grams) extra-virgin olive oil

1 medium (about 100 grams) onion, diced

1 pound (454 grams) loose breakfast sausage

10 eggs

3 cups (742 grams) whole milk

2 tablespoons (8 grams) finely chopped fresh sage

1 tablespoon fresh thyme leaves

1 tablespoon finely chopped fresh rosemary

3/4 teaspoon salt

1/2 teaspoon ground black pepper

2 cups (200 grams) shredded Gruyère cheese, divided

1 Preheat the oven to 350°F. On a baking sheet, arrange the bread in a single layer and bake until toasted, about 15 minutes. Set aside.

2 While the bread is baking, in a wide skillet over medium heat, warm the olive oil. Toss in the onion and cook for about 8 minutes, or until fragrant and translucent. Stir in the sausage and cook for about 10 minutes, or until well-browned. Turn off the heat and set aside.

3 In a large mixing bowl, whisk together the eggs, milk, sage, thyme, rosemary, salt, and pepper.

4 Arrange the toasted bread in a 9-by-13-inch baking dish or large cast-iron skillet. Stir 1 cup (100 grams) of the shredded Gruyère cheese and the sausage mixture into the bread. Pour the egg mixture into the baking dish, then spread the remaining 1 cup (100 grams) of shredded Gruyère cheese on top. Cover with foil and then transfer to the fridge overnight for at least 8 and up to 12 hours.

5 The next morning, preheat the oven to 350°F.

6 Transfer the foil-covered dish to the oven. Bake for 45 minutes, then remove the foil and continue baking for 15 minutes more, or until cooked through.

7 Serve warm. To store, cover the pan with foil and keep in the fridge for up to 5 days.

PREP TIME:
15 MINUTES

BAKE TIME:
45 MINUTES

RISE TIME:
0 MINUTES

YIELD:
MAKES ABOUT 12 SERVINGS

Cinnamon-Raisin Bread Pudding

When the pastures are frosty and the wood stove is bright with firelight, I crave simple, nourishing comfort food. I think we all do. Winter's cold weather calls to us that way. This bread pudding is perfect for those nights. It's soft and warm, infused with cinnamon and dotted with raisins.

It's also mercifully inexpensive to make. All you need is day-old bread and a little milk, sugar, and eggs. Yet, despite the simple, humble ingredients, it feels marvelously indulgent—especially on those cold nights.

FOR THE BREAD PUDDING

1 loaf Sourdough Brioche (page 150), cut into 2-inch cubes

3 cups (720 grams) whole milk

3/4 cup (144 grams) sugar

1/4 cup (57 grams) melted butter, plus more for the baking dish

1 teaspoon (5 grams) vanilla extract

1 teaspoon cinnamon

1/4 teaspoon salt

4 eggs, beaten

1 cup (200 grams) raisins

FOR THE SAUCE

1 cup (230 grams) heavy cream

1/2 cup (96 grams) sugar

2 tablespoons (15 grams) all-purpose flour

1 tablespoon (15 grams) vanilla extract

1. Preheat the oven to 350°F and butter a 9-by-13-inch baking dish.

2. **To make the bread pudding:** Arrange the bread in the prepared baking dish.

3. In a medium bowl, whisk together the milk, sugar, butter, vanilla, cinnamon, and salt, then whisk in the eggs. Pour the egg mixture over the bread, sprinkle with raisins, and bake for 45 minutes, or until golden brown and completely set.

4. **To make the sauce:** While the bread pudding bakes, in a small saucepan over medium heat, whisk the cream, sugar, flour, and vanilla. Stir constantly until there are no more lumps.

5. Turn the heat down to low and continue cooking for about 5 minutes, or until thickened. Allow the sauce to cool slightly, drizzle over the bread pudding, and serve warm. To store, cover the pan with foil and keep in the fridge for up to 1 week.

DON'T THROW IT AWAY!

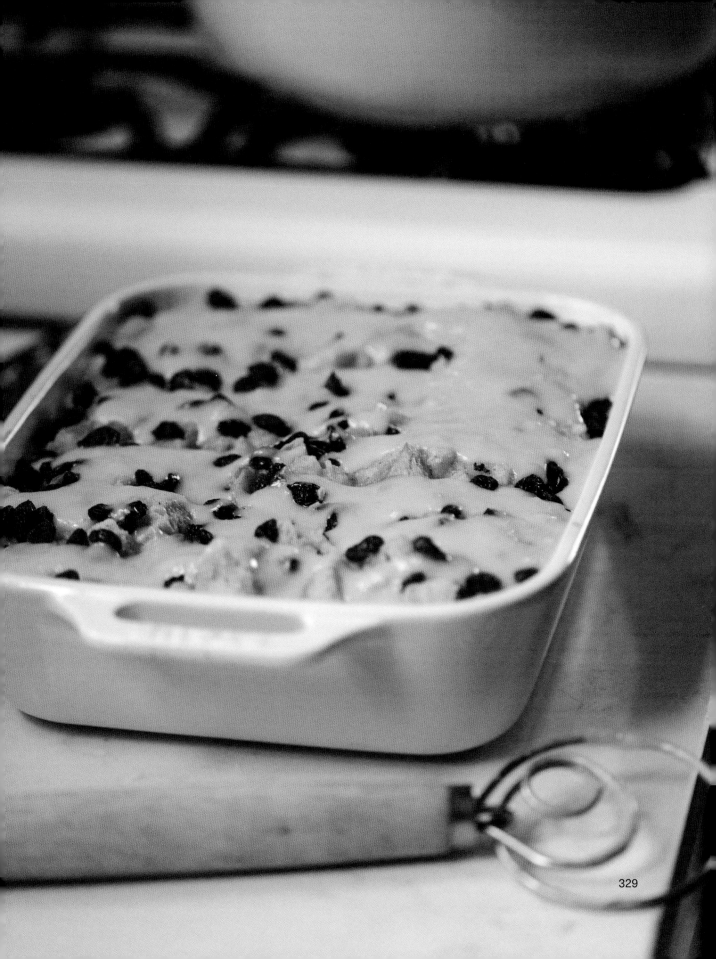

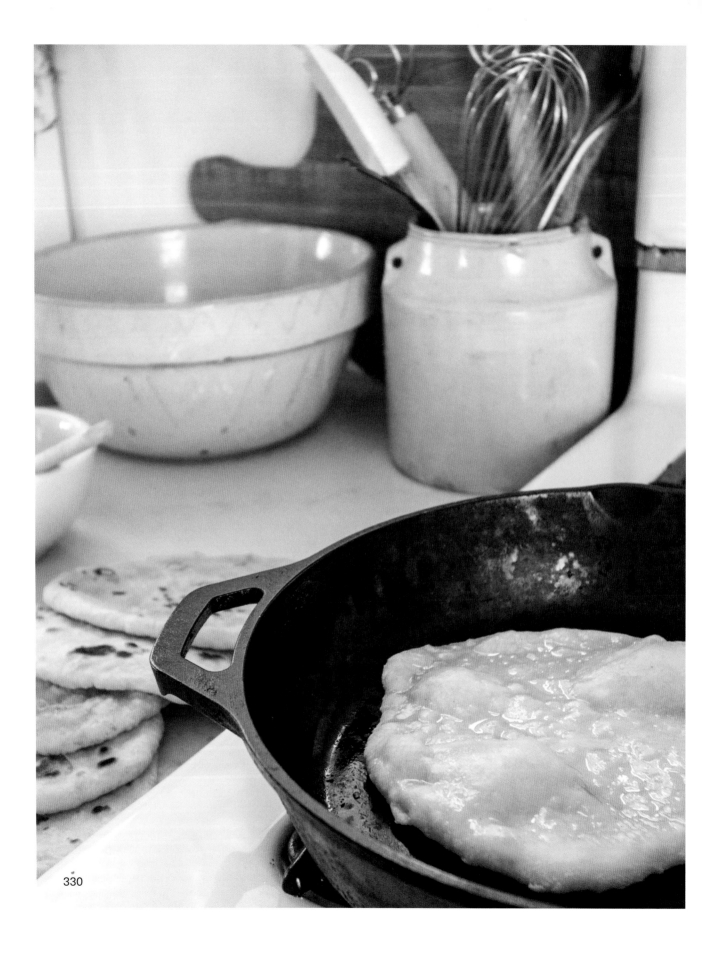

Troubleshooting

AS WITH ANY TYPE of baking, many factors affect the quality of your breads and treats. Sourdough is no different. It takes time to get to know your starter, hone your technique, and start making great bread. Plenty of practice builds great bakers.

Between creating your first starter, to proofing dough, to baking bread, there's a lot of room for error. Many new bakers experience a few stumbling blocks as they learn the process. And that's okay. I've outlined some of the most common challenges (and solutions) in this troubleshooting guide.

The Starter

Why is it taking so long for my starter to mature?
A starter needs this time to mature. For most bakers, the process takes a week. For some bakers, it takes two. Many bakers find that it takes three to four weeks before their starters are mature enough to consistently deliver good bread. Yeast and bacteria can take a long time to establish themselves. Many factors influence how long it takes your starter to mature. Temperature and water quality are especially important. Cold temperatures slow down fermentation. If you're working in a cold, winter kitchen, your starter will take longer to mature. Additionally, chlorinated water can impact fermentation. If you're having trouble, try filtering your water. Continue feeding your starter, and it will mature with time.

Can I use a different flour to feed my starter?
If you're out of your favorite flour, you can substitute another grain-based flour that you have. For example, if you're out of bread flour, you can use all-purpose. If you usually feed your starter whole-wheat flour, but you have only rye on hand, use that. You may notice some subtle differences in how the starter smells or how long it takes to rise when you change its food source. You can always switch back when you have your favorite flour in the pantry.

What is the liquid that forms on top of my starter?

Sometimes a yellow-gray liquid forms on the top of the sourdough starter. Sourdough bakers call it "hooch" because it is an alcoholic byproduct of fermentation. Hooch develops when your starter is hungry. The microbes have eaten their way through the flour in your starter and have begun producing alcohol. Pour off the liquid. Discard half of the remaining sourdough starter, and feed it equal parts flour and water. It may take a few feedings for your starter to return to its normal, bubbly self.

Why does my starter smell like nail polish or alcohol?

Starters can sometimes smell like acetone, beer, or liquor. Your starter is probably hungry. Discard half your starter, and feed it in an equal volume of flour and water to what you removed. It may take one or two feedings for your starter to bounce back.

If your starter smells putrid or so bad that you recoil when you open the jar, discard it and start over. A foul, putrid, or moldy smell is a good sign that your starter is unhealthy.

Is it possible to kill my starter?

Starters are resilient. More often than not, a little diligent care is all you need to bring a neglected starter back to life. If you've ignored your starter for months, discard all but a tablespoon or two at the bottom of the jar. Transfer this to a clean jar, and follow the instructions on creating a sourdough starter on page 80. It should revive within a week.

Use your best judgment here on whether it is "bad" or not. Its aroma and appearance will tell you if it truly is bad. If you see any signs of mold or discoloration, dump it and start over.

Exposing your starter to temperatures over 120°F can damage your starter. Temperatures over 140°F will kill your starter.

What if I see mold on my starter?

Sourdough starter is naturally acidic. This high level of acid helps protect the starter from mold. It is very rare for starters to develop mold, but it happens occasionally—especially in neglected starters. You might notice a musty smell when you open the jar or observe fuzzy spots of blue or black around the lip of the jar or on the surface of the starter. If you notice these signs, it's best to discard your starter entirely and start over with fresh water and flour in a clean jar.

Why is my starter bubbling, but not rising?

If your starter is bubbling but not rising, there are a few potential reasons. It could be a microbial imbalance, temperature fluctuations, or too much water.

If your starter erupts with a flurry of bubbles in the first few days before all activity stops, you have a bacterial imbalance. It's best to discard what you have and start over. A bit of established starter from a friend who bakes or that you buy from a shop can help set you on the right track

Hot temperatures favor bacteria and cool temperatures favor yeast development. So if it's summertime and your kitchen is warm, you might move your starter to a cooler space. It should start bubbling and rising when you control the temperature.

I recommend feeding your starter equal portions of flour and water. If you feed your starter more water than flour, you can create a very liquid starter. It may bubble but be too wet to rise. This is fine, and liquid starters can make great bread. To see if your starter is ready to bake, drop a spoonful into a glass of water. If it floats, your starter is ready for baking. If it sinks, feed it.

How often should I clean my starter's jar?

As long as there are no signs of mold or other forms of contamination, it's okay to keep your starter in the same jar indefinitely. I rarely clean mine. If it gets too crusty and unappealing, you can scoop your starter into a fresh jar, feed it, and then wash the old one. Switching jars every four to six weeks seems to work for many people, but you can also let it continue on in the same jar for months or even years. A well-tended starter doesn't need to switch jars; its bacteria and yeast are working in harmony.

The Dough

How do I know when my dough has risen enough?

During bulk fermentation it should just about double in volume. Doughs made with lots of whole-grain flours will rise a little less because the bits of bran and germ in the flour can puncture the air bubbles in the dough. Enriched doughs with lots of butter will also increase in volume but may not quite double.

For the final proof, gently press your finger into the dough. If it springs back immediately, it needs more time. If it slowly fills the indent left from your finger, it's ready for the oven. If the indent stays without filling, your dough is overproofed.

Why is my dough so stiff?

Sometimes your dough may just need a little more water—especially if it's too stiff right out of the mixer. Sometimes, it's too stiff because of overhandling. Handling and kneading the dough supports gluten development, but too much handling can stiffen the gluten and make the dough difficult to work with. Letting it rest for 30 minutes should help.

For many sourdough recipes, stretches and folds are gentle and should help, so when there is an option for stretch and fold, that is probably the better route. If your dough is still too stiff after doing stretches and folds, you may need to add more liquid to your dough.

Why is my dough so wet and sticky?

Sourdough often uses more liquid than many bread recipes. This is especially true for artisan-style breads. Time, kneading, and the stretch-and-fold technique can transform a dough from wet and shaggy to smooth and pliable. If the dough is too hard to handle, this is usually the case.

Sometimes, overproving your dough can make it sticky. This means you've allowed it to rise for too long during bulk fermentation. The extra time fermenting weakened the gluten bonds. Overproofed dough looks extremely puffy and also fragile. It deflates with very little pressure since the gluten has lost its strength. You might have luck dusting your working surface with flour and reshaping it.

Why didn't my dough rise very much during proofing?

Your dough will rise the most during bulk fermentation. Once you've shaped the dough for its final rise, it might grow a little bit. However, that growth won't be quite as dramatic as the first rise. In my experience, I see the greatest expansion in a shaped loaf during the first stage of baking (oven spring).

If you find your dough isn't rising at all, your kitchen might be too cold or your starter might be immature.

Why did my dough develop a crust while it was rising?

If you leave your dough uncovered, especially in a dry climate, it might dry out and form a crust. Always cover your dough while it rises unless the recipe instructs otherwise. During the bulk fermentation, you can cover the bowl with a lid or a square of plastic wrap. During the final proof, you can lay a damp tea towel over your dough or tuck it inside a loose plastic bag to keep it moist.

How do I know if I let my dough rise long enough?

The time your dough needs to rise during bulk fermentation depends on many factors. Everything from the time of year to altitude will affect how long your dough needs to ferment. Even the maturity of your starter plays a role. Dough will take longer to rise in a cold kitchen and less time to rise in a warm one. A lively, mature starter will make dough rise faster than an immature starter. Doughs that contain fats, such as butter or eggs, will take longer to rise and may not double at all.

During bulk fermentation look for a few telltale signs. You can tell your dough is ready when it has about doubled in size. For enriched doughs, it may not double, but it should grow significantly larger. A smooth surface marked by occasional bubbles is a good sign.

For the final proof, test the dough by gently pressing a fingertip into it. If it springs back immediately, your dough needs more time. If the dough slowly rises back into place, but a small indent remains, it's ready to bake. If the indent remains and does not fill at all, your dough is over-proofed. This is because the gluten structure is no longer strong enough to hold its shape.

How do I slow down the bulk fermentation?
If you have a scheduling conflict and feel a little worried that your dough might overproof, there's an easy solution. Tuck it into the fridge. Cold temperatures slow down fermentation. The dough will still rise, only it will take a little longer. Sometimes, bakers slow down fermentation intentionally by placing their dough in the fridge. This is called retarding the dough. It's a technique that encourages deeper and more complex flavors in your bread.

Why does my dough keep sticking to my banneton or proofing basket and tea towels?
Make sure you flour your tea towel really well. Don't be afraid of too much flour— absolutely coat it. You can always dust it off later. I recommend keeping a little jar of brown rice flour on hand. Brown rice flour is coarse and acts as a good barrier between your dough and your banneton or proofing basket or tea towels. It helps prevent sticking.

If, despite these extra measures, you find that your dough still sticks, you may have overproofed it.

Why did my dough deflate when I scored it?
If your bread deflates like a balloon when you score it, it has overproofed. Its gluten matrix has weakened and can no longer hold the structure of the bread, so it collapses. Next time, monitor the final rise a little more closely.

Baking

Why do my loaves keep burning on the bottom?

If your bread keeps burning on the bottom, it needs a better barrier to protect it from the oven's heat. Try moving the rack up, toward the center of the oven. Or place a baking sheet beneath your Dutch oven or loaf pan.

How do I know when my bread is ready?

Your bread should be a beautiful golden brown color. You can also take its internal temperature. For breads made without added fat, the internal temperature should be 190°F to 210°F. Sandwich breads should reach about 190°F, and enriched breads should reach 180°F to 190°F.

Why didn't my bread expand in the oven?

Poor oven spring is typically a sign that your dough either proofed too long or not long enough. Dough that overproofs during bulk fermentation will not expand much in the oven. Dough that hasn't risen enough after shaping and final proof may also not expand much in the oven.

Additionally, improper shaping can lead bread to lose its spring. It's important to shape your dough with a firm but gentle hand. This way you build adequate tension on the outside of the loaf. That tension helps the dough hold its shape and expand properly as it bakes.

The End Product

How do I know if the crumb is what it should be?

The "crumb" is the inside of your loaf. Artisan-style breads are made with a wet dough. They should have an open, airy crumb with evenly distributed holes. Sandwich loaves should have a tight crumb. Enriched breads should have a soft, tender crumb that pulls apart easily. Many sourdough lovers prefer the light airy loaves, but make what you love.

Why is my sourdough so flat?

Not allowing your bread to rise completely during bulk fermentation and letting it overproof are both culprits in flat, Frisbee-like sourdough. So is improper shaping.

If you don't allow your dough to double during bulk fermentation, then the yeast will not have had the opportunity to do all the work they need to do. Similarly, not allowing your bread to proof thoroughly during the final rise can also lead to flat, lifeless loaves.

Allowing your bread to overproof weakens the gluten and can make the dough sticky and prone to collapsing.

It's important to build tension as you shape your bread. This gives the dough's surface a tight, springy feel. Shaping builds the structure of the loaf, and if the structure is weak, the bread can weaken and lose its loft as it bakes.

Why hasn't my bread baked through?

If your bread looks done but is still wet or a little raw in the center, it might be because you didn't bake it long enough. Sometimes, underproofed dough will not cook all the way through, leaving a wet interior.

Why is my bread so gummy?

What a disappointment it is to slice into your bread only to find a dense, gummy mess. First, always let your bread cool completely before you slice it. Bread continues to bake even after you pull it out of the oven. The residual heat allows the starches to reorganize themselves into an appealing texture.

If you allowed the bread to cool completely, but it is still gummy inside, there are a few possible reasons. Uneven oven temperature can cause the outside of a loaf to brown while the interior turns gummy. Baking in a Dutch oven can help the bread keep an even temperature as it bakes. Both overproofing and underproofing can lead to a gummy crumb. Lastly, an immature starter is often the culprit. It may not have enough yeast activity to support proper crumb development.

Why are the holes in my bread so uneven?

Sometimes, you will slice open a gorgeous loaf of bread only to find one or two gaping holes. It's such a disappointment. If your starter is young and immature, it may not have enough yeast to develop properly. This can cause an uneven crumb. Keep feeding your starter, and it will soon be strong enough. Underproofing your dough, especially during bulk fermentation, can cause an uneven crumb.

Why does my bread keep tearing?

You need to score some types of bread before you put them in the oven, especially high-hydration dough. If you scored your bread, and it still tears, then a few things could have gone wrong. First, your expansion score may not have been deep enough to allow the bread to expand. Second, your bread may be underproofed, causing it to expand more than expected in the oven. Last, you may need to pay extra attention to shaping your loaves. This builds tension so that your bread expands properly in the oven.

How do I make my bread more sour?

Sourdough's flavor begins with the starter. White-flour starters will taste the mildest, while whole-grain starters have more intense flavors. So if you like extra-sour sourdough, feed your starter whole-grain flour. Dark flour will give it the most intense flavor. If your starter produces hooch, stir it into the starter when you feed it fresh flour and water. Additionally, keep your starter in a warmer spot. Warm temperatures favor lactic-acid bacteria, which will give your sourdough a distinctly sour taste.

You can also add more whole grains, especially rye flour, to your dough. Ferment your dough for a longer period of time, but be careful not to overproof your dough.

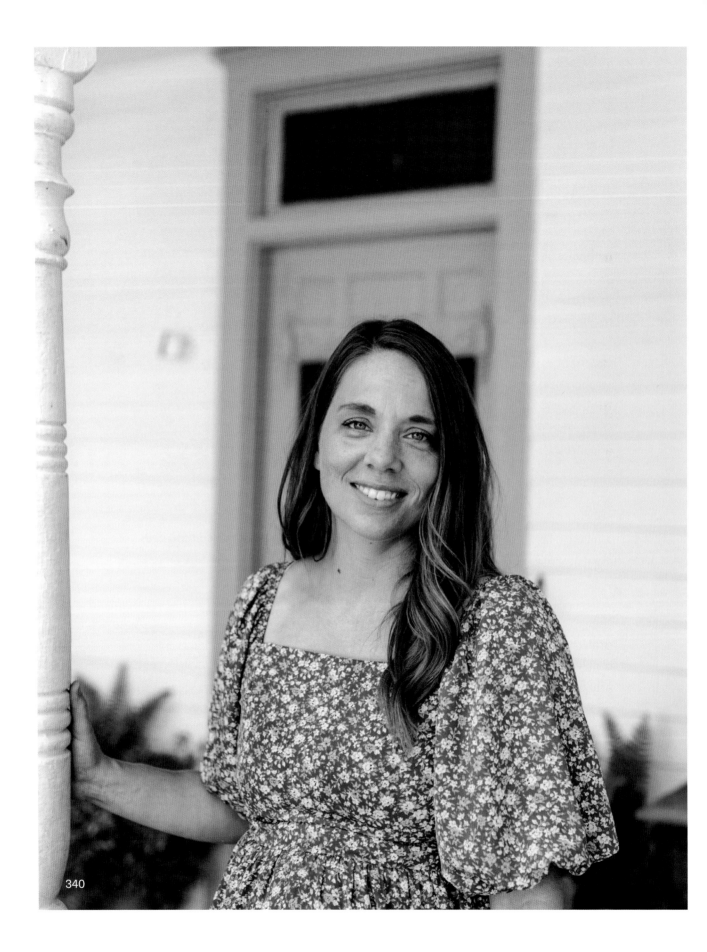

Final Thoughts

IF YOU ARE BRAND NEW to sourdough, I hope this book has given you the confidence you need to craft your very first loaves of wholesome bread. At first, you may need to follow the directions to a tee to get a loaf you're proud of, but over time it will become intuitive and straightforward.

You'll learn what your favorite recipes should feel like when the gluten is fully developed and how the dough bounces back when it isn't quite done with its final rise before baking. You'll see what the dough should look, smell, and feel like after a proper bulk fermentation, and how to manipulate the timing around your schedule, whether you're a stay-at-home mom or someone with a demanding career.

I encourage you to keep trying until you find your stride. If you have a few failures in your first several attempts, turn them into croutons, French toast casseroles, and bread crumbs. Nothing ever goes to waste, so start practicing without fear!

If you are a long-time baker, I hope you found something new you can add to your repertoire within these pages. Maybe you like working best with ancient grains, so you'll lean into einkorn and Khorasan wheat flour selections. Or maybe your family loves that artisan texture and taste of an all-purpose boule. In any kitchen, you will discover favorite recipes that you make over and over again while reserving other recipes for special occasions.

For more recipes and practical ways to incorporate sourdough into your daily life and schedule, head on over to my blog, Farmhouse on Boone (farmhouseonboone.com) and Youtube channel of the same name.

Happy baking!

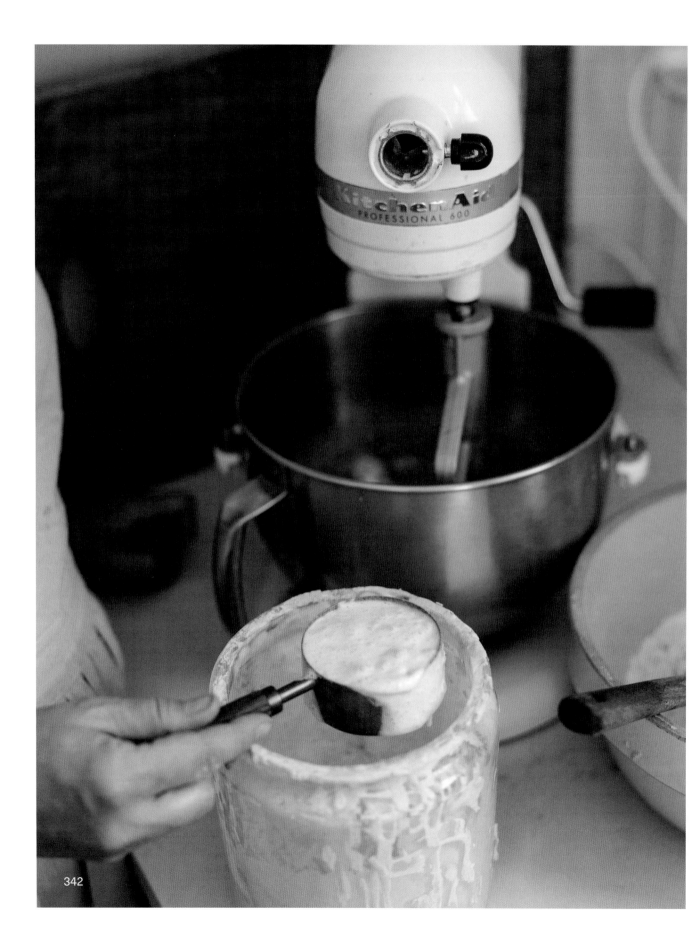

Resources

Flour and Grains

Azure Standard is a buying club that offers natural and organic foods in bulk at wholesale prices. It's a great place to pick up flour, grains, dried fruit, nuts, and chocolate in bulk. You can connect with a local group and order online at azurestandard.com.

Bluebird Grain Farms offers organically grown whole grains and freshly milled whole-grain flour. They specialize in heritage grains such as einkorn, spelt, and Sonoran white wheat. Order directly on their website at bluebirdgrainfarms.com.

Bob's Red Mill sells a wide variety of whole grains and flours, including high-protein bread flour, unbleached all-purpose flour, whole-wheat pastry flour, and others. You can find them in most grocery stores, natural foods shops, and online at bobsredmill.com.

Central Milling sells excellent high-protein bread flour and all-purpose flour. They also sell several types of specialty flours, including einkorn, spelt, and rye flour. Find them online at centralmilling.com.

Country Life Natural Foods offers grains, flour, dried fruit, and other pantry items in bulk. You can visit them at countrylifefoods.com.

Hayden Flour Mills offers artisan bread and all-purpose flour as well as specialty flours. They also offer various baking supplies. Order online at haydenflourmills.com.

Jovial Foods sells organic einkorn berries, whole-grain einkorn flour, and all-purpose einkorn flour. You can find them in well-stocked supermarkets, most health food stores, and online at jovialfoods.com.

King Arthur Flour sells high-quality flour and baking gadgets. They also offer many educational resources for bakers. Find them online at kingarthurbaking.com

Fats and Oils

Graza sells single-origin olive oil from Spain, including a light-tasting oil for cooking and a robust finishing oil. Find it online at graza.co.

Kerrygold sells delicious Irish butter from grass-fed cows. They also make good cheese, too. Kerrygold is widely available in most grocery stores. You can also visit them online at kerrygoldusa.com.

Sierra Nevada Cheese sells gorgeous butter from grass-fed cows. It has a rich flavor and smooth character. You can buy it in many natural foods markets as well as online at sierranevadacheese.com.

Thrive Market sells a wide variety of natural and organic foods, and offers coconut oil as well as chocolate at a great price. Visit them at thrivemarket.com.

Salt

Baja Gold Salt Co. makes sea salt that is rich in trace minerals and has a mild flavor. Find them at bajagoldsaltco.com.

Jacobsen Salt Co. produces American-made sea salt with a beautiful, delicate crystalline structure. It's good for adding finishing touches to baked goods. Find them online at jacobsensalt.com.

Redmond Life sells minimally processed salt from ancient sea deposits in Utah. You can find both coarse and finely ground salt. They are widely available in stores as well as online at redmond.life.

Sweeteners

Just Panela sells minimally processed, organic, and unrefined cane sugar. You can order from them online at justpanela.com.

Wholesome Sweeteners offers minimally processed sugars, including rapadura, which they sell under the name Sucanat. They also sell excellent organic brown sugar, granulated sugar, and powdered sugar. Their products are widely available in stores, and you can also purchase them online at wholesomesweet.com.

Sourdough Baking Supplies

Cultures for Health offers heirloom sourdough starter cultures. They also sell various baking supplies including bread lames, bannetons, and proofing boxes. Order online at culturesforhealth.com.

MadeTerra sells high-quality proofing baskets and sourdough kits. Find them online at madeterra.com.

Mockmill sells beautiful grain mills and several types of whole grains. Order online at mockmill.com.

NutriMill sells a wide variety of grain mills, stand mixers, and attachments. Order online at nutrimill.com.

Pleasant Hill Grain sells grain mills, loaf pans, pizza stones, bannetons, and many other pieces of baking equipment. Order online at pleasanthillgrain.com.

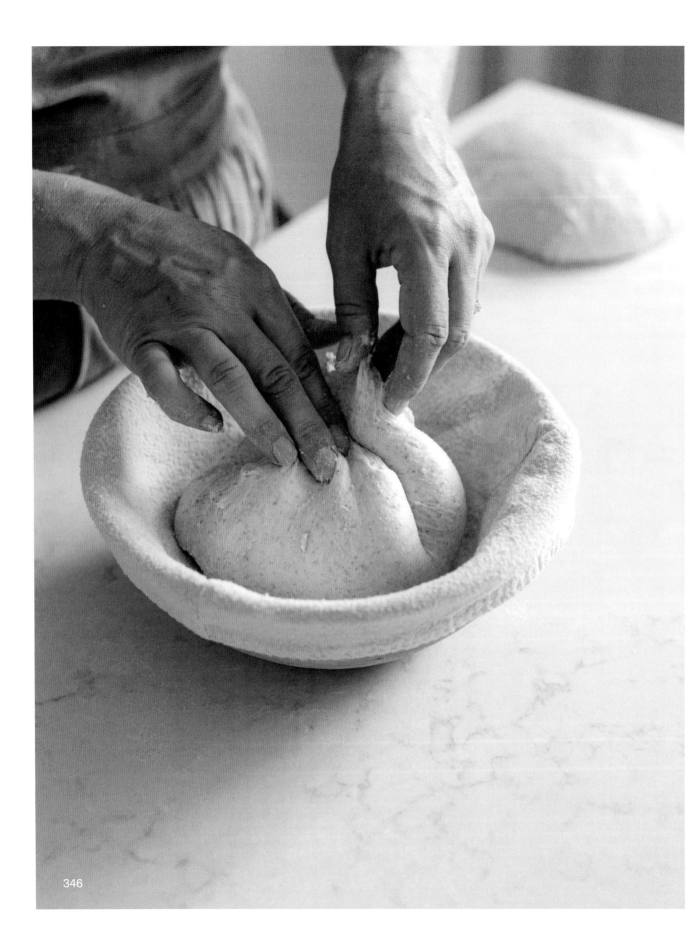

Index

347

INTERESTED IN LEARNING HOW TO PRESERVE FOOD AT HOME?

ADD THESE TOOLS TO YOUR ARSENAL WITH

EVERYTHING WORTH PRESERVING FROM MELISSA K. NORRIS AND

FREEZE-DRYING THE HARVEST FROM CAROLYN THOMAS

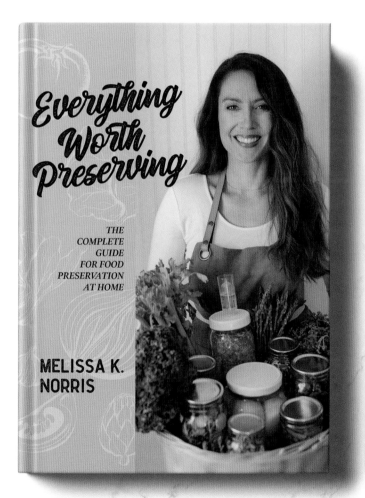

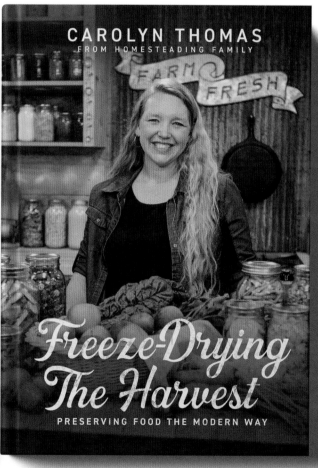

 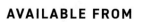 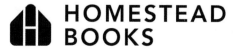

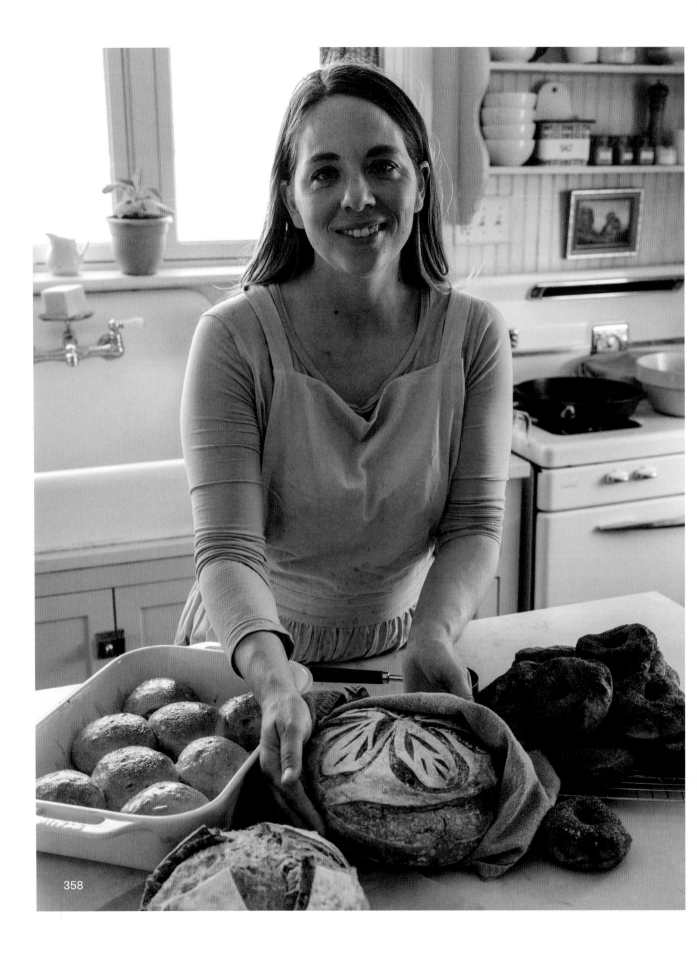

About the Author

Lisa Bass is a homeschooling mother of eight, from-scratch cook, baker, and entrepreneur. She has nurtured a sourdough starter in her Missouri farmhouse for over a decade and loves the everyday ritual of creating something beautiful and nourishing for her large family.

For the first 11 years of their marriage, she and her husband, Luke, lived in a little craftsmen bungalow in town on Boone Street. Lisa always craved that homestead life and spent those years learning how to bake bread, garden, preserve the harvest, sew simple projects, and take care of backyard chickens.

She and her family now live on a small farm and are able to work side by side and share their life and recipes with the world via their blog and YouTube channel both named *Farmhouse on Boone*. Every recipe is tested in their farmhouse kitchen and well loved by her large family.

Daily Sourdough covers the benefits of sourdough and the tools, flours, pantry items, and recipes you'll need to make sourdough recipes.